ABC of Behavior Change

A guide to successful disease prevention and health promotion

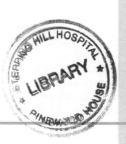

Edited by

Jacqueline Kerr BA MSc PhD
Senior Researcher, Munich Cancer Registry, Ludwig-Maximilian University, Munich, Germany

Rolf Weitkunat Dipl-Psych PhD Privatdozent
Senior Lecturer, School of Public Health, Ludwig-Maximilian University, Munich, Germany, and Senior Lecturer, School of Public Health, University of Health Informatics and Technology, Tyrol, Innsbruck, Austria

Manuel Moretti Dipl-Psych
Research Assistant, Bavarian Public Health Research Center, Munich, Germany, and Management Consultant, dankermoretti Institute for Marketing Communication GmbH, Göppingen, Germany

Foreword by
Dr Rafael Bengoa
Director, Management of Noncommunicable Diseases and Mental Health, World Health Organization, Geneva, Switzerland

Cartoons by **Katz & Goldt**
Cover illustration by **dankermoretti**

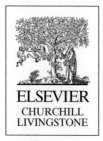

ELSEVIER
CHURCHILL
LIVINGSTONE

EDINBURGH LONDON NEW YORK OXFORD PHILADELPHIA ST LOUIS SYDNEY TORONTO 2005

ELSEVIER
CHURCHILL LIVINGSTONE

First published 2005

ISBN 0 443 07428 3

British Library Cataloguing in Publication Data
A catalogue record for this book is available from the British Library

Library of Congress Cataloging in Publication Data
A catalog record for this book is available from the Library of Congress

Notice
Knowledge and best practice in this field are constantly changing. As new research and experience broaden our knowledge, changes in practice, treatment and drug therapy may become necessary or appropriate. Readers are advised to check the most current information provided (i) on procedures featured or (ii) by the manufacturer of each product to be administered, to verify the recommended dose or formula, the method and duration of administration, and contraindications. It is the responsibility of the practitioner, relying on their own experience and knowledge of the patient, to make diagnoses, to determine dosages and the best treatment for each individual patient, and to take all appropriate safety precautions. To the fullest extent of the law, neither the publisher nor the editors assume any liability for any injury and/or damage.

The Publisher

 ELSEVIER
your source for books,
journals and multimedia
in the health sciences
www.elsevierhealth.com

The publisher's policy is to use paper manufactured from sustainable forests

Printed in China

Contents

Contributors

Rafael Bengoa MD
Rafael Bengoa is Director of the Department of Management of Noncommunicable Diseases at the World Health Organization. This department includes programs dealing with the management of cancer, cardiovascular diseases, diabetes, and chronic respiratory diseases, as well as programs managing disabilities, blindness, and deafness, and human genetics. Dr Bengoa's main interests are linking community resources and public health. Before joining WHO, Dr Bengoa was director of planning and organization of health care in the Basque Country in Spain.

Jacqueline Kerr BA MSc PhD
Jacqueline Kerr received her PhD from the University of Birmingham. She is currently a Researcher at the Munich Cancer Registry, in Germany. Her main interests are psychooncology, the environment, communication and the media, and physical activity promotion.

Rolf Weitkunat Dipl-Psych PhD Privatdozent
Rolf Weitkunat received his Psychology diploma and PhD from the Social and Behavioral Sciences Faculty of the University of Tübingen and his postdoctoral lecture qualification in Biostatistics and Epidemiology from the Medicine Faculty of the University of Munich. He is currently a Senior Lecturer at the Schools of Public Health of the Ludwig-Maximilian University in Munich, Germany, and the University of Health Informatics and Technology, Tyrol, Innsbruck, Austria. His main interests are behavioral epidemiology and causal modeling.

Manuel Moretti Dipl-Psych
Manuel Moretti received his degree in Psychology from the Ludwig-Maximilian University of Munich. He is currently a Research Assistant at the Bavarian Public Health Research Center, Munich, Germany, and a Management Consultant at the dankermoretti Institute for Marketing Communication. His main interests are health promotion, health communication, advertising psychology, and consumer behavior.

Tim Barnett BScEcon(Government)
Tim Barnett received a BScEcon(Government) with Honours from the London School of Economics (University of London) in 1981. He is currently a Member of the New Zealand Parliament. His main interests are politics, travel, indigenous rights, and change.

Mel Bartley BA MSc(Econ) PhD
Mel Bartley received her PhD from Edinburgh University. She is currently Professor of Medical Sociology at the International Centre for Health and Society, Department of Epidemiology and Public Health, University College London, England. Her main academic interests are health inequality, international comparative studies of health, and social demography.

Adrian Bauman MBBS MBH PhD FAFPHM
Adrian Bauman is Professor of Epidemiology and Public Health at the University of New South Wales and Research Director in the Australian Center for Health Promotion. He received his PhD from the University of Sydney. His main interests are understanding influences upon physical activity participation and evaluating the impact of environmental, transport, mass media, and primary care interventions to promote physical activity.

Nicola W Burton BSc(Hons) MPsych(Clinical)
Nicola Burton received a Master's in Clinical Psychology from the University of Queensland. She is currently a Research Officer in the School of Public Health, at the Queensland University of Technology, Australia. Her main interests are understanding the psychological, social, and environmental correlates of health-related behavior and self-management practices.

Donald J Cegala BA MA PhD
Donald Cegala received his PhD from Florida State University. He is currently a Professor at Ohio State University, USA. His main interests are physician–patient communication and communication skills training interventions for patients and physicians.

Alan J Christensen PhD
Alan Christensen received a PhD from the University of Utah. He is currently a Professor at the University of Iowa, Departments of Psychology and Internal Medicine. His main interests are patient adherence to medical regimens and adaptation in chronic disease.

Robert B Cialdini PhD
Robert Cialdini received his PhD from the
University of North Carolina. He is currently
Regents Professor of Psychology at Arizona State
University, USA. His main interests are persuasion,
social influence, and altruism.

Mark Conner BSc PhD
Mark Conner received his PhD from the University
of Birmingham. He is currently a Reader in
Psychology at the University of Leeds. His main
interests are attitudes and health behaviors.

Richard A Crosby PhD
Richard Crosby received his PhD from Indiana
University. He is currently Assistant Professor,
Department of Behavioral Sciences and Health
Education, Rollins School of Public Health, Emory
University, USA. His main interests are prevention
of sexually transmitted infections, adolescent
health, behavioral theory, and research methods in
health promotion.

Jamie Cvengros BSc
Jamie Cvengros received a BSc from Loyola
University of Chicago. She is currently a graduate
student at the Department of Psychology,
University of Iowa, USA. Her main interest is
clinical health psychology with an emphasis on
adjustment to chronic illness.

Mark G Davis MSc MPhil
Mark Davis received his MPhil from the
University of Bristol. He is currently a 'Better
Aging' Project Manager in the Department of
Exercise and Health Sciences, at the University of
Bristol, England. His main interests are blood
pressure management through exercise,
counseling to promote behavior change, and
measurement of physical activity.

Elinor Devlin BA(Hons)
Elinor Devlin received a BA(Hons) degree in
Marketing and Economics from the University of
Strathclyde. She is currently a Research Officer at
the Centre for Social Marketing at the University
of Strathclyde, Scotland. Her main interests are
social marketing, mass media, youth smoking
prevention, and the impact of commercial tobacco
marketing on smoking behavior.

Ralph J DiClemente PhD
Ralph DiClemente received his PhD from the
University of California, San Francisco. He is
currently the Charles Howard Candler Professor of
Public Health and Medicine (Pediatrics) and
Associate Director of the Center for AIDS Research,
Rollins School of Public Health, Emory University,
USA. His main interest is sexually transmitted
disease prevention among youth.

Robert J Donovan PhD
Robert Donovan received his PhD from the
University of Western Australia. He holds the
Cancer Foundation Chair in Behavioral Research at
Curtin University, Perth. His main current interests
are cancer prevention, intimate partner violence,
and mental health promotion.

Mary A Gerend MA PhD
Mary Gerend received her PhD from Arizona
State University. She is currently an Assistant
Professor in the Department of Medical
Humanities and Social Sciences in the College of
Medicine at Florida State University. Her main
interests are in women's health, prevention, and
risk perception.

Jochen Haisch DrPhil DrBiolHumHabil
Jochen Haisch received his PhD from the
University of Mannheim. He is currently Professor
of Social Psychology in Medicine in the
Department of General Medicine at the University
of Ulm, Germany. His main interests are
prevention, health promotion, and theories of
medicine.

Gerard Hastings BSc PhD
Gerard Hastings received his PhD from the
University of Strathclyde. He is currently Director
of the Centre for Social Marketing at the
University of Strathclyde, Scotland. His main
interests are social marketing and the impact of
commercial marketing of tobacco, alcohol, and
food on health behavior.

Rainer Hornung Dipl-Sociol DrPhil
Rainer Hornung received his PhD from the
University of Zurich. He is currently Professor of
Social and Health Psychology in the Department
of Psychology at the University of Zurich,
Switzerland. His main interests are health behavior,
health promotion, and evaluation research.

Christian Janßen MA DrPhil
Christian Janßen received his PhD from the
University of Düsseldorf. He is currently working as
a scientific collaborator in the Department of
Medical Sociology at the University of Cologne,
Germany. His main interests are social
epidemiology, health-care research, and methods
of empirical social research.

Aleksandra Luszczynska PhD
Aleksandra Luszczynska received her PhD from
Warsaw University. She is currently a Senior
Lecturer at Warsaw University, Poland, and an
Alexander Von Humboldt Fellow at the Free
University of Berlin, Germany. Her main
interests are behavior change and coping with
stress.

Lynn MacFadyen BA(Hons) PhD
Lynn MacFadyen received a PhD from the University of Strathclyde in Scotland, where she worked as a Senior Research Fellow in the Centre for Social Marketing. Her main research interests were tobacco marketing communications, smoking cessation, and social marketing.

Jon K Maner MA PhD
Jon Maner received his PhD from Arizona State University. He is currently an Assistant Professor in the Department of Psychology at Florida State University. His research focuses on the relationship between motivation and social cognition, primarily in the areas of mating, power, and risk taking.

Elizabeth McDade-Montez BA
Elizabeth McDade-Montez received a BA from Stanford University. She is currently a graduate student at the Department of Psychology, University of Iowa, USA. Her main interest is clinical health psychology.

Jim McKenna PhD
Jim McKenna received his PhD from the University of Bristol. He is currently a Senior Lecturer and acting Head of Department in the Department of Exercise and Health Sciences, at the University of Bristol, England. His main interests are counseling for behavior change (especially in medical settings), and social and psychological aspects of exercise behavior.

James F McKenzie BS MEd PhD MPH CHES
James McKenzie received his PhD from Ohio State University. He is currently a Professor in the Department of Physiology and Health Science at Ball State University, Muncie, USA. His main interests include health promotion program planning, community health, and patient education.

Brian R W McMillan BSc PhD
Brian McMillan received his PhD from the University of Leeds, England, where he is currently a Research Fellow. His main interests are the application of sociocognitive theories to health behaviors, the relationship between stress and eating, and the social psychology of drug use.

Brian Oldenburg BSc(Hons) MPsych PhD
Brian Oldenburg received his PhD from the University of New South Wales, Australia. He is currently a Professor of Public Health at Queensland University of Technology at Brisbane, Australia. His main interests are primary and secondary prevention of chronic diseases and associated risk factors, and developing, implementing, evaluating, and disseminating public health interventions in a range of settings, including general practice, work organizations, and schools.

Holger Pfaff DrPhil
Holger Pfaff received his PhD from the University of Berlin. He is currently Professor of Medical Sociology at the University of Cologne, Germany. His main interests are work and health, health services research, and health promotion.

James O Prochaska BA MA PhD
James Prochaska received his PhD from Wayne State University, Detroit, Michigan in 1969. He is currently the Director of the Cancer Prevention Research Center and Professor of Clinical and Health Psychology at the University of Rhode Island, USA. His main interests are grandchildren, traveling, and golf.

Constanze Rossmann MA
Constanze Rossmann received a Master's degree from the University of Munich. She is currently a teaching assistant at the Institut für Kommunikationswissenschaft, University of Munich, Germany. Her main interests are media effects, health communication, and methodology.

Laura F Salazar PhD
Laura Salazar received her PhD in Community Psychology from Georgia State University. She is currently Director of Research Projects at the Department of Behavioral Science and Health Education, Rollins School of Public Health, Emory University, USA. Her main interests are in women's and adolescent health issues, such as sexually transmitted diseases, domestic and dating violence, and obesity.

Michael D Slater MpA PhD
Michael Slater received a PhD from Stanford University (1988). He is currently Professor of Journalism and Technical Communication (joint appointment in Psychology) at Colorado State University, USA. His main interests are in health communication, media effects, persuasion processes, and communication campaigns.

Ben J Smith MPH PhD
Ben Smith received his PhD from the University of Sydney. He is currently a Lecturer in Health Promotion in the School of Public Health at the University of Sydney, Australia. His main interests are in the design and evaluation of population-wide strategies to promote behavior change, including health communications and marketing campaigns, primary care interventions, and environmental and policy initiatives.

Vivian M Stevens PhD
Vivian Stevens received her PhD from the University of Health Sciences/The Chicago Medical School. She is currently a Professor of Behavioral Sciences in the Department of Psychiatry and

Behavioral Sciences, Oklahoma State University College of Osteopathic Medicine, USA. Her main interests are in behavioral medicine and smoking cessation.

Stephen Sutton BA MSc PhD

Stephen Sutton received his PhD from the University of London. He is currently Professor of Behavioural Science at the University of Cambridge, England. His main interests are risk communication and behavior change.

Bas Verplanken PhD

Bas Verplanken received his PhD from the University of Leiden. He is currently a full Professor of Social Psychology at the University of Tromsø, Norway. His main interests are attitude theory, attitude–behavior relations, and decision making.

Claus Vögele Dipl-Psych CPsychol PhD

Claus Vögele received his PhD from the University of Hamburg and his professional qualification (Habilitation) from the University of Marburg. He is currently Professor of Clinical and Health Psychology at the School of Psychology and Therapeutic Studies, University of Surrey, Roehampton, London. His main interests are cardiovascular psychophysiology, eating disorders, and health effects of and adherence to physical activity across the lifespan.

Gina M Wingood ScD MPH

Gina Wingood received her ScD from Harvard School of Public Health. She is currently Associate Professor in the Department of Behavioral Sciences and Health Education at the Rollins School of Public Health, Emory University, USA. Her main interest is sexually transmitted disease prevention among women.

Foreword

This millennium will be one of chronic disease. The world is facing a double burden of disease, both chronic communicable and chronic non-communicable diseases. Today chronic conditions account for almost 60% of the global disease burden. 52% of the global disease burden is due to non-communicable conditions, and chronic communicable diseases such as HIV/AIDS add another 7% to this estimate. Interestingly, it is not only the diseases that are becoming chronic; it is also the risk factors and the behaviors that cause them. Given the trends resulting from the more negative aspects of globalization, this is likely to get worse.

Fortunately, the world is not passively looking at this trend and this *ABC of Behavior Change* is an example of that attitude and action. We can be optimistic since we now know how to deal with risks at a population level in a more powerful way than before. Furthermore, we know that when we intervene on several risk factors like tobacco, diet, and physical exercise simultaneously we are potentially preventing several diseases at the same time. In addition, within the formal health-care systems and personal medical care we have learned how to better manage the diseases and their risk factors by reorganizing health care so that it is proactive, more integrated, and patient-centered.

All these advances at both the population and individual level are an enormous opportunity. We know how to intervene across the prevention and care continuum. Some advances are in the health promotion domain, some in the disease prevention domain, and yet others are in the disease management domain. When we look at them in an integrated manner we can see the enormous opportunity and potential of a multipronged attack of health promotion, disease prevention, and management.

Most policy makers intuitively know that injecting new funds into the health system is not the only solution; deeper interventions need to be undertaken to get beyond the status quo. Consequently, there is a growing realization that most countries require deep transformations towards pursuing a public health agenda in which health promotion and disease prevention take a more relevant role. Although there is nothing new in this concept, what is new is that the need is getting much greater, that there is more awareness that funds alone will not help us cope with that complexity, and especially that we know today how to move forward on the health promotion front. This book is a clear exponent of those advances in both population and individual health promotion.

It is well known that the response from countries to the shifting pattern of disease is still one of reactive downstream policies and treatments and it is often said that existing health-care delivery systems cannot handle today's complexity. This text will help the reader to understand that, although challenging, there are tools to handle that complexity in health promotion.

Furthermore, it will be a great guidance for WHO and other international organizations which have to ensure that less developed nations do not repeat the same mistakes as developed ones, one of the most important ones being the dramatic underestimation of the potential of health promotion, disease prevention, and proactive chronic care as well as the total lack of linkage of community resources with care delivery.

Developing countries are often faced with the further complexity of insufficient resources combined with inadequate access to necessary drugs and technologies. Given this context, one could be led to believe that health promotion and behavior interventions would not be a priority for less developed nations. Quite the contrary. They need them more than developed nations. For example, worldwide, only 5% of those in need have access to essential HIV/AIDS health care; in Africa, this figure drops to 1%. There are major initiatives under way to improve access to drugs but access *will not be enough*. Complex situations such as HIV/AIDS will require complex interventions and most of them will call for behavior-type interventions. Again, health promotion will have to play a key role.

The magic bullet approach launched by well-meaning policy makers tends to take the world towards vertical programs which frequently achieve short-term results and after some months simply break down because of the lack of sustainability. Very little attention is given to the basic infrastructure required to ensure that the right incentives and behaviors are present. For example, in the case of HIV/AIDS the potential short-term gains of improved access to drugs programs may be far outweighed by the potential spread of drug resistance if prescribing practices are inconsistent and there is poor monitoring of adherence to therapy. The only certain way to avoid drug resistance will be to ensure that all programs improving access to drugs are complemented by strong adherence programs. We cannot afford to encourage transmission of the drug-resistant HIV/AIDS virus within a community because we have not set up appropriate health promotion support systems.

The tools in this book will help planners decide which approaches are best adapted for their purposes, even for such dramatic circumstances as the one described above. It is therefore extremely relevant also for middle-income and low-income countries.

Typically, policy makers acknowledge the magnitude and burden of lifestyle-related diseases. Many, however, resist allocating more resources to health promotion because they are skeptical about the potential results. They believe there is insufficient evidence in favor of health promotion.

In other words, health promotion would take off and fulfill its full potential if only we could prove its impact at individual and population level! That naive scenario is highly unlikely as clearly demonstrated by the tobacco epidemic or the asbestos/cancer problem. In both those cases very little action happened, despite overwhelming evidence. Other barriers are at work; most are external, the main one being industrial 'misbehavior'. Progress does not depend simply on more evidence. Scientific evidence is obviously needed but health promotion must go further. This is the reason why the WHO, together with member states, has recently been developing new political and legal environments, especially those related to the control of the tobacco industry. This book also covers very successfully these important external factors required for effective health promotion and consequently not only makes it extremely relevant for practitioners but also for decision makers responsible for shifting the agenda to broader public health goals.

For the World Health Organization it is most important for this type of guidance to be developed and released with this quality and at this time, in view of the challenging international agendas it is developing which require new approaches to health promotion. I wish to congratulate the authors and promoters of this initiative and guarantee that the WHO will support its active dissemination around the globe.

Rafael Bengoa

Preface

Our health is strongly determined by what we do or don't do, what we eat, what we drink, how we live and work, and how our society is structured. Changing behavior is not a simple matter. Most people have problems giving up the things they enjoy or are accustomed to. They may not be in control of their behavior or society may not support a healthier lifestyle. This is the challenge of behavior change: providing the right framework – mental, physical, or social – in which an individual or group can change.

Currently, national health targets are not being met and some unhealthy behaviors are on the increase. This may partly be due to poorly planned and suboptimally executed interventions to change health behavior. Considering we are only seeing the tip of the iceberg of failed interventions, because non-significant results are less likely to be published, we should be concerned. Behavior change interventions are often inappropriate for the depth of the problem, are not relevant to the target audience, or only address one variable of change without considering other factors that also influence behavior. Other interventions blindly follow a theoretical framework without considering practical issues, such as competing behaviors, communication options, and media channels. This is not to dismiss all behavior change efforts up till now; some have been very successful and those that have been unsuccessful have been well intentioned. We recognize that behavior change is not an easy task. This is why the *ABC of Behavior Change* aims to help preventive medicine, health promotion, and behavior change practitioners, whether they are professionals or students, to better design and evaluate behavior change interventions.

The *ABC of Behavior Change* addresses the basics of behavior change, covering the range of behavior change possibilities, demonstrating their theoretical foundations, but also focusing on the practical implications of what to change and how. It outlines both personal and environmental influences in behavior change and is applicable to both individual and community interventions. It approaches the problem of behavior change from a variety of angles and theoretical standpoints, summarizing and prioritizing, while also highlighting pitfalls to avoid.

This book brings together the work of over 40 authors from the USA, Europe, Australia, and New Zealand. We are delighted to present the thoughts of those often considered the top experts in their field. The aim of this book is to demonstrate the multiple influences on health and health behavior and thus the many ways of implementing change. To this end, we have assembled authors from many disciplines including psychology, sociology, cancer research, journalism, marketing, communication, research methods, public health, epidemiology, psychiatry, and politics.

This book can be approached by the reader in several ways. Naturally, readers will want to explore their main topic of interest, and we encourage them to do so, as the chapters present very comprehensive and up-to-date reviews written by the best. In addition, we challenge readers to discover chapters on topics that they would not normally consider. We want health promoters and intervention designers to succeed in changing health behavior and suggest that they try to respond to the questions posed in the *Vademecum*. If a question highlights an issue not yet addressed in an intervention plan, follow the matrix and read the chapters relating to that topic. The matrix not only questions your assumptions but provides a more interactive indexing system. Further, within each chapter, cross-references to other chapters are provided; please follow these and explore alternative ways of creating behavior change.

The first section of the book – **A** – presents the background to health promotion, disease prevention, and intervention planning. In particular, Chapters A2 and A3 suggest reasons for the limited success we have seen so far in this field. Section **B** then provides details of intrapersonal and interpersonal factors that affect health, health behavior, and behavior change. The different factors are grouped into chapters according to their theoretical foundations. These chapters describe, prioritize, and demonstrate how to measure variables of change. Section **C** outlines the range of external and environmental determinants of health and behavior. The aspects described in these chapters are often overlooked when considering individual behavior change. Section **D** then summarizes how to translate theory into practice. It shows the multiple ways of changing intrapersonal and interpersonal factors as well as external and mediated factors. Chapters D3–D6 are relevant to the former and Chapters D7–D10 to the latter. However, techniques from both apply across all fields.

We do not mean to frighten or dishearten practitioners, students, or researchers with the seemingly endless possibilities and multiple complexities of behavior change. Nor are we suggesting that health promoters try to include all these variables in their interventions. Quite the opposite: an intervention needs a clear focus. With this book, we want to encourage intervention designers to question their assumptions. We want health promoters to ask themselves whether the proposed intervention is the best possible solution considering the nature of the problem. We would like people to spend more time in the planning stage, investigating a wider range of behavior determinants and establishing which the key variables are. Then we hope that decision makers thoroughly consider the various possible intervention strategies and communication channels, making sure that the intervention is appropriate for the scale and complexity of the problem.

Compared to many other sciences, health promotion is in its infancy. We have so much to learn and discover. It is important that people realize how complex health behavior change is and that identifying health behavior determinants is as challenging as genetic research, for example. Unfortunately, health behavior research is not as well funded as biomedical research. Nor is it considered as important. Both have similar aims, however: to stop disease before it starts. These are exciting times when governments, policy makers, and the public are starting to recognize the need to avoid illness and its costly consequences. It is therefore important that interventions are properly designed and evaluated and, ultimately, that they are effective in changing behavior at a population level.

We would like to thank all those who have supported us and contributed to this book.

Munich 2004   JK, RW, MM

The Scope of Behavior Change

Overview of health promotion

A1

Richard Crosby, Laura Salazar,
Ralph DiClemente, and Gina Wingood

INTRODUCTION TO HEALTH PROMOTION

The influence of behavioral and psychological factors, as well as social and ecological factors (e.g. political, cultural, and economic factors) has become a well-recognized source of disease etiology and, therefore, disease prevention (Berkman & Kawachi 2000). It is increasingly recognized that morbidity and mortality are linked to both behavioral and social factors (McGinnis & Foege 1993, McKinlay & McKinlay 1977). Health promotion transcends these, focusing specifically on an individual's behavior by seeking to influence structural changes, e.g. changes in families, communities, workplaces, and political aspects of society that encourage and maintain health promotion practices (Green 1984).

As health promotion has become an integral part of public health practice, its goals have been defined by primary and secondary prevention of disease and health-compromising conditions. Primary prevention efforts are designed to either prevent acquisition of a pathogen or (for chronic disease) to lower known risk factors for disease onset. For example, several large-scale trials of community-wide efforts designed to reduce risk for cardiovascular disease have been conducted. Each is an example of health promotion focused on primary prevention (Carleton et al 1995, Luepker et al 1994, Winkleby et al 1996), whereas secondary prevention efforts are intended to enhance early detection of disease and reduce adverse psychosocial sequelae of disease. A classic example of secondary prevention is the administration of the Pap test, a widely used indicator of cervical dysplasia (the precancerous stage of cervical malignancies). When detected early, appropriate surgical procedures can significantly reduce the likelihood of subsequent carcinogenesis (Kiviat et al 1999).

THE VALUE OF HEALTH PROMOTION

Health promotion may enhance containment of medical costs

One particularly important reason why health promotion has become a focal point in public health is that it has a tremendous potential to relieve economic burdens imposed by the spiraling cost of medical care. Medical care, by definition, is provided to people after disease pathologies have manifest symptoms. Clearly, reversing the disease process at such an advanced stage is problematic and therefore labor and resource intensive. Applying medical models to health has often been referred to as a 'downstream' approach because it metaphorically focuses intervention efforts on pulling drowning individuals from the river's

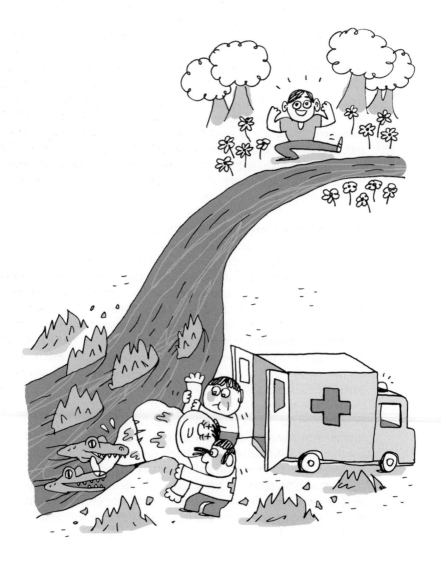

currents. Conversely, health promotion has been referred to as an 'upstream' approach due to its focus on early intervention so people do not fall into 'dangerous rivers' in the first place.

Acquired immune deficiency syndrome (AIDS) is a poignant example of the 'downstream and upstream' metaphor and serves as an excellent illustration of how health promotion can dramatically reduce medical care burdens. Costs associated with caring for a person who has AIDS are considerably greater than costs associated with massive health promotion programs designed to prevent people from becoming infected by the human immunodeficiency virus (HIV). A recent cost–benefits analysis demonstrated that prevention programs designed to decrease incidence of HIV infection have resulted in substantial savings in medical and other AIDS-related costs that would have otherwise been incurred, given a lack of prevention efforts (Holtgrave & Pinkerton 2000).

Recognizing that cost-effectiveness is a critical determinant of whether health promotion programs are implemented, the Centers for Disease Control and Prevention (CDC) recently published a comprehensive review of evidence regarding the cost-effectiveness of various prevention programs, addressing health issues such as breast and cervical cancer, bicycle-related head injuries, childhood lead poisoning, chlamydia-related infertility, colorectal cancer, diabetic retinopathy, dental caries, pneumococcal disease, influenza among the elderly, and tuberculosis (CDC 1995). Generally, favorable cost-effectiveness evaluations for health promotion programs have contributed to the emergence of health promotion as a viable strategy for augmenting the practice of medicine.

Health promotion addresses emerging epidemics

As new and previously unrecognized pathogens become an increasing source of global disease (Garrett 1994), medical models of intervention may be less efficient compared with health promotion approaches that focus on disease prevention. Thus, health promotion interventions can be employed during early phases of an epidemic, potentially averting geometric or exponential increases in the number of people infected. One such example is Ebola, a highly contagious and fatal disease without a medical remedy. When Ebola outbreaks have occurred, health promotion strategies have been effective in tempering the results (Garrett 1994). Health promotion strategies applied include:

- education of community members regarding the dangers of practicing traditional funeral rituals
- education of hospital staff members regarding the dangers of reusing needles and syringes
- the provision of adequate supplies of clean needles and syringes
- the provision of culturally acceptable alternative burial rituals (Garrett 1994).

Health promotion increases quality of life

Health promotion also has a profound impact on the quality of life as experienced by a community. Consider the prevention of diabetes, for example. Promoting a healthy diet and regular exercise can prevent adult onset (type II) diabetes. When people acquire and maintain these health behaviors, not only does their risk of diabetes decrease, thereby averting potential morbidity and mortality, but they also experience a host of collateral health benefits (e.g. reduced risk of obesity, cardiovascular disease, and possibly some forms of cancer). Moreover, they may experience a sense of increased energy and capacity for performing and enjoying life's physical tasks (recreational or labor) and feel better about their appearance. This increased capacity may, in turn, extend to improved mental and social well-being (Smedley & Syme 2000). Figure A1.1 illustrates this concept by showing that health promotion is capable of achieving much more than merely the prevention of somatic disease.

Health promotion programs that seek to decrease neonatal morbidity are also an excellent example of programs that address quality of life issues in addition to contributing to decline in mortality. Diarrheal disease is a primary cause of infant mortality. One solution is to promote breastfeeding among new mothers who may otherwise choose to feed formula to their infants (Condran & Preston 1994). Evidence suggests that women who breastfeed their infants may have substantially lower risk of developing ovarian cancer or post-menopausal breast cancer (Eaton et al 1992, Speroff et al 1989) and tend to return to their pre-pregnancy weight faster than those who do not breastfeed. Further, the hormonal changes that accompany lactation may provide a degree of temporary protection against rapid repeat pregnancy among women who breastfeed (Hatcher et al 1994). Thus, programs that promote breastfeeding exemplify the value of

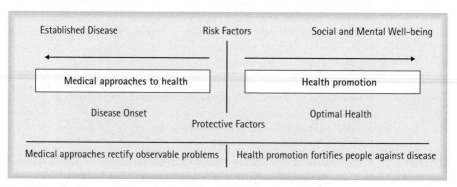

Fig A1.1   Health promotion extends far beyond disease prevention

health promotion from a holistic perspective. Although breastfeeding serves an important purpose at multiple physical levels, it may also have positive psychological effects for both mother and infant, thereby exemplifying how health promotion can increase quality of life.

PRINCIPLES OF EFFECTIVE HEALTH PROMOTION

Table A1.1 displays several principles of health promotion stratified by primary versus secondary prevention efforts. It also displays the benefits of health promotion.

Audience segmentation

Several principles can be applied to increase the effectiveness of health promotion efforts. For example, successful programs are tailored to a narrowly defined (homogeneous) audience. This may be challenging from a design and implementation perspective, as differences among subgroups often exist. Differences in socio-economic status, gender, race, and religion represent common factors that may define homogeneous segments of a population.

 see D2, C1

Table A1.1 Benefits and principles of prevention			
Primary prevention		**Secondary prevention**	
Benefits	**Principles**	**Benefits**	**Principles**
Reduced medical cost	Audience segmentation	Reduced medical cost	Audience segmentation
Control of epidemics	Formative research	Control of epidemics	Formative research
Increased quality of life	Measurable objectives	Increased length of life	Measurable objectives
	Community involvement		Theory-guided practice
	Ecologic perspective		
	Theory-guided practice		

Formative research

Given the importance of a psychographic assessment, another essential principle is that health promotion programs can benefit from the initial use of formative research. Formative research provides practitioners with an ethnographic understanding of how members of the target audience think and behave in relationship to the health practice under consideration.

 i see D9

Clearly defined health objectives

It is essential to prioritize the identified health promotion objectives. A useful strategy is to consider two parameters. The first is the potential impact of the objective on a measurable health outcome (Green & Kreuter 1999). It is important for those engaged in the planning process to ask the question, 'Will changing health behavior X result in a substantial reduction in disease outcome Y?'. At this juncture in the planning process, epidemiological evidence largely drives decision making. The second parameter to consider is the likely degree of success in changing any given health risk behavior (Green & Kreuter 1999).

Community involvement

An often overlooked principle of health promotion is the inclusion, sponsorship, and guidance of members within the target audience in the design of the program (note: the target audience is often referred to as a community and may consist of geographically or socially defined groups of people). In the absence of this sponsorship and guidance, health promotion programs may fail altogether or (if they do succeed) may fail to be sustained beyond an initially defined period. The development of community coalitions is therefore essential to successful *i* see D8 health promotion practices (Butterfoss & Kegler 2002).

Adopting an ecological perspective

Perhaps the most essential element of health promotion is the adoption of an ecological perspective when thinking about disease prevention (Smedley & Syme 2000). An ecological perspective suggests that health promotion should be multifaceted, with boundaries that reach far beyond the immediate influences on individuals' health behaviors (Berkamn & Kawachi 2000, Crosby et al 2002). As opposed to placing sole emphasis on the individual as the primary agent of change, an ecological perspective conceptualizes the individual as enmeshed in a complex system of *i* see D1 interrelated influences that inevitably shape health behavior.

Theory-guided practice

Behavioral, social, and ecological theories provide a basis for under-standing why people engage in behaviors that may place them at risk of premature morbidity and mortality. Theory also provides a lens for viewing and understanding how people successfully adopt health-protective behaviors. Thus, a cornerstone of health promotion is the selection of theories that can best guide program development (Crosby et al 2002, Green & Kreuter 1999, Smedley & Syme 2000).

 see B2-B5

EXAMPLES OF SUCCESSFUL PROGRAMS

Several different studies suggest that health promotion programs can be effective. For example, the Community Intervention Trial for Smoking Cessation (COMMIT) was a 4-year intervention conducted in randomly assigned cities within 11 matched city-pairs. Unlike other projects targeting multiple risk factors, COMMIT was designed specifically to get people to quit smoking, particularly heavy smokers. The trial demonstrated that a community-level health promotion program could produce significant declines in tobacco use among people who originally reported light to moderate cigarette use. Extended analyses revealed a correlation between level of exposure to the intervention activities and quitting cigarette use (COMMIT Research Group 1995).

A gender and culturally appropriate program for African-American women is another example of a successful health promotion effort. The aim of this program was to reduce African-American women's vulnerability to acquiring HIV, by enhancing their partners' use of condoms (DiClemente & Wingood 1995). Women randomized to the HIV health promotion program received a five-session educational curriculum that emphasized women's ethnic and gender pride, fostered self-esteem, acknowledged their self-worth and identified positive role models in their lives. To resist high-risk sexual situations, this education curriculum also sought to enhance women's decision-making skills, condom application skills and sexual communication skills. Compared with women who were randomized to the HIV education control condition, women who were randomized to the HIV health promotion program reported greater control over their sexual lives, were more likely to ask their partner to practice safer sex, were more likely to initiate a discussion on using condoms, reported having partners whose norms were supportive of consistent condom use, and, most importantly, were more likely to use condoms consistently when they did have sexual intercourse.

Successful programs span topics ranging from preventing cancer morbidity (e.g. screening homes for radon, colorectal cancer screening programs, promoting mammography use, and Pap testing) to promoting compliance with flu vaccine, and recommendations to programs designed to help people adopt and maintain exercise and dietary routines that can prevent diabetes, heart disease, and stroke. Despite this diversity and the intuitive appeal of such programs, health promotion efforts nonetheless have a few limitations.

LIMITATIONS

As is true with many disciplines that involve service to people, the effects of health promotion can be very difficult to evaluate. Efficacy trials (such as those described earlier in this chapter) determine whether programs have a *statistically significant* effect when contrasted with a control or comparison group. However, the ultimate question is whether health promotion programs have *public health significance.* For example, a Pap testing program that achieves a statistically significant effect in screening rates must also demonstrate reduced incidence of cervical carcinoma among women receiving the program, compared with women not receiving the program. This magnitude of evaluation clearly requires a substantial investment in following and assessing cohorts of women over protracted periods of time. The same can be said of programs that seek to reduce behaviors that may contribute to the prevention of heart disease, obesity, stroke, diabetes, hypertension, etc. Establishing public health significance is also important when preventing infectious disease is the goal of health promotion. For example, a program that achieves a statistically significant increase in condom use may or may not translate into meaningful reductions in incidence of sexually transmitted infections, including HIV infection.

A key difference between establishing statistical and public health significance is the temporal order of when effects can be measured. The former is generally evaluated soon after completion of the health promotion program, whereas the latter may be assessed long after the program has concluded. This difference raises another limitation of health promotion: program effects may produce temporary rather than long-term changes in risk behavior and the environment. Indeed, a central theory of health promotion practice (i.e. the Transtheoretical Model) suggests that behavior change is a slow and evolving process that involves iterative cycles of success, followed by regression to unhealthy behaviors. Clearly, the identification of effective approaches for promoting the long-term maintenance of health behaviors represents an unmet and vital challenge facing the field of health promotion.

A primary, and perhaps inevitable, limitation of health promotion is that prevention can be difficult to quantify. Unlike the practice of medicine (where cure rates and number of lives saved can be easily documented), the end-product of health promotion is far less tangible. Indeed, an unfortunate reality of health promotion is that successful prevention efforts may obviate public perception of a need to have any program at all. In an attempt to counter this perception and provide empirical evidence in support of health promotion efforts, Durlak & Wells (1997) conducted a metaanalysis of 177 primary prevention programs designed to prevent behavioral and social problems in children and adolescents. Findings indicated that participants in programs surpassed the performance of those in control groups by between 59% to 82%, with revealed dual benefits of problem reduction and competency enhancement. Thus, although making connections between effects of health promotion programs and corresponding reductions in morbidity and mortality is inherently problematic, other desirable outcomes (i.e. intermediate markers of success) may be realized and measured.

CURRENT AND FUTURE CHALLENGES

Integrating health promotion into medical practice

A seamless integration of health promotion (prevention focused) and medical practice (treatment focused) may have potential synergistic effects on morbidity and mortality. Indeed, one form of this integration is termed preventive medicine. Preventive medicine recognizes that clinical encounters represent valuable opportunities to intervene with respect to the etiology of the disease process. For example, a recent review article concluded that counseling and structured training of hypertension patients produces superior declines in blood pressure compared with the declines occurring with only medical treatment (Ebony et al 2001). A recent multisite study sponsored by the CDC is also a good illustration of this principle. The project demonstrated that brief, interactive, counseling protocols effectively reduced patients' risk of sexually transmitted disease (STD) acquisition over a 1-year period of follow-up assessments (Kamb et al 1999).

Clinical encounters may also represent opportunities to screen for disease or risk behavior unrelated to the initial clinical visit. A novel version of this concept is exemplified by a recent study that investigated the utility of enrolling tobacco-using parents of children, admitted to a hospital unit, in a smoking cessation program (Winickoff et al 2001). Clinical encounters may also be ideal opportunities to screen for other forms of risk factors, such as domestic violence victimization (McCaw et al 2001).

Preventive medicine also addresses policy issues that relate specifically to health care and health promotion practices. For example, the American College of Preventive Medicine issues policy statements on multiple health issues, such as the fortification of grain products to reduce the incidence of neural tube defects (Bentley et al 1999). Despite the parallels between preventive medicine and health promotion and the apparent success of preventive medicine (Messonnier et al

1999), it should be noted that widespread acceptance has not been realized, attributed in large part to either a lack of resources (financial and otherwise) or a lack of will (meaning that the traditional practice of medicine is philosophically preferred over an integration of medicine and health promotion), or both.

Designing research in health promotion

When health promotion programs target the individual (as opposed to communities, workplaces, or policy initiatives), research agendas can easily follow a sequence beginning from observational studies and concluding with randomized controlled trials. However, this level of simplicity does not characterize health promotion research designed to evaluate programs delivered beyond the individual level. Community-level interventions, for example, cannot readily adopt randomized designs because the unit of randomization would be an entire community. Randomly assigning communities to treatment conditions presents practical challenges and political barriers and clearly necessitates large financial costs, given the need to analyze study findings by the unit of randomization (i.e. communities) rather than by individuals. Even so, research designs that assess community-level effects of a health promotion program may be more generalizable than programs that follow a specified cohort of individuals, because the former is a better approximation of 'real world' effects and therefore has greater external validity.

Because health promotion programs should be designed to enhance quality of life (as well as reduce morbidity and mortality), researchers also need to create and incorporate quality of life indicators into their study designs. Similarly, health promotion programs that seek to change a specified set of risk factors may benefit from evaluations designed to determine:

- whether the program also has an impact on unspecified risk behaviors (i.e. risk behaviors that were not part of the planned approach to health promotion)
- whether the specified risk behaviors change as a consequence of the health promotion program or whether a single risk factor changes and then creates a cascading effect with regards to adoption of the remaining risk behaviors.

In addition, researchers should continue to refine their repertoire of measures designed to determine the impact of health promotion programs on morbidity and mortality. Although self-report measures are often necessary, they are seldom preferable to objective measures (e.g. laboratory-confirmed diagnosis of a pathogen or clinically confirmed diagnosis of a disease or condition). Yet, objective measures may be costly and pose multiple logistic complications when applied in the context of large-scale health promotion studies. The use of objective measures also obligates the researcher to provide standard-of-care treatment to any study participant diagnosed as positive. The emergence of highly sensitive and specific screening tests (particularly those that can be applied in the field) combined with the availability of single-dose (or single-visit) treatments may greatly enhance the ability of health promotion researchers to use objective markers of program success.

Finally, researchers need to continue their search for constructs that measure environmental or contextual attributes that can contribute to explanations of health behavior. Social capital, for example, may be an overarching construct with unending implications for health promotion practice (Berkman & Glass 2000). Social capital, defined as trust and cohesiveness within communities that promotes common welfare, has been associated with public health measures such as STDs/HIV, violent behavior, child welfare, mortality and health status (Holtgrave & Crosby 2003, Kawachi & Berkman 2000). In general, social capital is positively associated with health indicators.

Influencing public health policy

Finally, at the dawn of the 21st century, it has become readily apparent that health promotion efforts, without corresponding policy changes, may not be optimally effective. Given that a basic premise of health promotion is to provide structural support (e.g. changes in families, communities, workplaces, and political aspects of society) for behavior changes, policy changes are inextricably linked with health promotion practice. Policies related to abortion, intimate partner violence, contraceptive cost, employment, and education are strong determinants of women's health worldwide (Caldwell & Caldwell 1994, LeVine et al 1994). Policy related to tobacco production and distribution, especially tobacco exported from developed nations to developing nations, represents a prominent factor in the success or failure of health promotion programs designed to prevent the onset or cessation of tobacco use (Warner 2000). Policy support for harm reduction programs, such as those providing bleach kits or new injection equipment to drug users at risk of HIV infection, is an essential aspect of health promotion. Policy related to managed care is also a potentially critical determinant of whether (and how extensively) health promotion practices can be integrated into medical settings.

CONCLUSION

Health promotion is a multifaceted discipline that can have a substantial and lasting impact on key morbidity and mortality indicators in any given nation. Grounded in theory and guided by research findings, health promotion not only serves as an entity in its own right, but also enhances traditional medical care. Moreover, health promotion has an established track record of cost-effectiveness and can be mobilized quickly in response to emerging epidemics. Viewed from an ecological perspective, health promotion embodies changes in community infra-structures, as well as policy-level changes. Like the larger field of pub-lic health, the discipline of health promotion faces many challenges for the future. These challenges should be embraced as they represent opportunities to improve substantively the health and well-being of countless individuals, their families, and their communities.

References

Bentley J R, Ferrini R L, Hill L L 1999 American College of Preventive Medicine public policy statement: folic acid fortification of grain products in the U.S. to prevent neural tube defects. American Journal of Preventive Medicine 16:264-266

Berkman L F, Glass T 2000 Social integration, social networks, social support, and health. In: Berkman L F, Kawachi I (eds) Social epidemiology. Oxford University Press, New York, pp 137-173

Berkman L F, Kawachi I 2000 Social epidemiology. Oxford University Press, New York

Butterfoss F D, Kegler M C 2002 Toward a comprehensive understanding of community coalitions: moving from practice to theory. In: DiClemente R J, Crosby R A, Kegler M C (eds) Emerging theories in public health practice and research. Jossey-Bass Wiley, New York, pp 157-193

Caldwell J, Caldwell P 1994 Patriarchy, gender and family discrimination, and the role of women. In: Chen L C, Kleinman A, Ware N C (eds) Health and social change in international perspective. Harvard University Press, Boston, pp 339-374

Carleton R A, Lasater T M, Assaf A R et al 1995 The Pawtucket Heart Health Program: community changes in cardiovascular risk factors and projected disease risk. American Journal of Public Health 85(6):777-785

Centers for Disease Control and Prevention (CDC) 1995 Assessing the effectiveness of disease and injury prevention programs: costs and consequences. Morbidity and Mortality Weekly Report 44(RR-10):1-10

COMMIT Research Group 1995 Community Intervention Trial for Smoking Cessation (COMMIT): II. Changes in adult cigarette smoking prevalence. American Journal of Public Health 85:193-200

Condran G A, Preston S H 1994 Child mortality differences, personal health care practices, and medical technology: the United States, 1930–1990. In: Chen L C, Kleinman A, Ware N C (eds) Health and social change in international perspective. Harvard University Press, Boston

Crosby R A, Kegler M C, DiClemente R J 2002 Understanding and applying theory in health promotion practice and research. In: DiClemente R J, Crosby R A, Kegler M (eds) Emerging theories in health promotion practice and research. Jossey-Bass Wiley, New York, pp 1-15

DiClemente R J, Wingood G M 1995 A randomized controlled trial of an HIV sexual risk-reduction intervention for young adult African-American women. Journal of the American Medical Association 274(16):1271-1276

Durlak J A, Wells A M 1997 Primary prevention mental health programs for children and adolescents: a meta-analytic review. American Journal of Community Psychology 25:115-152

Eaton S B, Pike M C, Short R V et al 1992 Women's reproductive cancers in evolutionary context. Department of Radiology, Emory University, Atlanta

Ebony B L, Daumit G L, Frick K D et al 2001 An evidence-based review of patient-centered behavioral interventions for hypertension. American Journal of Preventive Medicine 21:221-222

Garrett L 1994 The coming plague: newly emerging diseases in a world out of balance. Farrar, Straus, and Giroux, New York

Green L 1984 Research and evaluation. In: Rubinson L, Alles W F (eds) Health education foundations for the future. Waveland Press, Prospect Heights, pp 195-230

Green L W, Kreuter M W 1999 Health promotion planning: an educational and ecological approach, 3rd edn. Mayfield, Mountain View

Hatcher R A, Trussell J, Stewart F et al 1994 Contraceptive technology, 16th edn. Irvington Publishers, New York

Holtgrave D R, Crosby R A 2003 Social capital, poverty, and income inequality as predictors of gonorrhea, syphilis, chlamydia and AIDS case rates in the United States. Sexually Transmitted Infections 79:62-64

Holtgrave D R, Pinkerton S D 2000 Assessing the economic costs and benefits of behavioral interventions. In: Schneiderman N, Speers M A, Silva J M et al (eds) Integrating behavioral and social sciences with public health. American Psychological Association, Washington, pp 249-265

Kamb M L, Fishbein M, Douglas J M Jr et al 1999 Efficacy of risk-reduction counseling to prevent human immunodeficiency virus and sexually transmitted diseases: a randomized controlled trial. Project RESPECT Study Group. Journal of the American Medical Association 280:1161-1167

Kawachi I, Berkman L 2000 Social cohesion, social capital and health. In: Berkman L F, Kawachi I (eds) Social epidemiology. Oxford University Press, New York, pp 174-190

Kiviat N B, Koutsky L A, Paavonen J 1999 Cervical neoplasia and other STD-related genital tract neoplasias. In: Holmes K K, Sparling P F, Mardh P et al (eds) Sexually transmitted diseases, 3rd edn. McGraw-Hill, New York, pp 811-832

LeVine R A, LeVine S E, Richman A et al 1994 Schooling and survival: the impact of maternal education on health and reproduction in the third world. In: Chen L C, Kleinman A, Ware N C (eds) Health and social change in international perspective. Harvard University Press, Boston, pp 303-338

Luepker R V, Murray D M, Jacobs D R et al 1994 Community education for cardiovascular disease prevention: risk factor changes in the Minnesota Heart Health Program. American Journal of Public Health 84:1383-1393

McCaw B, Berman W H, Syme S L, Hunkeler E F 2001 Beyond screening for domestic violence: a systems model approach in a managed care setting. American Journal of Preventive Medicine 21:170-176

McGinnis J M, Foege W H 1993 Actual causes of death in the United States. Journal of the American Medical Association 270:2207-2211

McKinlay J B, McKinlay S M 1977 The questionable contribution of medical measures to the decline of mortality in the United States in the twentieth century. Milbank Memorial Fund Quarterly 55:405-428

Messonnier M L, Corso P S, Teutsch S M et al 1999 An ounce of prevention... What are the returns? American Journal of Preventive Medicine 16:248-263

Smedley B D, Syme S L 2000 Promoting health: intervention strategies from social and behavioral research. National Academy Press, Washington

Speroff L, Glass R H, Kase N G 1989 Clinical gynecologic endocrinology and infertility. Williams and Wilkins, Baltimore

Warner K E 2000 The need for, and value of, a multi-level approach to disease prevention: the case for tobacco control. In: Smedley B D, Syme S L (eds) Promoting health: intervention strategies from social and behavioral research. National Academy Press, Washington, pp 417-449

Winickoff J P, Hibberd P L, Case B et al 2001 Child hospitalization: an opportunity for parental smoking intervention. American Journal of Preventive Medicine 21:218-220

Winkleby M A, Taylor C B, Jatulis D et al 1996 The long-term effects of a cardiovascular disease prevention trial: the Stanford Five-City Project. American Journal of Public Health 86:1773-1779

Health and behavior

Rolf Weitkunat and Manuel Moretti

All men's miseries derive from not being able to sit in a quiet room alone. (Blaise Pascal)

HEALTH

From an epidemiological point of view, human life can be considered as a sexually transmitted disease with a 100% fatality rate. Whereas its etiology, diagnosis, and outcome are clear, neither its pathology nor its progression is sufficiently understood. In theory, epidemiology can help us to identify appropriate risk factors. Even if some of epidemiology's methodological nuggets (like the formidable case control study) cannot be used (due to the lack of an appropriate control group), some encouraging findings are available today. One conclusion we can draw is that there is no natural history of life and no notion of a 'natural death'. Instead, we know there are a variety of ways to gradually or abruptly accelerate life's development. Although to date no way of avoiding the lethal outcome is known, considerable progress has been made in prolonging the time to event, at least in Western countries.

The major opponent of longevity is disease. Traditionally, absence of disease was considered health. Since 1948, the World Health Organization (WHO) has insisted on 'a state of complete physical, mental and social well-being and not merely the absence of disease'. Although this adds some positive, albeit 'subjective' element, health remains essentially a concept that we consider from a negative perspective. Even if there are (mostly vague) conceptualizations of 'positive health' and its (saluto)genesis (e.g. Antonovsky 1979), disease-related research dominates. A detailed criticism of 'positive health' approaches would lengthen this text intolerably. Suffice it to say that such definitions do not add much to our specific, objective understanding and our ability to improve health. Our habitual 'perception' of 'health' is mostly a blur and often a literally unfelt, static, interoceptive background: if we don't feel it, it's health. In contrast, we have myriad ways to perceive illness symptoms. Additionally, we often successfully identify specific causes of symptoms, whereas we cannot easily identify causes of health.

Up to the beginning of the 20th century the main causes of early demise were infections, such as tuberculosis and pneumonia (Armstrong et al 1999). Even before effective medical interventions became available, many viruses and bacteria were suppressed by improved living conditions, hygiene, and nutrition (McKinlay & McKinlay 1981). Age did not then take over as the main threat to survival. Rather, we nowadays simply survive long enough to die from non-infectious diseases, such as cardiac infarction, stroke, and cancer. Often chronic diseases, such as diabetes, hypertension, hyperlipidemia, and arteriosclerosis, precede these.

As with infectious diseases, preventing rather than curing chronic disease is most likely to bring the greatest health benefits. Understanding the pathophysiology of diseases, or at least conjecturing intelligently, was often helpful historically. Avoiding drinking infected water resulted in reduced cholera incidence (Snow 1860) and immunization against germs led to lowered infection rates (CDC 1997). Even if our current comprehension of the biopsychosocial causation (Engel 1977) of many chronic diseases is limited, it is known that chronic diseases increase in frequency when people behave in certain ways.

The WHO's world health report in 1995 stated:

Lifestyle-related diseases and conditions are responsible for 70–80% of deaths in developed countries and about 40% in the developing world. Examples are cardiovascular diseases, cancer, diabetes, chronic bronchitis, obesity, malnutrition, mental and behavioral disorders, accidents and violence, alcohol and drug dependency, HIV/AIDS and other sexually transmitted diseases, vaccine-preventable infectious diseases, vectorborne and foodborne diseases, and low birth weight. (p. 12)

This indicates that, although genes and the environment might play a certain role, behavior is by far the most dominant risk factor for morbidity and mortality. According to Fries et al (1998), chronic diseases related to lifestyles account for 70% of the health-care costs in the USA. They also play a crucial role in the context of absenteeism, early retirement, and reduced quality of life.

A careful look at health-related behavior is therefore an urgent and challenging research aim. Whereas specific germs cause infections, chronic diseases usually have multiple causes, operating for long periods of time. Behaviors related to chronic diseases include diets high in fat and low in fruit and vegetables, little physical activity, smoking, alcohol and drug consumption, risky sports, or dangerous driving. Most of these behaviors have multiple health effects or can act together in pathogenetic synergy. Behaviors are even part of the causal network of new or newly identified infections, such as AIDS (having unprotected sex) or variant CJD (eating beef). As can be seen from the coronary heart disease (CHD) example contained in Figure A2.1, the type of causation and the

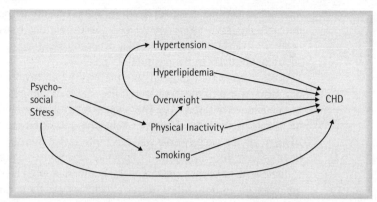

Fig A2.1 Simplified example of multiple causes contributing to coronary heart disease

interrelation of different causes can be complex. Regrettably, such causal networks are hard to identify empirically (Weitkunat & Wildner 2002).

Because the major chronic diseases are associated with lifestyles, the term 'preventable diseases' is frequently used. The crux of the matter is, however, that they are not easy to prevent in practice. The prevalence of chronic diseases is still high or even increasing. Talking of preventable diseases has, in spite of its questionable validity, the 'advantage' that the victims can be blamed (Crawford 1977).

In the chronic disease arena, science and public health do seem to reflect aspects of cultural fashions, being sensitive to a variety of 'isms' (like healthism, ecologism, vegetarianism, etc.) and hidden agendas. Scholars need to carefully watch the demarcation between benevolent (or self-interested) health paternalism and science, to avoid ideological and political corruption. For example, epidemiologic evidence has yet to be gathered on whether reduced use of preservatives and increased natural food consumption (accompanying a continued 'back to nature' trend in public opinion) will have positive or negative public health effects, due to increasing incidence of foodborne illnesses. It might be enlightening to remember that technology has largely contributed to food safety and that there are presumably very few life-savers as effective as that most common appliance: the fridge.

BEHAVIOR

Life is dangerous. In fact, we all die from it. Although life affects both animals and humans, only the latter are aware of the seriousness of the condition and understand that certain health-related behaviors increase their odds of dying prematurely. The question arises: why then do people behave in unhealthy ways? One rationale could be that they don't want to suffer from life any longer. In fact, suicide is one of the risks competing with infections and other causes of death for the premature termination of life. In reality, are not smokers and drinkers also committing a suspended form of suicide? Yet, at the same time, they often consider their behavior as contributing positively to the pleasure of life.

If we assume that most people prefer life and health to death and disease, the will to preserve sacred life seems to compete with the fun of behaving in a 'sinful' way. This allows us to ask more specifically: why do people prefer the pleasures of behaving unhealthily to the pleasures of longevity? If we seriously want to try to tackle this question, we first have to look into the nature of behavior at a more general level.

There is no conclusive answer to the question of what behavior is. There are many angles from which to look at behavior, e.g. the sociological, ethological, ethnological, cultural, biological, and psychological. What degree of complexity should be regarded: large (molar) or small (molecular) units of behavior? What level of willfulness should be considered – reflexes, habits, or deliberate acts? A pragmatic approach, preferred by many research psychologists, is that any functional activity beyond mere vital signs must be conceived as behavior. But even then, behavior is more than one-dimensional. In addition to the commonsense conception of overt behavior, there are physiological as well as cognitive activities not only accompanying it but being part of it (Lang 1978), especially in emotional contexts.

Is this breaking down of 'behavior' to the dimensions of verbal reports, cognitions, physiological responses, and overt or motor responses academic sophism? No. If, for example, a certain intervention addresses only one level of behavior, say the cognitive one, any effect is extremely unlikely to last. Convincing smokers of the fact that smoking is not contributing to their health is as easy as all compassionate health education. If, however, the habitual aspects of their behavior and their physiological cravings are not changed, then the chances of 'sustainable' quitting are subzero. One long-known reason is that behaviors and attitudes are bound to be consistent within individuals (Festinger 1957). It is also wise to remember that the assumption that changing people's attitudes must necessarily change their behaviors is by no means coercive. Furthermore, there is a difference between initiation and maintenance of behavior change. This point was made by William James in 1887 who noted that new habits must become firmly rooted in daily life to gain something like 'sustainability'.

i see B4, B5

In addition to the strange situation that we must address behavior with respect to a phenomenon – health – that is not defined other than heuristically, there is another paradox associated with behavior itself. Whereas in the physical world consequences succeed causes, in behavior this order is reversed. Without going into the details of behaviorism, it is a consistent finding that behaviors that were rewarded in the past tend to occur more frequently in the future.

Even if we narrow our perspective to health-relevant behavior, definitions and concepts do not get any easier. Health-relevant behavior can be health promoting (i.e. positive) or detrimental (i.e. negative). And it can be both – depending on the circumstances and the health outcome under consideration (e.g. jogging or alcohol consumption). Other predicates of health-related behavior are its legality (it can be legal as well as illegal), individuality (it can occur either unaccompanied or in groups), and singularity (behavior can occur once or repeatedly).

Also, behaviors do not occur in isolation but come in packages. These packages, usually denoted as patterns, do not occur in people at random. Rather, certain behaviors occur in some kinds of people more often than in others. How do such 'kinds of people' differ, other than in their behavior? They do so in conditions like sex, age, health status, social class, familial status, education, living area, country, society, as well as biography and epoch of living. They also do so in terms of psychologic resources like intelligence, personality, attitudes, and skills. These factors do have a relation to how people perceive themselves and their physical and social surroundings, i.e. to their world-view. Patterns of behavior in the context of the above factors are denoted by the term 'lifestyles'. Although the word suggests that we have choice, there is no agreement on this. Also, there are different conceptions of whether the above factors are determinants or even constituents of lifestyles (see Weitkunat 1998 for an overview). Besides these open questions, attending to lifestyles in the context of health-related behaviors can help us to understand which subpatterns we have to address in which sequence.

From all of this we see that the reasons for unhealthy behavior are diverse: biological, social, environmental, educational, habitual, lifestyle-related, or reward-dependent. But the most influential reason seems to be our limited cognitive capability; we often do not act rationally. Deviations from rationality become evident from our overestimation of losses compared with gains, our preference for security, or the dependence of our behavioral choices on others (Kahneman & Tversky 1984). Additionally, health-related behavior suffers from a very basic asymmetry. Overall, positive health behavior is immediately costly (just think of health food here) and eventually beneficial, whereas the reverse is true for negative health behaviors. Smoking a cigarette right now can be extremely rewarding, whereas the (potential) penalty in terms of a respiratory disease is light-years away. In other words, positive health behavior is often synonymous with delayed gratification, while risk behavior often provides instantaneous satisfaction. This is why the prevention of negative and the promotion of positive health behaviors are often unsuccessful 'shelf warmers'. In contrast, the concept of 'wellness' (usually associated with pleasant but not necessarily health-promoting consequences) has been very popular (Svenson 1984).

HEALTH AND BEHAVIOR

There are two general pathways leading from behavior to health (see Fig A2.2). The first is the psychosomatic pathway, which is addressed

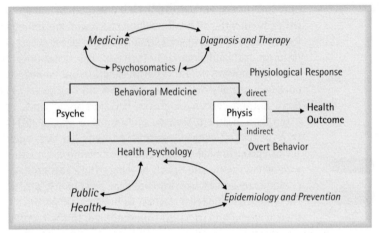

Fig A2.2 Two main pathways connecting the psychological with the physiological dimension

by behavioral medicine (Schwartz & Weiss 1978). The second, more indirect one is addressed by health psychology (Matarazzo 1980) from the behavior-oriented and more individual-based angle, but also by social and behavioral epidemiology (e.g. Marmot et al 1997, Weitkunat & Wildner 2002) from the more outcome-oriented and population-based angle. It is concerned with overt behaviors and their health consequences.

In contrast to our discussion of the overwhelming role of behavior in health outcomes, many epidemiological findings suggest only weak associations between health and behavior. The first reason for this phenomenon is that the latency between a certain behavior and its health outcome might be long, possibly extending over decades. The second reason is that some health outcomes are seemingly only weakly related to risk behaviors, because the latter are not necessary or sufficient, but component causes in complex causal networks. The third reason is that behavioral risks are rarely as clearly cut and one-dimensional as the case of active smoking and its association with lung cancer. These reasons alone make the identification of behavioral risk factors through epidemiology rather unlikely. Moreover, epidemiology generally does not do too well when causes are weak and diseases are rare (Rose 1992).

This situation, the fourth reason, is drastically aggravated when different causes have different proximities to a specific health outcome in causal chains (Weitkunat & Wildner 2002). Unfortunately, behavioral causes usually, if not generally, play a distal part in the concert of risk factors. For example, if lack of physical activity and arteriosclerosis of coronary arteries are both analyzed with respect to cardiac infarction, the latter risk factor is literally closer to the outcome than the former. Regrettably, proximity of risk factors is not often accounted for in epidemiological analyses. It seems to be likely that a large proportion of findings from studies which investigate behaviors (and sometimes even their psychosocial causes, which makes the investigation even more difficult) along with clinical, physiological, and laboratory measures must, for purely statistical reasons, dismiss the former for the latter. It therefore does not seem to be a surprise, but rather a consequent methodological artefact, that currently there is a profound hype towards subcellular and genetic risk factor research in epidemiology. There is a danger that this programmatic trail may lead to perplexity and disappointment (along with more medicalization, of course). The reason is that genetic risk factors, although studied with great enthusiasm, are, in much the same way as behavioral risk factors, excessively penalized during traditional statistical analysis by their long causal distance from the health outcome. If rough and ready multiple regression analyses remain dominant, both types of factors will preponderantly fail to be identified as relevant to health and disease. Despite providing little insight as yet, epidemiology continues to perform much mechanistic 'risk-factorology' (Skrabanek 1991, Smith 2001).

To avoid these flaws, a more sophisticated form of epidemiology is required, which is sensitive to the complex causal relations between certain key behaviors and health outcomes. We suggest this is called behavioral epidemiology (Fig A2.3). It looks at health-related behaviors as mediators, which are in turn under the influence of a wide variety of second-order causes, i.e. causes of (behavioral) causes of diseases. These include (as contained in the lifestyle concept) the behavioral context of the key behaviors under investigation, but also factors like culture, legislation, social norms, values, beliefs, social status, social networks and support, personality, education and skills, habits, innate and learned motives and needs, sex, age, health, job strain, addiction, choices, reward systems, self-perception, locus of control, self- and outcome-efficacy expectation, cues to action, temporal discounting, and others.

 see B, C

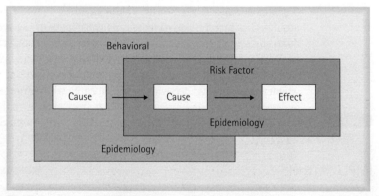

Fig A2.3   Causes of behaviors are distal causes of diseases (from Weitkunat & Wildner 2002)

BEHAVIOR CHANGE

The sheer number of possible causes outlined in the behavioral epidemiology approach gives us a good clue to why lifestyle-oriented prevention is often unsuccessful. If key behaviors are interwoven in complex lifestyles and are influenced by complex causal networks themselves, simplistic behavior change approaches simply must fail. The major error of public health prevention planning (often ignorant of concepts of behavioral sciences to the greatest possible extent) seems to be the unsinkable superstition of health-related behavior being straightforwardly controlled by reason, attitudes, and 'will' (see Ainslie 2001). Health education, aimed at information and attitude change, is quite naively assumed to be sufficient – an assumption that has a good chance of easily winning the most frequently falsified hypothesis trophy. Rather, in most instances, desired behaviors must be modeled, rehearsed, and reinforced – not explained. This implies (as does the complexity of behavioral determination altogether) tailored intervention, which brings us to another grandiose error: the one-size-fits-all approach to health promotion, cherished by all bureaucrats of the world. There is much evidence that, for many behaviors, prevention is only effective if properly tailored (e.g. Orleans et al 1999). This does not include passive prevention (protection) and prevention by legislation, which may, however, not be readily acceptable in a liberal society.

Developing tailored programs of effective health behavior modification is a major research endeavor. It requires two main ingredients. First, rigorous methodology for efficacy evaluation of specific interventions known from the field of controlled clinical trials; there is a large arsenal of methods available for different levels of intervention eagerly awaiting assessment, as described in this book and elsewhere (e.g. Smedley & Syme 2000). Second, as outlined above, we have to incorporate insights from behavioral research concerning the final target of prevention and the carrier of the key behavior to be changed: the individual. When planning campaigns, at both the community and individual level, it is necessary to understand that individual risk assessment is dominated by the perceived individual absolute risk and the aim of increasing the quality of the present life. This differs grossly from epidemiological risk assessment (blandly linking health and behavior), which is essentially based on relative and attributable risk (Jeffrey 1989) and aims to increase population survival time. Overall, whenever preventive behavior is advanced by a 'watering can' principle, by advice, rule, bad conscience, threat, explanation, paternalism, and devaluation, we should not be surprised if it fails dramatically.

IMPLICATIONS

'Life' is a difficult thing, from whatever angle it is looked at. Conceptually, it is very close to 'existence', which according to Kant is not a logically valid predicate. Using it as one, therefore, leads to antinomies. Looking at life as a disease is not a convincing solution and implies even more logical problems. Nonetheless, it has some enlightening aspects. It becomes clear why Russell suggested not confusing conceptual levels in order to avoid paradoxes. Obviously, the concept (or set in the logical sense) of life contains the set of all diseases (which would not exist if there was no life). Considering life itself as a disease leaves us with a set, which is part of itself. Due to life's definition problems, we often focus on a health proxy, when we actually seek to improve life. Unfortunately, health is also not easily defined.

Currently, lifestyle-related diseases are threatening human life (i.e. health) to a serious degree. Part of our problem with the lifestyle concept arises from the fact that we unfortunately do not understand its fundamental constituent: behavior. At least, we can identify some psychological reasons why it is more pleasurable to add life to years than years to life.

In order to control behavior-related health problems, the most widely applied approach in the past has been benevolence. It has failed badly and we understand that hard scientific work lies ahead. There are several specific insights about the matter and we are gradually improving in fighting lifestyle-related diseases at a pragmatic level. For example, vaccinations prevent many premature deaths every day. The same holds true for seatbelts, preservatives and refrigerators, and, to a much lesser degree, even community-based health education. It is encouraging to see that as old a science as physics has made much improvement without understanding its possibly most basic concept – gravity. The comparably young metaphysical and empirical (and thereby intricate) science of behavioral epidemiology should have a careful look at venerable physical sciences like astronomy and how improved understanding was achieved there. It was not achieved mainly by Baconean empiricism but rather by interplay between rationality (i.e. conception of theories) on the one hand and quantification and testing on the other.

It seems that the importance of theories is the most underestimated epistemic aspect of current epidemiology. The dual notion of conjecture and refutation, i.e. of the testing of models, has been shortened to the testing branch. Popperian philosophy of science (e.g. Popper 1963) is not called rational empiricism but critical rationalism, because research results, data, and statistics alone do not add to our understanding of life. They are only useful in relation to theories and concepts. It is this very point that elevates Popper's eminence to the pinnacle of philosophy. (Behavioral) epidemiology should try very hard to understand this point. Otherwise there is a danger of drowning in meaningless exploratory analyses and non-reproducible and mostly ineffective campaigns. In the broad field of health and behavior, there are several black boxes to be filled with appropriate contents, i.e. with testable theories.

References

Ainslie G 2001 Breakdown of will. Cambridge University Press, Cambridge

Antonovsky A 1979 Health, stress, and coping: new perspectives on mental and physical well-being. Jossey-Bass, San Francisco

Armstrong G L, Conn L A, Pinner R W 1999 Trends in infectious disease mortality in the United States during the 20th century. Journal of the American Medical Association 281:61-66

Centers for Disease Control and Prevention (CDC) 1997 Status report on the childhood immunization initiative. Morbidity and Mortality Weekly Report 46:665-671

Crawford R 1977 You are dangerous to your health: the ideology and politics of victim blaming. International Journal of Health Services 7:663-680

Engel G L 1977 The need for a new medical model. Science 196:129-136

Festinger L A 1957 A theory of cognitive dissonance. Stanford University Press, Stanford

Fries J F, Koop C E, Soklov J et al 1998 Beyond health promotion: reducing need and demand for medical care. Health Affairs 17:70-84

James W 1887 The laws of habit. Popular Science Monthly 30:433-451

Jeffrey R W 1989 Risk behaviors and health: contrasting individual and population perspectives. American Psychologist 44:1194-1202

Kahneman D, Tversky A 1984 Choices, values and frames. American Psychologist 39:341-350

Lang P J 1978 Toward a psychophysiological definition. In: Akiskal H S, Webb W L (eds) Psychiatric diagnosis: explorations of biological predictors. Spectrum, New York, pp 365-389

Marmot M G, Bosma H, Hemingway H et al 1997 Contribution of job control and other risk factors to social variations in coronary heart disease incidence. Lancet 350:235-239

Matarazzo J D 1980 Behavioral health and behavioral medicine: frontiers for a new health psychology. American Psychologist 35:807-817

McKinlay J B, McKinlay S M 1981 Medical measures and the decline of mortality. In: Conrad P, Kern R (eds) The sociology of health and illness. St Martins Press, New York, pp 12-30

Orleans C T, Gruman J, Ulmer C et al 1999 Rating our progress in population health promotion: report card on six behaviors. American Journal of Health Promotion 14(2):75-82

Popper C R 1963 Conjectures and refutations: the growth of scientific knowledge. Routledge and Kegan Paul, London

Rose G 1992 The strategy of preventive medicine. Oxford University Press, Oxford

Schwartz G E, Weiss S M 1978 What is behavioral medicine? Psychosomatic Medicine 39:377-381

Skrabanek P 1991 Risk-factor epidemiology: science or non-science? In: Anderson D C (ed) Health, lifestyle and environment. Social Affairs Unit, London, pp 47-56

Smedley B D, Syme S L 2000 (eds) Promoting health: intervention strategies from social and behavioral research. National Academy Press, Washington

Smith G D 2001 Reflections on the limitations to epidemiology. Journal of Clinical Epidemiology 54:325-331

Snow J 1860 On the mode of communication of cholera, 2nd edn. John Churchill, London

Svenson O 1984 Time perception and long term risk. Canadian Journal of Operations Research and Information Processing 22:196-214

Weitkunat R 1998 Computergestützte Telefoninterviews als Instrument der sozial- und verhaltensepidemiologischen Gesundheitsforschung. Logos, Berlin

Weitkunat R, Wildner M 2002 Exploratory causal modeling in epidemiology: are all factors created equal? Journal of Clinical Epidemiology 55:436-444

World Health Organization (WHO) 1995 World health report 1995: bridging the gaps. World Health Organization, Geneva

The problem of behavior change

Jim McKenna and Mark Davis

INTRODUCTION

Kurt Lewin is famously credited for suggesting that a test for anyone who thinks they understand something is to try to change it. Clearly this whole book is about behavior change, and within it this chapter will argue that looking more closely at change perspectives may help to develop more potent and long-lasting programs, whether they are individual, interpersonal, or community based.

There is also a need to prevent the negative, and unintended, impact of well-intentioned programs. There are numerous examples of such interventions across a range of health-related areas, including heroin reduction programs that increased heroin use or cycling safety campaigns that reduced levels of cycling. The Cochrane Library records that only 26 of 56 alcohol reduction interventions and only five of 17 smoking cessation interventions were 'effective'. In the UK, a nationwide physical activity intervention was associated with no change in behavior at a cost of £3 million (Hillsdon et al 2001). Two further factors limit how published research can inform health promotion practice: many non-significant studies are not published and some study methods are not considered suitable to judge effectiveness.

We argue that personal and professional ethics, ontology, intention, epistemology, and training may merely serve as 'formalized prejudices' (McKenna & Riddoch 2003, p. 2). Further, this is compounded by a relative lack of interest in the self-reflection they require. Attention to these issues addresses 'the theory of the intervention' as much as it does 'the theory of the problem' (MacDonald & Green 2001, p. 244), which helps deliverers to refine intervention design and improve treatment fidelity. It also fosters professional development. For these reasons this chapter poses questions that encourage readers to consider why they know what they think they know (Cutliffe & McKenna 2002).

WHAT MAKES YOU THINK THAT CHANGE IS NEEDED?

One starting point for assessing perspectives on change is to consider how we know that change is needed. Obviously, interventions are driven by proven or assumed need. Implicit in this are perceptions of risk, which can shape the style of any subsequent intervention.

Even allowing for changes proposed by any growing evidence base, a strong sense of personal responsiveness underpins what is done and why. Scenarios considered unacceptable, like head injuries among child cyclists, often precipitate an intervention by health promoters or vested professional groups, including teachers (Bergman et al 1990) or practice nurses (Lee et al 2000). Severity of risk clearly drives the need for change, supported by the morality of adult generativity (McAdams & de St Aubin 1998). Given this road safety scenario, the different responses that may be made by a physical education teacher, a practice nurse, or a road safety specialist illustrate how professional ethics, values, and norms combine to influence decision making.

Urgency, dread, and vulnerability are other factors that promote action. This is illustrated by the recent outbreak of sudden acute respiratory syndrome (SARS) (Hesketh 2003). Perceptions of risk that affect clients who appear to have low levels of clinical 'suffering' rarely secure the levels of resource allocated to, say, an outbreak of foot and mouth disease. Such decisions also support the disparity between budgets allocated to prevention versus treatment.

 see B3, C5

Health promoters also need time to reorient their actions. Updating practice to incorporate innovations with proven value (e.g. Machold et al 2002) is also an important issue. However, remarkably little is known about how to refine behavior change training, even within in-service training (Rimer et al 2001). Armstrong et al (1996) uncovered informal mechanisms that influenced general practitioners' drug prescribing. Personal interactions with influential others, like colleagues or patients, lead to change. Recommendations from a 'flagship' journal and the 'drip-drip' effect of accumulating evidence were also important. Different professional groups may capitalize on these, and other, processes. However, these elements also risk reinforcing the status quo and lead to the next question...

WHY DO YOU THINK CHANGE IS POSSIBLE (OR NOT)?

Green et al (1980) suggested that targeted interventions benefit from considering how a target population has responded to previous approaches. This can be a valuable tool for prioritizing populations when resources are scarce (Rimer et al 2001), although it may lead to ignoring the hardest-to-reach or most resistant populations, in favor of especially responsive groups.

Previous experience with groups can lead staff and participants to have expectations for support. Resistance (characterized by reluctance to talk, to suggest options, or to make any effort to work with the helper) or denial (acting as though there is no problem) represent significant impediments, not least because they can undermine the deliverers' motivation. Worse, these clients can repel subsequent health promoters and their interventions. Social marketing suggests the value of developing interventions that make these clients 'defenseless' (Andreasen 1995).

Another concern that supports our 'working' rules for estimating changeability is the weight given to numerical evidence. Interventions can have positive effects that are lost in empirical investigation. For example, in a recent randomized controlled trial (RCT), the mean change in blood pressure was achieved by fewer than 10 of 80 participants (Cooper et al 1999). Focusing on the numbers of participants who achieve benefits, and then exploring their experiences of the intervention, may offer alternative insights into the question that deliverers typically ask: 'Who responds to what?'.

Health promoters may look to published literature to answer another question: 'What works?'. However, many studies do not have accurate measurements of their key outcomes. When the variability implicit to an outcome measurement exceeds the intervention effect, important and meaningful differences go undetected. This may explain why epidemiologists place such faith in mortality as a major outcome. Seligman (1993) urged health promoters to be cautious in 'privileging' evidence from RCTs. He notes five design limits that may contribute to misunderstanding of their implications.

ℹ see A4

The first point refers to program duration, which in health promotion is often flexible and determined by progress or termination. Second, RCTs focus on delivering a few techniques in a fixed order, whereas delivery in the field is self-correcting and innovative (Rimer et al 2001), with techniques being adopted as needed. Participants in behavior change initiatives are often actively involved; they leave when they want to, unlike the passivity required to accept randomization and the behavior of the treatment arm. Behavior change clients can have parallel or interacting problems, unlike the RCT participants who are carefully screened for a single problem. Finally, behavior change interventions often aim to improve general functioning of people who are variously colleagues, friends, clients, or patients (rather than subjects). In contrast, RCTs focus on reducing specific symptoms or ending a disorder.

Proposing the value of experiential evidence, MacDonald & Green (2001) show how qualitative studies can address delivery issues within a specific context. Their findings show what many health promoters already know; that behavior change often hinges on its compatibility with the politics of the local setting. Illustrating this, a recent editorial about improving preventive cardiovascular care was entitled 'Achieving organizational change in general practice: gently simmer for two years' (Elwyn 2002).

ℹ see D8

Hard-to-reach populations often have most to gain from effective interventions and may include people whose behaviors can have severe consequences (e.g. unprotected sex, injecting drugs). However, even the label of 'hard-to-reach' suggests that health promoters shape their cognitive narratives (probably their spoken narratives too) before their consultations begin. This has implications for their expectations of consultations. Doctors use the label 'heart sink' (Silagy et al 1993) to describe unresponsive and recurrent patients. Considering the client groups that are labeled as hard-to-reach may help individual health promoters to address the cascade of effects that this may initiate. Levinas (1969) describes how professionals can involve themselves with their clients. By 'opening' to the experience of the other person, a working relationship is created with individuals who might otherwise be seen as nuisances or pests. In this way, helpers can also live more fulfilled professional lives, which stems from working with the person as much as with their 'problem'.

WHY DOES 'PROBLEMING' HELP?

This part questions the assumption that understanding a problem helps to develop appropriate support. In the prevention of work-, sport-related, or road traffic accidents, the Haddon matrix identifies pre-, in-, and post-event features that contribute to injury mechanisms (Runyan 1998). However, uncovering such mechanisms does not necessarily yield change-responsive elements.

A further problem exists when practice is based on dated bodies of evidence. In a UK study of children's play (Hillman et al 1991), the parental 'licence' (freedom) offered to 9 year olds in 1979 was only available to 13 year olds in 1997. From 80% of 7–8 year olds going to school on their own in the 1970s, this had fallen to fewer than 1 in 10 in 1990. Not only is there an ongoing need to revise and refine models that support contemporary interventions, we also need to conduct research that reminds us of what has been forgotten or overlooked through familiarity (Barritt 1986). This is a particular issue for recurrent or worsening problems.

Although many theoretical arguments surround the impact of 'naming' a problem (Madjar & Walton 1999), many health promoters find that it offers important avenues to improve their practice. However, given an ongoing fear about creating an unintended intervention backlash (Witte & Allen 2000), alternatives may encourage clients to focus beyond their past and their 'problem'. Solution-focused approaches (Iveson & Ratner 1999) are thought to foster empowerment and directions for positive change. Practitioners encourage clients to talk about solutions, while avoiding discussions or explanations of 'why'. The underpinning professional epistemology is that knowing why problems occur does not matter to either the client or the helper. Neither does it matter that the helper can see the 'logic' of the solution. This is central to the solution-focused concept of client-centered care.

With behaviors that are situated in dynamic social contexts, the role of agents who encourage 'non-change' is rarely considered. This effect is strong enough to prevent even well-intentioned sedentary employees from becoming more active (McKenna & Francis 2003). These individuals will play a role in many behavior change settings. Damping the negative influence of these individuals may become an important target in preparing for subsequent interventions.

Value systems also influence understanding of cause and effect; success is due to effort, strategy, and ability, and failure due to luck and task difficulty (Hewstone 1989). Consistent with current approaches to harness environmental factors to promote health, Shinn & Toohey (2003) use the term 'context minimization error' to show how these factors support non-change. Faced with clients who attribute their (unhealthy) behavior to their environment, health promoters may need to resist dismissing these clients as unresponsive. This whole issue suggests a greater need to address social validity (Winett et al 1991), which describes how interventions are made relevant and viable. The related, but distinct, qualitative concept of 'credibility' leads into the next question...

WHY DO THAT FIRST?

Lawrence Green once described health promotion as 'toiling in the darkened goldmine'; Rimer et al (2001, p. 231) describe how intuition guides the 'feel' of what works best. This also directs the order of intervention content, as it is tailored to meet the needs of individual clients. There remains a need to understand the optimum intervention sequence for change. Existing theories tend to prioritize some approaches over others. These decisions typically go unexplained in research papers. Close attention to research design and methods is underlined here, since these features contribute to the outcomes that health practitioners value (Raphael 2000). In an attempt to create the capacity for waves of change, addressing particularly obstructive behaviors, including antisocial lifestyles (Farrington 2003), may be an important priority to optimize intervention outcomes.

Sequential interventions rely on participant development. In the stages of change model, the maturation of the client helps to accept change and support it through lapse and relapse. Defensiveness is one unwanted form of client maturity that may result when fear appeals are used to motivate change. Strong negative, defensive emotions, including resistance ('Yes, but I can't do that...'), reactance ('You're manipulating me, so I'll ignore you ...'), or denial ('This has nothing to do with me...'), can result from interventions that fail to support the efficacy of change once fear has been generated (Witte & Allen 2000). Further, helpers may dislike creating, or even witnessing, negative emotions in their clients. The evidence base is unclear about how persuasive messages can be effective in the face of unstable emotion-states like anxiety, confusion, powerlessness, disgust, or irritation (Witte & Allen 2000, p. 605). An alternative approach involves developing interventions that capitalize on the energizing effects of positive emotions, such as excitement, surprise, and enjoyment.

i see B5

Health promoters will be familiar with, but also dread, clients who reject well-intentioned support. The backlash to any well-intentioned campaign can take many defensive forms. These include avoidance ('This is too much for me right now – I can't think about it...'), wishful thinking ('Isn't that everybody's dream?'), and searching for absolute certainty ('You have to have the right plan, built to suit you...') (McKenna & Francis 2003). For others it encourages reveling in their current behavior ('Yeah, great, isn't it?...'). These responses may reflect decision making about the 'fit' of suggested changes into preexisting behavioral patterns, which the next question addresses.

WHAT ARE THE PARTICIPANTS' REAL-LIFE CHOICE 'CONTESTS'?

A fundamental issue facing most health promoters is their focus on single behaviors, such as smoking, drinking, or drug reduction. In contrast, clients' lifestyles involve choosing between behaviors, as well as about behaviors. Although data are scarce, it is clear that the choice between eating a salad or drinking a cold beer can be made when opening the fridge door. Equally, the purchase of low-fat foods may be best encouraged where these decisions are taken – in the aisles of the supermarket. There is a growing need to address such decision making and deliver campaign messages at the points where decisions are made. Recently, interventions showing people how to cook foods and make them tasty to their families, have made important changes in the diets of target groups (Kennedy et al 1998). Interventions may also question: 'Why is this program delivered here?'.

Another tool to help identify important issues is the 'needs analysis'. While this has an intuitive logic, Hawe (1996) has suggested a refocusing on change, rather than on needs. Focusing on change triggers the active decision making encouraged by many client-centered counseling approaches. In this way, the responsiveness to elements of any possible intervention can be carefully estimated. Further, while client-centered approaches are typically limited to the front end of program development, Tallon et al (2000) have reported on using individualized client-centered outcomes to evaluate interventions. This approach may be useful in developing a better understanding of how to support individuals who maintain successful behavior changes, who may not be the center of attention within intervention programs.

WHICH MESSAGES CHANGE WHAT?

For the management of hypertension, a 'rule of halves' (Hart 1992) has been accepted for some time in medical circles. In this rule, half of patients with high blood pressure are diagnosed, half of those diagnosed are treated, of whom only half take their medication and respond. The relevance of this rule to health promotion efforts had gone unrecognized until Donovan & Owen (1994) hypothesized how it might affect media-based health promotion campaigns. First the target audience is 100%, from there the halving begins: 50% are exposed to a campaign message, of whom only half listen to the message and then only 50% accept the message. Intention, success, repetition, and coping with relapse further amplify the loss of campaign effects.

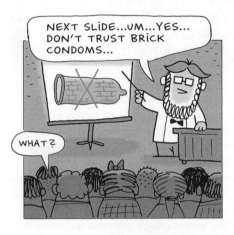

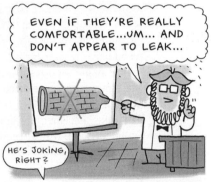

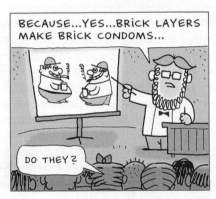

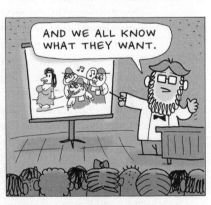

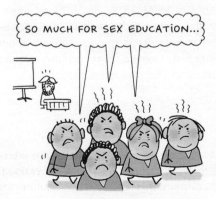

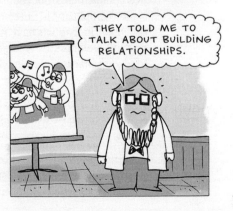

What is clear is the need to identify the influences that optimize client responsiveness to the different elements in this pernicious cascade. This places a greater priority on inclusiveness of campaigns from the outset to maximize the initial pool of participants. Extending 'program reach' will widen the impact of health promotion interventions. Marketing experts can guide the optimizing of exposure and uptake of campaign messages (e.g. Slater 1996).

Yet some practice – even active decision making – appears to contradict recent evidence. Despite being endorsed by UK government agencies, the '5-a-day campaign' has been delivered at the same time as a 7% fall in adult consumption of fresh fruit and vegetables (ONS 2002). Although the explanations are not currently available, there may be good reasons for this. Perhaps the '5-a-day' is a good message – it is recognized by over 50% of polled adults – but the rule of halves may reduce population responses. Statistical modeling of trends may show that the campaign slowed a pattern of temporal decline. These and other issues may affect many domains where new behavioral problem areas are emerging, including becoming overweight (especially in young people), use of recreational drugs, or increases in work–home conflict.

Of course, individualized intervention outcomes hinge on the qualities of interactions. Counseling effectiveness literature suggests that the client–practitioner relationship accounts for up to 40% of outcome variability (Goldfried et al 1990). Here 'rapport' generates this working relationship, which is characterized by mutual acceptance and respect for autonomy. However, few interventions demonstrate achieving this essential criterion, nor how it changes across sequential involvement. Working relationships may even be contrary to this idea: weight management literature is replete with examples of how health professionals stigmatize and are biased against their clients (Puhl & Brownell 2001). This may be avoided by answering the question: 'What am I doing that might impede change for this client?'. Practitioner-researchers who adopt RCT designs in their work risk their efforts to be objective being seen as lack of interest. Either way, it is hard to see how this complements the counselors' need to establish rapport.

The complexity of interactions is deepened by the different intentions that individuals have for their meetings. Pronk et al (1998) distinguished readiness to change from willingness to communicate about lifestyle change. Rudebeck (2001) showed that patients attend consultations with different concerns that may combine:

- personal understanding of their symptoms
- the meaning of symptoms
- how to communicate about symptoms.

Further, with an understanding of symptoms, responses may be internalized and stimulate self-care. Where this encourages an external approach, it may encourage recruiting others who might help.

Finally, clients may also be sensitive to time within consultations even before they begin. Patients intentionally curtailed consultations with family doctors if they thought the doctor was facing intense time pressures (Pollock & Grime 2003). This resulted in interactions that 'got to the point', which reduced the chances of receiving the opportunistic health promotion interventions that doctors like to offer (Silagy et al 1993). Strict control of consultation duration requires careful consideration as it risks establishing a working relationship with an individual client, and with it the chance of delivering an intervention that makes a difference.

CONCLUSION

Although acts of faith may support many of the positive effects of health promoters, these may also support interventions that have negative effects. The maxim 'the road to hell is paved with good intentions' is worth considering. Helping to know where that hell lies has been a central purpose of this chapter. Box A3.1 provides a summary.

Box A3.1   Summary of key questions to assist intervention planning

- **What makes you think that change is needed?**
  Implication: Be sure that change in a particular group is a priority health need and not motivated by emotional reactions.
- **Why do you think change is possible (or not)?**
  Implication: Realize that the ability to change is seen differently by different groups and individuals.
- **Why does 'probleming' help?**
  Implication: Do not necessarily focus on the problem or its roots; solutions may generate a more positive outlook for interventions.
- **Why do that first?**
  Implication: Consider which steps to take first, assess whether they have been successful or not, and how to capitalize on this in subsequent stages of the intervention.
- **What are the participants' real-life choice 'contests'?**
  Implication: Find out the participants' competing issues and priorities. These priorities may not be directly associated with health, in the way you understand 'health'.
- **Which messages change what?**
  Implication: Consider how, and who, will respond to different health-related messages. What is the main obstacle to behavior change? Does the message address that obstacle? Remember, not everyone will hear and respond.

This chapter has explored how our 'mis'-understanding of behavior change 'problems' may be at the heart of interventions that do not succeed. This, in turn, is underpinned by how willing helpers are to change their own approaches to behavior change, particularly to look more closely at unresponsive individuals and groups. A range of perspectives have been used to show how health promoters can firstly understand and respond to the many forms of evidence and secondly understand and develop their understanding of clients and target groups.

References

Andreasen A R 1995 Marketing social change: changing behaviour to promote health, social development, and the environment. Jossey-Bass, San Francisco

Armstrong D, Reyburn H, Jones R 1996 A study of general practitioners' reasons for changing their prescribing behaviour. British Medical Journal 312:949–952

Barritt L 1986 Human science and the human image. Phenomenology and Pedagogy 4:14–22

Bergman A B, Rivara F P, Richards D D et al 1990 The Seattle Children's Bicycle Helmet Campaign. American Journal of Disorders in Children 144:727–731

Cooper A C, Moore L, McKenna J et al 1999 What is the magnitude of blood pressure response to a programme of moderate intensity exercise? Randomised controlled trial among sedentary adults with mild-moderate hypertension. British Journal of General Practice 50:958–962

Cutliffe J R, McKenna H P 2002 When do we know that we know? Considering the truth of research findings and the craft of qualitative research. International Journal of Nursing Studies 39:611–618

Donovan R J, Owen N 1994 Social marketing and population interventions. In: Dishman R K (ed) Advances in exercise adherence. Human Kinetics, Champaign, Illinois, pp 249–290

Elwyn G 2002 Achieving organizational change in general practice: gently simmer for two years. Preventive Medicine 35:419–421

Farrington D 2003 The impact of anti-social lifestyle on health (editorial). British Medical Journal 326:834–835

Green L W, Kreuter M W, Deeds S G et al 1980 Health education planning: a diagnostic approach. Mayfield, Palo Alto

Goldfried M R, Greenberg L, Marmar C 1990 Individual psychotherapy: process and outcome. In: Rosenweig M R, Porter L W (eds) Annual review of psychology, volume 41. Annual Review, Palo Alto, pp 659–688

Haddon W 1999 The changing approach to the epidemiology, prevention, and amelioration of trauma: the transition to approaches etiologically rather than descriptively based. Injury Prevention 5:231–236

Hart J 1992 Rule of halves: implications of increasing diagnosis and reducing dropout for future workload and prescribing costs in primary care. British Journal of General Practice 42:116–119

Hawe P 1996 Needs assessment must become more change-focused. Australian and New Zealand Journal of Public Health 20:473–478

Hesketh T 2003 China in the grip of SARS. British Medical Journal 326:1095

Hewstone M 1989 Causal attribution: from cognitive processes to collective beliefs. Blackwell, Oxford

Hillman M, Adams J, Whitelegg J 1991 One false move . . . a study of children's independent mobility. Policy Studies Institute, London

Hillsdon M, Cavill N K, Nanchahal K et al 2001 National level promotion of physical activity: results from England's Active for Life campaign. Journal of Epidemiology and Community Health 55:755–761

Iveson G E, Ratner H 1999 Problem to solution, 2nd edn. BT Press, London

Kennedy L, Hunt C, Hodgson P 1998 Nutrition education programme based on EFNEP for low income women in the UK, 'Friends with Food'. Journal of Nutrition Education 30:89–99

Lee A J, Mann N P, Takriti R 2000 A hospital led promotion campaign aimed to increase bicycle helmet wearing among children aged 11–15 living in West Berkshire 1992–98. Injury Prevention 6:151–153

Levinas E 1969 Totality and infinity (trans. A Lingis). Dusquenes University Press, Pittsburgh

MacDonald M A, Green L W 2001 Reconciling concept and context: the dilemma of implementation in school-based health promotion. Health Education and Behaviour 28:749–768

Machold W M, Kwasny O, Eisenhardt P et al 2002 Reduction of severe wrist injuries in snowboarding by an optimized wrist protection device: a prospective randomized trial. Journal of Trauma 52:517–520

Madjar I, Walton J A 1999 Nursing and the experience of illness. Routledge, London

McAdams D P, de St. Aubin E 1998 Generativity and adult development: how and why we care for the next generation. APA, Washington

McKenna J, Francis C 2003 Exercise contemplators: unravelling the processes of change. Health Education 103:41–53

McKenna J, Riddoch C J 2003 Introduction. In: McKenna J, Riddoch C J (eds) Perspectives on health and exercise. Palgrave, Basingstoke, pp 1–6

Office for National Statistics (ONS) 2002 Expenditure and food survey. Office for National Statistics, London

Pollock K, Grime J 2003 Patients' perceptions of entitlement to time in general practice consultations for depression: qualitative study. British Medical Journal 325:687–692

Pronk P P, Tan A W H, O'Connor P 1998 Obesity, fitness, willingness to communicate and health care costs. Medicine and Science in Sports and Exercise 31:1535–1543

Puhl R, Brownell K D 2001 Bias, discrimination and obesity. Obesity Research 9:788–805

Raphael D 2000 The question of evidence in health promotion. Health Promotion International 15:355–367

Rimer B K, Glanz K, Rasband G 2001 Searching for evidence about health education and health behaviour interventions. Health Education and Behaviour 28:231–248

Rudebeck C E 2001 Grasping the existential anatomy: the role of bodily empathy in clinical communication. In: Toombs S K (ed) Handbook of phenomenology. Kluwer Academic, Dordrecht, pp 297–316

Runyan C W 1998 Using the Haddon matrix: introducing the third dimension. Injury Prevention 4:302–307

Seligman M E P 1993 The effectiveness of psychotherapy. American Psychologist 50:965–974

Shinn M, Toohey S M 2003 Community context of human welfare. Annual Review of Psychology 54:427–459

Silagy C, Muir J, Coulter A et al 1993 Cardiovascular risk and attitudes to lifestyle: what do patients think? British Medical Journal 306:1657–1660

Slater M D 1996 Theory and method in health audience segmentation. Journal of Health Communication 1:267–283

Tallon D, Chard J, Dieppe P 2000 Priorities of patients with knee OA. Arthritis Care and Research 13:312–319

Winett R A, Moore J F, Anderson E S 1991 Extending the concept of social validity: behaviour analysis for disease prevention and health promotion. Journal of Applied Behavioural Analysis 24:215–230

Witte K, Allen M 2000 A meta-analysis of fear appeals: implications for effective public health campaigns. Health Education and Behaviour 27:591–615

Planning and evaluating interventions

A4

James McKenzie

As has been noted in other chapters, the process of behavior change is very complex and is influenced by a number of personal and environmental factors. Because of the complexity of the behavior change process, planning and evaluating interventions can be very challenging. Even the most experienced health promotion specialists find the process of program development demanding because of the constant changes in settings, resources, and priority populations (McKenzie & Smeltzer 2001). Successful interventions do not occur by chance; detailed planning is a must! In this context, planning is defined as a process in which an intervention is developed that meets the needs of the targeted audience and is designed in such a way that the outcomes of the program can be measured.

MODELS FOR PLANNING PREVENTION PROJECTS

It is generally accepted that the process of intervention development can take many different forms. In fact, a number of planning models are available (e.g. Anspaugh et al 2000, Bartholomew et al 2001, CDC 1999, Green & Kreuter 1999, McKenzie & Smeltzer 2001, Neiger 1998, Simons-Morton et al 1988, Timmreck 2002). Though each of the planning models may be slightly different, and use different labels to identify the steps in the planning process, all approaches usually center on a generic set of tasks. These tasks are presented in the Generalized Model (McKenzie & Smeltzer 2001).

The generalized model

The Generalized Model is composed of six generic tasks that need to be addressed when planning and evaluating interventions.

41

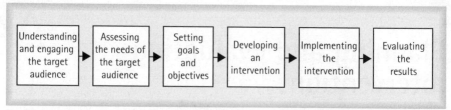

Fig A4.1   A Generalized Model for program development (McKenzie & Smeltzer 2001, p. 10. Reprinted by permission of Pearson Education, Inc.)

UNDERSTANDING AND ENGAGING THE TARGET AUDIENCE

The first step in this model is to understand and engage the people in the target audience, those whom the intervention is intended to serve. Understanding the target audience means finding out as much as possible about the people and the environment in which they exist. Engaging the target audience means getting them involved early in the planning process and keeping them involved throughout. Also as a part of this first step, planners should form a planning committee with representation from the various subgroups of the target audience to further engage the target audience and ensure they feel some 'ownership' in the project.

ASSESSING THE NEEDS OF THE TARGET AUDIENCE

In order to create an effective intervention, planners, with assistance of the planning committee, must determine the needs and wants of those in the target audience. This step is referred to as a needs assessment and defined as the process of collecting and analyzing information, to develop an understanding of the issues, resources, and constraints of the target audience, as related to the development of the intervention (Anspaugh et al 2000).

SETTING GOALS AND OBJECTIVES

Once the needs have been identified and prioritized, the planners must write the goals and objectives for the intervention. Goals and objectives should be thought of as the foundation of the intervention. The remaining portions of the programming process will be designed to achieve the goals by meeting the objectives.

The words 'goals' and 'objectives' are often used interchangeably, but there is a significant difference between the two. Neiger (1998) has defined goals as general statements of intent. Goals include two basic components – who will be affected and what will change because of the project. Here are two examples.

- To reduce the number of unintended pregnancies in the community.

- To help cancer patients and their families deal with lifestyle changes after diagnosis.

Objectives are more precise and can be considered as the steps neces-sary to achieve the project goals. They comprise four parts (who, what, when, and how much) and outline changes that should result from the implementation of the intervention. Since some goals are more com-plex than others, the number and level of objectives needed to reach a goal will vary. In general, the more comprehensive a goal, the greater the number of objectives needed. Table A4.1 presents a hierarchy of the different levels of objectives first created by Deeds (1992) and adapted by McKenzie & Smeltzer (2001).

From the examples presented in Table A4.1, note that the complexity of the levels increases as one goes down through the hierarchy. It takes fewer resources to increase awareness in the target audience than to improve its health status. Also, note that the objectives are written in specific terms (observable and measurable).

DEVELOPING AN INTERVENTION

This step of the planning process includes designing activities and strategies that will help achieve the objectives and goals. These activi-ties are collectively referred to as the intervention or treatment.

The number of activities/strategies in an intervention may vary. Although no minimum number has been established, it has been shown that multiple activities/strategies are often more effective than a single activity/strategy. Few people change a behavior based on a single expo-sure (or dose); instead, multiple exposures (doses) are generally needed to change most behaviors.

The choice of activities/strategies for an intervention depends on a number of factors. McLeroy et al (1988) have indicated that different levels of influence need to be considered when developing interven-tions. These levels include:

- intrapersonal (individual) factors
- interpersonal (small group) factors
- institutional or organizational factors
- community factors
- public policy factors.

Thus, interventions can be developed to 'attack' an identified need of a target audience at any or all of these levels. Regardless of the number activities/strategies included in an intervention and at what levels of influence the intervention is aimed, planners need to be able to accu-rately describe the intervention in writing. This process is referred to as preparing a written protocol. See Box A4.1 for commonly used intervention activities/strategies.

Table A4.1 Hierarchy of intervention objectives (Reprinted with permission from McKenzie et al 2002, p. 127)

Type of objective	Program outcomes	Possible evaluation measures	Type of evaluation	Example
Process administrative objectives	Activities presented and tasks completed	Number of sessions held, exposure, attendance, participation, staff performance, appropriate materials, adequacy of resources, tasks on schedule	Process (form of formative)	On June 12 2002, the breast cancer brochure will be distributed to all female customers over the age of 18 at the Ross grocery store.
Learning objectives	Change in awareness, knowledge, attitudes, and skills	Increase in awareness, knowledge, attitudes, skill development/acquisition	Impact (form of summative)	When asked in class, 50% of the students will be able to list at least four risk factors for heart disease.
Behavioral and environmental objectives	Behavior adoption, change in environment	Change in behavior, hazards, or barriers removed from the environment	Impact (form of summative)	During a telephone interview, 35% of the residents will report having had their blood cholesterol checked in the last 6 months.
Program objectives	Change in quality of life (QOL), health status or risk, and social benefits	QOL measures, morbidity data, mortality data, measures of risk (i.e. HRA)	Outcome (form of summative)	By the year 2000, infant mortality rates will be reduced to no more than 7 per 1000 in Franklin County.

> **Box A4.1** Intervention activities and examples (Reprinted with permission from McKenzie et al 2002, p. 120)
>
> 1 **Communication activities**
>   Examples include: mass media, flyers, newsletters, pamphlets, posters, video and audio materials.
> 2 **Educational activities**
>   Examples include: printed educational materials, teaching strategies and techniques.
> 3 **Behavior modification activities**
>   Examples include: modifying behavior to stop smoking, managing stress, regulating diet.
> 4 **Environmental change activities**
>   Examples include: no-smoking signs, putting only 'healthy' foods in vending machines.
> 5 **Regulatory activities**
>   Examples include: laws, policies, rules to change health behavior.
> 6 **Community advocacy activities**
>   Examples include: mass mobilization, social action, community advocacy, such as a letter-writing campaign.
> 7 **Organizational culture activities**
>   Examples include: activities that work to change norms and traditions.
> 8 **Incentives and disincentives**
>   Examples include: money and other material items, fines.
> 9 **Health status evaluation activities**
>   Examples include: health risk appraisals (HRAs), health screenings (both self- and clinic-administered).
> 10 **Social intervention activities**
>   Examples include: support groups, social networks.
> 11 **Technology-delivered activities**
>   Examples include: educating or informing people by using technology (e.g. computers, telephones).

IMPLEMENTING THE INTERVENTION

Implementation is the actual carrying out of the activities/strategies that make up the intervention. Parkinson & Associates (1982) have identified three different levels of implementation: pilot testing, phasing-in, and total implementation. If resources are available, the use of all three levels is likely to ensure a more successful implementation.

A pilot test is a trial run. It occurs when the intervention is presented to just a few individuals who are either from the targeted audience or from a very similar group. The purpose of pilot testing is to determine whether there are any problems or concerns with the intervention so they can be corrected.

After pilot testing, an intervention is ready to be disseminated and implemented. Rather than implementing the intervention to the entire targeted audience at once, it is advisable for planners to phase it in gradually. Phasing-in refers to implementation in which the number of people receiving the intervention gradually increases. Common means by which interventions are phased in include by participants' ability, number of participants, program offerings, and program location. Phasing-in continues until total implementation is completed.

EVALUATING THE RESULTS

The final step in the Generalized Model is evaluation which is the process of determining the value or worth of the object of interest by comparing it against a standard of acceptability (Green & Lewis 1986). Common standards of acceptability include, but are not limited to, mandates (policies, statutes, laws), values, norms, and behavior of comparison/control groups. The standards of acceptability should be reflected in the 'what' and 'how much' of the objectives.

The rigor of the evaluation will depend on the purpose and scope of the intervention. When the stakes of evaluation are high (i.e. much is riding on the outcome of an intervention) evaluation procedures need to become formal, explicit, and justifiable (CDC 1999). Formal evaluation processes are characterized by systematic well-planned procedures (Williams & Suen 1998). As such, the evaluation is designed to control the extraneous variables that could produce evaluation outcomes that are incorrect. When stakes are not as high and proving the worth of an intervention is not as critical, evaluation is often more informal. Informal evaluation is characterized as impromptu unsystematic procedures (Williams & Suen 1998). Such evaluation processes are used when making small changes in interventions, like changing the time it is offered, adding an additional class session, consulting colleagues about a program concern, or making intervention changes based on participant feedback.

Evaluation can be further categorized into summative and formative evaluation. Formative evaluation is done during the planning and implementing processes to improve or refine the program. For example, validating the needs assessment and pilot testing are both forms of formative evaluation. Summative evaluation begins with the development of goals and objectives and is typically conducted after implementation to determine the impact of the intervention.

PROCESSES TO ENSURE THE QUALITY OF AN INTERVENTION

Planning a quality intervention is not an easy process. In working through the six-step model presented in this chapter, planners will be faced with a number of decisions and processes that will have a lot to say about the final quality of the intervention. Some of these are presented next.

Selecting an evaluation design

Typically, because of limited resources, it is most difficult, if not impossible, to create the perfect evaluation. Thus, the challenge for planners is to devise the optimal evaluation for their intervention (CDC 1999). The basic design decision facing planners is whether to use a quantitative or qualitative design or a combination of the two. A quantitative design generally produces numeric data, such as counts, ratings, scores, or classifications, while qualitative designs produce narrative data, such as descriptions. Figure A4.2 provides a few examples of quantitative designs commonly used for health promotion interventions. Those designs that include a control (i.e. experimental designs) or comparison (i.e. quasi-experimental) group are the most powerful, and thus the most desired.

Commonly used qualitative designs include: participant–observer methods, ethnographic methods, various forms of interviewing (i.e. in-depth, elite, and focus groups), content analysis, case studies, nominal group process, Delphi techniques, and quality circles. (See McDermott & Sarvela (1999) for an in-depth explanation of these methods.) While a specific situation may dictate the use of just a quantitative or

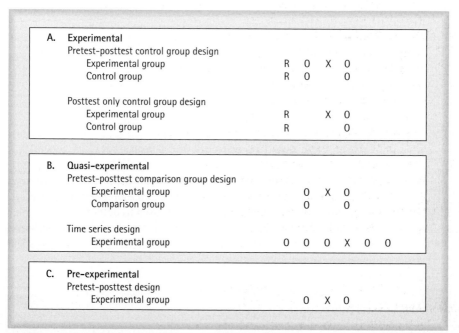

Fig A4.2   Commonly used quantitative evaluation designs. R = random assignment, O = observation/measurement and X = intervention/treatment

qualitative design, there are times when the strongest evaluation design is a combination of the two methods. Steckler et al (1992) have presented a rationale for integrating the two methods since, to a certain extent, the weaknesses of one method are compensated for by the strengths of the other.

Data collection

While planning and evaluating an intervention, planners will be faced with the task of collecting data. This task is most often encountered during the processes of needs assessment and evaluation. Because these are such critical processes to a successful intervention, much care needs to be taken when collecting the data. In the next part of this chapter, several key data collection concepts are presented.

LEVELS OF MEASUREMENT

A fundamental question of the data collection process is determining how something should be measured (McDermott & Sarvela 1999). In other words, what type of measuring stick should be used? For example, suppose planners were interested in collecting 'age' data from the priority population. They could ask the participants their age in several different ways.

- **Question:** *Are you old enough to have a driver's license?*
- **Question:** *Which category best describes your age?*
  - <20 years old
  - 21–40 years old
  - 41–60 years old
  - 61+ years old
- **Question:** *How old were you on your last birthday?*

Each of these questions will elicit the person's age, but generates a different form of data.

Thus, when planners begin to think about data collection, they need to consider the form(s) of data (or levels of measurement) they want to use. There are four levels of measurement used to determine how something can be assessed: nominal, ordinal, interval, and ratio measures. These levels are hierarchical in nature and determine what statistical analyses can be used.

Nominal

Nominal level measures, the lowest level in the measurement hierarchy, enable planners to put data into categories.

The two requirements for nominal measures are that the categories have to be mutually exclusive so that each case fits into one of the categories, and the categories have to be exhaustive so that there is a place for every case. (Weiss 1998, p. 116)

Example questions that generate nominal data include:

- **Question:** *What is your sex?*
- **Question:** *In what country were you born?*

Ordinal

Ordinal level measures, like nominal level measures, allow planners to put data into categories that are mutually exclusive and exhaustive, but also permit them to rank-order the categories. 'The different categories represent relatively more or less of something' (McKenzie & Smeltzer 2001, p. 97). However, the distance between categories cannot be measured. Example questions that generate ordinal data include:

- **Question:** *How would you describe your level of health?*
  - Good
  - Fair
  - Poor
- **Question:** *Which category best represents your age?*
  - 20–35
  - 36–50
  - 51+

Interval

Interval level measures enable project planners to put data into categories that are mutually exclusive and exhaustive, rank-order the categories, and measure the distance between the categories. There is, however, no absolute zero value. Example questions that generate interval data include:

- **Question:** *What was the temperature this morning when you got up?*
- **Question:** *What was the student's z-score on the standardized test?*

Ratio

Ratio level measures, the highest level in the measurement hierarchy, enable project planners to do everything with data that can be done with the other three levels of measures; however, they are done using a scale with an absolute zero. Example questions that generate ratio data include:

- **Question:** *How high is your temperature?*
- **Question:** *What is the gross income of your family for a year?*

CHARACTERISTICS OF DESIRABLE DATA

The results generated from the interpretation of the collected data are only as good as the data that were used to produce the results. If the collected data are inaccurate, biased, or ambiguous, there is a good chance that the results of the needs assessment will not reflect the true needs of the target audience or the evaluation will not provide a clear picture of the worth of the intervention. Therefore, it is of vital importance that planners ensure that the collected data are reliable, valid, unbiased, and culturally appropriate (McKenzie & Smeltzer 2001).

Reliability

'Reliability refers to consistency in the measurement process. A reliable instrument gives the same (or nearly the same) result every time' (McKenzie & Smeltzer 2001, p. 98). Several different methods can be used to establish instrument reliability, depending on the type of instrument. They include internal consistency reliability, stability reliability, rater reliability, and parallel forms reliability.

Validity

A valid data collection instrument measures what it intends to measure. That is, it correctly measures the concepts under investigation. For example, if planners want to create a needs assessment instrument and collect data about the health behavior of the target audience, the questions need to be oriented towards those behaviors and not towards health knowledge. Like reliability, there are several different methods for establishing the validity of a data collection instrument. They include face validity, content validity, criterion-related validity, and construct validity.

Unbiased

'Biased data are those data that have been distorted because of the way they have been collected' (McKenzie & Smeltzer 2001, p. 101). In order to effectively create and evaluate interventions, planners must work to eliminate bias. Examples of data collection bias include: when participants do not feel comfortable answering a sensitive question, when participants act differently (e.g. in a manner to please the observer) because they know they are being watched, or when certain characteristics of the interviewer (e.g. body language) influence a response (Windsor et al 1994). Examples of steps that can be taken to limit bias include using unobtrusive observation, collecting sensitive data using anonymous, techniques, or using a representative sample when selecting project participants.

Culturally appropriate

'Culture shapes the way of life shared by members of a population. It is the sociocultural adaptation or design for living that people have worked out (and continue to work out) in the course of their history' (Ogbu 1987, p. 156). Because of the importance of culture in people's lives, planners need to be sensitive to the impact culture plays when collecting data from the target audience. Thus, questions on data collection instruments need to be worded in ways that are consistent with the culture or cultures of the target audience. For example, culturally insensitive questions may not take into account that people from some cultures see some foods as an important part of their diet, while others see the same foods as dirty and not to be consumed.

METHODS OF DATA COLLECTION

There are a number of different methods that can be used to collect data; the primary means of doing so are described below.

Self-report

Self-report data are those that are generated by having individuals report about themselves. Such data can be collected using written questionnaires, face-to-face interviews, telephone interviews, or electronic means, such as email or fax questionnaires.

Observation

Data can be collected using either direct or indirect observation. Direct observation means seeing someone actually doing something, while indirect observation uses a proxy measure to 'observe' behavior. An example of indirect observation would be counting empty beverage bottles/cans as a means of measuring alcohol consumption. As noted earlier, bias in observation can be reduced through using unobtrusive methods of observing.

Existing records

Records that exist for another purpose often provide a rich data source for planners. Often such data are inexpensive to collect. Examples include epidemiological data collected by governmental agencies, medical records held by health-care providers and health insurance claims data. Major disadvantages of using these data include gaining access due to privacy issues and, after gaining access, finding incomplete or inaccurate data.

Meetings

Getting people to respond to a data collection instrument, sent through the mail or email or collected over the phone, can often become a barrier to data collection. Thus, meetings become a convenient face-to-face setting for collecting data.

Subject selection/recruitment

Subject selection and recruitment is always a concern when planning and evaluating interventions. Collecting data from individuals who 'represent' those in the target audience is important to avoid selection bias, which can generate biased data. Depending on the purpose of the intervention and the size of the target audience, the planners need to decide from whom and how many they will need to collect data.

CENSUS AND SAMPLES

If adequate resources (i.e. time, money, and person-power) are available and the target audience is not too large, planners may want to collect data from everyone. This is called a census. However, if resources are not great and/or the target audience is overly large, a sample of the participants will need to be used. There are two types of samples: probability and non-probability.

Probability sampling

A probability sample is one in which each person in the population has an equal chance and known probability of being selected. Such criteria increase the chances that the selected sample is representative of the population, which in turn increases the chances that the data collected from these individuals will be free from sampling bias. Different forms of probability sampling include: simple random sampling (SRS), systematic sampling, stratified random sampling, and cluster sampling.

Non-probability sampling

A non-probability sample is one in which each person in the population does not have an equal chance and/or known probability of being selected. Such a sample is used when all in the population cannot be identified, when resources are limited, and for purposes of convenience. If such a process is used for sampling, planners need to be aware of the limitations of this type of sample and the chance for sampling bias. Examples of non-probability sampling techniques include convenience, volunteer, grab, homogeneous, judgmental, snowball, and quota (McDermott & Sarvela 1999).

SAMPLE SIZE

An often-asked question associated with sampling is, 'How many individuals are needed for planners to feel confident that sampling error is within an acceptable range so that reasonable conclusions can be drawn from the data analyzed?'. There is not an easy answer to this question. Appropriate sample size is determined by considering both statistical and practical considerations. Space in this chapter does not permit a discussion of sample size determination. See Dupont & Plummer (1990) for a good explanation of items that must be considered when determining sample size.

CONCLUSION

There are a number of different models that can be used to plan and evaluate interventions. The Generalized Model (McKenzie & Smeltzer 2001) was presented because it includes the six basic steps of intervention planning and evaluating. The reader was also introduced to several other processes that need to be considered to ensure a successful intervention, including evaluation design, levels of measurement, characteristics of good data, methods of data collection, sampling procedures, and sample size.

References

Anspaugh D J, Dignan M B, Anspaugh S L 2000 Developing health promotion programs. McGraw-Hill, Boston

Bartholomew L K, Parcel G S, Kok G et al 2001 Intervention mapping: designing theory and evidenced-based health promotion programs. Mayfield, Mountain View

Centers for Disease Control and Prevention (CDC) 1999 Framework for program evaluation in public health. Morbidity and Mortality Weekly Report 48(RR-11):1-40

Deeds S G 1992 The health education specialist: self-study for professional
    competence. Loose Canon, Los Alamitos

Dupont W D, Plummer W D 1990 Power and sample size calculations: a review
    and computer program. Controlled Clinical Trials 11:116-128

Green L W, Kreuter M W 1999 Health promotion planning: an educational and
    ecological approach, 3rd edn. Mayfield, Mountain View

Green L W, Lewis F M 1986 Measurement and evaluation in health education
    and health promotion. Mayfield, Palo Alto

McDermott R J, Sarvela PD 1999 Health education evaluation and
    measurement, 2nd edn. WCB/McGraw-Hill, New York

McKenzie J F, Smeltzer J L 2001 Planning, implementing, and evaluating
    health promotion programs: a primer, 2nd edn. Allyn and Bacon, Boston

McKenzie J F, Pinger R R, Kotecki J E 2002 An introduction to community
    health, 4th edn. Jones and Bartlett, Boston

McLeroy K R, Bibeau D, Steckler A et al 1988 An ecological perspective for
    health promotion programs. Health Education Quarterly 15(4):351-378

Neiger B L 1998 Social marketing: making public health sense. Paper
    presented at the Annual Meeting of the Utah Public Health Association,
    Provo

Ogbu J 1987 Cultural influences on plasticity in human development.
    In: Gallagher J L, Ramey C T (eds) The malleability of children. Paul H
    Brooks, Baltimore, pp 155-169

Parkinson R S and Associates 1982 Managing health promotion in the
    workplace: guidelines for implementation and evaluation. Mayfield, Palo
    Alto

Simons-Morton D G, Simons-Morton B G, Parcel G S et al 1988 Influencing
    personal and environmental conditions for community health: a multilevel
    intervention model. Family and Community Health 11(2):25-35

Steckler A, McLeroy K R, Goodman R M et al 1992 Toward integrating
    qualitative and quantitative methods: an introduction. Health Education
    Quarterly 19(1):1-8

Timmreck T C 2002 Planning, program development, and evaluation, 2nd edn.
    Jones and Bartlett, Boston

Weiss C H 1998 Evaluation, 2nd edn. Prentice-Hall, Upper Saddle

Williams B, Suen H 1998 Formal vs. informal assessment methods. American
    Journal of Health Behavior 22(4):308-313

Windsor R, Baranowski T, Clark N et al 1994 Evaluation of health promotion,
    health education, and disease prevention programs, 2nd edn. Mayfield,
    Mountain View

Personal Factors

Personality and individual differences

Elizabeth McDade-Montez, Jamie Cvengros, and Alan Christensen

The goal of this chapter is to provide an overview of the research involving the relationship of personality and individual difference characteristics to health behavior and health behavior change. In this initial part, we provide an introduction to some of the individual difference characteristics of central empirical interest in the health behavior literature. In the subsequent part, we examine common models of health behavior change and the role that individual differences play in moderating the effectiveness of health behavior change programs.

INDIVIDUAL DIFFERENCES

Social

ETHNICITY

Demographic factors have long been known to be associated with distinct patterns of health-related behavior. Different patterns of positive and negative health behaviors have clearly been noted for different ethnic groups (Dowda et al 2003, Fardy et al 2000, Penn et al 2000, Sharkey & Haines 2001). For example, significant differences in eating habits, weight, and alcohol consumption have been noted among Black or African-American, Caucasian, and Hispanic populations. Data from the United States indicate that Hispanic Americans consume less alcohol than other demographic groups, while Black Americans consume diets higher in saturated fat and cholesterol. Moreover, Caucasian American women maintain lower body weight relative to individuals from other ethnic or cultural backgrounds.

Cultural differences have also been noted in levels of physical activity between ethnic groups, with Black men and Caucasian women often found to engage in the highest levels of physical activity and Hispanic men and women engaging in the least amount of moderate to vigorous physical activity (see, for example, Dowda et al 2003). In contrast, additional research has found that both Black and Hispanic men and women are less physically active than Caucasians, even after controlling for the effects of socio-economic status (see, for example, Yen & Kaplan 1998). Finally, among adults with diabetes, one study found no ethnic differences in physical activity levels (Wood 2002). This area of research has generated considerable attention, but variable results, and firm conclusions regarding ethnic differences in physical activity are not yet apparent.

Ethnic differences have also been noted in international cross-cultural comparisons, including levels of smoking among Russian and Finnish youth (Kemppainen et al 2002), and Bangladeshi and Pakistani adults (Bush et al 2003), and in drinking patterns among Jewish immigrants to Israel (Aharonovich et al 2001). For example, in a study of 9th-grade smoking behavior, 29% of young men and 7% of young women surveyed in the Pitkaranta district in Russia were daily smokers as compared to 19% of young men and 21% of young women in Eastern Finland (Kemppainen et al 2002). Explanations for such ethnic distinctions in smoking and alcohol use, as well as other health behaviors, have included socio-economic status, religion, and family influence.

i see C1

AGE

Research has generally shown that promoting one's own health and engaging in certain positive health behaviors (e.g. diet, dental care, sun protection) typically increases with age (Amir 1987, Cockerham 1997, Jensen et al 1992). Adolescents, for example, typically perceive less risk from engaging in negative health behaviors than adults (Cohn et al 1995). However, certain positive health behaviors, such as exercise, may decline with age (see, for example, Burton et al 1999). In a study of initiation and maintenance of physical activity among those 65 years and older, Burton et al (1999) found that, over a 4-year period, the majority (41.3%) of participants maintained their initial level of physical activity (brisk physical activity at least three times per week), yet 21.6% declined in activity and only 12% increased their activity level during this time period. While age generally correlates positively with engagement in health-promoting behaviors, some such behaviors, such as exercise, may decrease over time.

GENDER

Researchers have found different patterns of health behaviors among men and women in a number of domains. For example, gender differences have been noted regarding smoking (Ross & Bird 1994), alcohol consumption (McDonough & Walters 2001), and dieting (Stronegger et al 1997), with women typically smoking and drinking less and following healthier diets than men. Since the 1990s, however, smoking among young women has increased steadily (US DHHS 2001) and has been decreasing among young men (CDC 2002), which may eventually change the current patterns of gender differences in smoking. Regarding exercise and physical activity, men typically engage in more such activity than women (James et al 2003, Ross & Bird 1994, Stronegger et al 1997, Waldron 1997). While traditional thinking has associated healthier behaviors with women, closer examination reveals that patterns of positive health behaviors may vary depending on type of behavior.

Psychological

PERSONALITY

Health behavior researchers have increasingly become interested in the relationship between personality and health behaviors. The Five Factor Model (FFM) of personality, which includes the domains of neuroticism, extraversion, openness, agreeableness, and conscientiousness (Costa & McCrae 1992), has proven particularly instructive in health behavior research and in identifying protective and risk factors for disease and wellness. Neuroticism refers to an individual's tendency to experience and display negative emotions, extraversion refers to an individual's degree of sociability and interest in others, openness relates to creativity, imagination, and willingness to try new experiences, agreeableness is the tendency to trust others and to express positive affect towards them, and conscientiousness reflects the tendencies toward reliability, perseverance, and self-discipline (McCrae & Costa 1997). While some researchers have pointed out the shortcomings of relying solely on the FFM (Marshall et al 1994), many agree on the benefits of using a common, organizing framework for understanding the effects of personality on health behaviors (Wiebe & Smith 1997).

Booth-Kewley & Vickers (1994) found all five major personality dimensions, as measured through the NEO Personality Inventory (Costa & McCrae 1985), to be significantly associated with at least one of four major health behavior domains. Specifically, individuals high in neuroticism were less likely to report positive health behaviors and accident control behaviors and more likely to report substance risk-taking. Individuals high in extraversion were more likely to report wellness behaviors and accident control and were also more likely to report substance risk-taking. Individuals high in conscientiousness and agreeableness were more likely to report wellness behaviors and accident control and fewer traffic risk-taking behaviors. Finally, individuals high in openness reported more substance use.

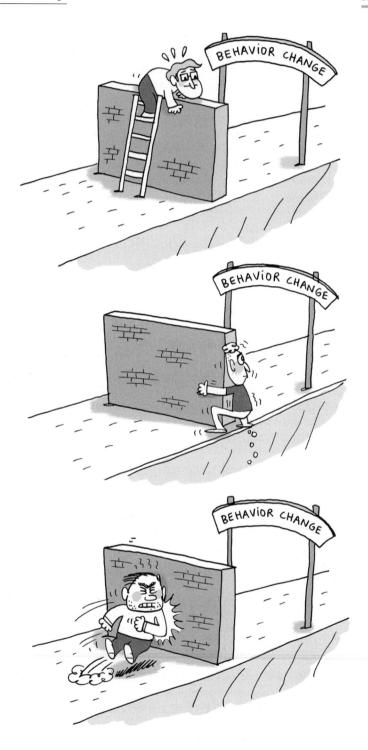

In a second study that investigated the relations between the FFM and health behaviors (Lemos-Giraldez & Fidalgo-Aliste 1997), neuroticism predicted engaging in fewer positive health behaviors and conscientiousness predicted engaging in more positive health behaviors (e.g. not smoking, not drinking alcohol, consuming fruit, etc.). Other research has found a similar effect for conscientiousness and positive health behaviors, such as instituting indoor smoking bans in the home (Hampson et al 2000) and avoiding alcohol intoxication, smoking, and risky sexual behavior (Vollrath et al 1998). In addition, Vollrath et al (1998) found that individuals high in neuroticism were not more or less likely to engage in risky negative health behaviors, yet were more likely to perceive themselves as susceptible to alcohol dependency, drunk driving, HIV/AIDS, and other sexually transmitted infections. Vollrath et al also found that those individuals high in extraversion and openness were more likely to engage in negative health behaviors, such as taking sexual risks and drinking to the point of intoxication.

To summarize, health behaviors have been found to be significantly influenced by personality traits, as measured by the Five Factor Model. In particular, higher levels of conscientiousness and agreeableness have been found to be associated with more positive health practices and fewer negative health behaviors, and neuroticism has generally been associated with fewer positive health behaviors. Higher levels of extraversion and openness to experience have been associated with more negative health practices in certain domains (e.g. substance use).

Dispositional optimism

While the Five Factor Model of personality presents one useful method through which to conceptualize personality and study health behaviors, research has also illustrated the utility of other constructs of personality, such as dispositional optimism, in the study of health behaviors. Ouellette & DiPlacido (2001) define dispositional optimism as 'an individual's stable, generalized expectation that they will experience good things in life' (p. 179). Dispositional optimism is thought to influence health behaviors in two possible ways. First, an individual's expectations regarding an outcome (e.g. pessimistic or optimistic) determine behavior. Therefore, optimistic outcome expectations lead individuals to pursue health-related behaviors more than pessimistic outcome expectations (Scheier & Carver 1987). Secondly, optimistic individuals may have more adaptive coping mechanisms when faced with stress (Mulkana & Hailey 2001). Dispositional optimism has been linked to taking vitamins in coronary artery bypass patients (Scheier & Carver 1992), to exercising and lowering levels of saturated fat and body fat in cardiac rehabilitation patients (Sheppard et al 1996), and to having fewer anonymous sexual partners (Scheier & Carver 1992). Optimism has also been found to predict similar patterns for different ethnic groups, including African-Americans (Mulkana & Hailey 2001).

Hostility and Type A Behavior

Clinical researchers have observed for decades a potential connection between coronary heart disease (CHD) patients and a particular personality type, labeled the 'type A behavior pattern' (Friedman & Rosenman 1974). This behavioral pattern includes a tendency toward impatience, competitiveness, high-achievement striving, and hostility or anger proneness. Recently, researchers have begun to deconstruct the relationship between the multifaceted 'type A' pattern and health (Smith 1992). The general consensus has been that hostility, or the tendency to mistrust or feel anger towards others, is more directly connected to health behaviors than other 'type A' behaviors. For example, higher trait hostility, assessed using the Cook-Medley Hostility Scale (Cook & Medley 1954), has been found to correlate with decreased exercise, decreased dental care, increased alcohol consumption, and increased smoking (Smith 1992). In a study of rural Western Europeans, individuals high in hostility, as measured with the California Psychological Inventory (Gough 1957), were found to have poorer eating and sleeping habits and exercised less (Vingerhoets et al 1990). The influence of hostility on health behaviors and outcomes remains of considerable interest to researchers in this area and is deserving of further attention.

PRINCIPLES OF LEARNING

In this part, we will review some of the major models of learning that have been applied to understanding health behavior change. Specifically, the classical conditioning paradigm and the operant conditioning paradigm have been employed in health behavior change theory and research and will be examined here.

Classical conditioning

In the classical conditioning model (also called respondent learning) the natural association between a stimulus and a response is modified such that an ambiguous stimulus will now elicit the same response. Within the classical conditioning paradigm, there are two types of stimuli (unconditioned and conditioned) and two types of responses (unconditioned and conditioned). An unconditioned stimulus is one that naturally elicits an unconditioned response. For example, the smell of food naturally elicits salivation. Through conditioning, this unconditioned stimulus is repeatedly paired with an ambiguous stimulus (e.g. a bell). Eventually, the ambiguous stimulus will also elicit the unconditioned response. Thus, the ambiguous stimulus becomes the conditioned stimulus and the response it elicits becomes the conditioned response. In the previous example, the bell will eventually elicit the salivation without the smell of food.

Classical conditioning principles both maintain poor health behaviors and are used to elicit health behavior change. For example, smoking is often maintained by classical conditioning principles and these same principles are employed in smoking cessation programs. In smoking behavior, ambiguous stimuli such as certain environments (e.g. the office break room), situations (e.g. immediately after a meal), or objects (e.g. an ashtray) are repeatedly paired with nicotine craving, the unconditioned stimulus, and eventually become conditioned stimuli. Thus, the office break room, mealtimes, and ashtrays elicit the conditioned response (e.g. smoking a cigarette). These associations are often quite powerful and make smoking cessation very difficult.

Recognizing and modifying these conditioned stimuli–response pairs is called stimulus control. In stimulus control, the conditioned stimulus–response association is broken by separating the conditioned stimulus (e.g. office break room) from the ability to smoke. For example, if the break room filled with other smokers consistently elicits smoking, a client would be encouraged to take their break elsewhere. For example, he could spend his break in the building lobby, where smoking is prohibited, or taking a walk in a nearby park. By limiting exposure to smoking-inducing stimuli, the desire to smoke may be decreased.

Operant conditioning

In the operant conditioning model a behavior is increased or decreased by the application of environmental consequences. There are two broad categories of environmental consequences: reinforcement, which increases the behavior, and punishment, which decreases the behavior. Within these categories, consequences can be positive or negative. Specifically, positive reinforcement is the application of a positive, environmental attribute following a behavior that increases the desired, target behavior. Negative reinforcement is the removal of an unpleasant, environmental attribute following a behavior, which then serves to increase the frequency of the target behavior. Positive punishment is the application of an aversive consequence that decreases the undesired behavior. Negative punishment, also known as 'response cost', is the removal of a pleasant or valued attribute when a target behavior occurs.

Operant conditioning procedures are also useful in eliciting and maintaining health behavior change. For example, exercise programs often capitalize on positive reinforcement principles and failure to exercise may be maintained by operant principles. Often, the initial attempts at exercise produce positive punishment outcomes, such as sore muscles and fatigue, decreasing the likelihood that the exercise behavior continues. However, if these initial hurdles can be overcome, exercise programs may be maintained using operant conditioning. For example, positive reinforcements for exercise include increased positive mood and increased energy level. Negative reinforcements include decreased poor self-image and decreased fatigue. A positive punishment for not exercising could be increased weight gain and a negative punishment could be clothes that no longer fit.

INDIVIDUAL DIFFERENCES AS MODERATORS IN HEALTH BEHAVIOR CHANGE

Although models of behavior change are widely applied to health behaviors, the results may vary based on the individual difference characteristics of those engaging in the change. It is not surprising that individual variances in attitudes, personality, and motivation can greatly impact the efficacy of a health behavior change intervention. However, there is surprisingly little research on this issue. A review by Dance & Neufeld (1988) explored the role of the individual difference ('aptitude') by treatment interaction in health behavior change programs. The goal of these studies was to determine how an individual difference may affect the outcome or effectiveness of a particular treatment. More specifically, the goal was to determine if individual differences moderate the effectiveness of treatment on health behavior change and, if so, to determine a method of assigning clients to an intervention approach based on these characteristics. In general, this research has produced mixed results. In some studies, a clear individual difference by treatment pattern emerged. In other studies, outcome did not vary as a function of individual differences. One individual difference variable that did show promise in this literature review was active versus passive coping style. Briefly, active coping involves employing strategies directly aimed at reducing the stress. For example, if one is actively coping after myocardial infarction, one may take steps such as cardiovascular rehabilitation to prevent future attacks. There is a suggestion that those people with characteristically more active coping strategies show greater success in self-directed, as opposed to therapist-directed, interventions (Dance & Neufeld 1988). Specific studies that demonstrate this finding will be reviewed below.

Another individual difference variable that has been studied is locus of control (LOC). Control expectancies, or locus of control, in the health context, refer to the degree of control that individuals feel they have over their health. An internal locus of control refers to the belief that individuals control their own health and an external locus of control refers to the sense that either powerful others (e.g. physicians) or no one (i.e. chance) control their health (Wallston & Wallston 1978).

Smoking cessation

Best & Steffy (1971) examined the role of locus of control in smoking cessation treatment. Locus of control, measured by the Rotter LOC scale (Rotter 1966), is defined as the extent to which a person adopts an internal control approach to change versus an external or environmental control approach. Participants were divided between two broad treatment categories. The 'internal' treatment emphasized the role of a participant's own control over their smoking cessation. Participants in this group were encouraged to make a conscious decision to quit smoking and to envision possible obstacles to smoking cessation. The 'external' treatment emphasized the role of tailoring one's environment to control smoking. Participants in this group were given tools to help manipulate their environment such as an '*I Am Quitting Smoking*' button and wall signs that said '*Don't Smoke Now*' (Best & Steffy 1971). Despite the theoretical link between personal locus of control and treatment focus, there was not a significant interaction effect on smoking cessation. In other words, a match between participant locus of control and treatment focus did not predict more effective treatment in this study.

In contrast, Best (1975) found a significant interaction between participant individual differences and treatment conditions in predicting smoking cessation. Participants were divided into treatment groups based on three factors: treatment focus (either internal or external), application of punishment (either punishment was applied or not), and timing of attitude change manipulation (either just before or just after behavior change). Relevant participant characteristics were measured using the Rotter LOC scale (relevant to the treatment focus) and two motivation measures (relevant to the timing of attitude change). Participants were grouped according to match or mismatch on focus and match or mismatch on timing of attitude change. For example, a match on focus could mean that the participant reported internal focus on the Rotter scale and was placed in the internal focus treatment condition. A match on timing of attitude change could mean that the participant demonstrated high motivation to change and received the attitude manipulation early in treatment. Those participants whose attitudes (i.e. locus of control and level of motivation) matched their treatment conditions (i.e. internal versus external focus and early versus late attitude manipulation) on both factors demonstrated the highest levels of smoking cessation (Best 1975). This finding supports the importance of individual characteristics in health behavior change effectiveness.

Weight reduction

Rozensky & Bellack (1976) examined the match between degree of self-reinforcement and treatment style. Tendency to provide oneself with positive reinforcement, defined as a positive self-evaluation, has been linked to behavior change in previous research (Rozensky & Bellack 1974). Participants were classified as either high or low self-reinforcers, using an assessment procedure previously employed by Bellack and colleagues, and were randomly placed in treatment that focused on self-control, therapist-control, or minimal contact (control condition). All participants were exposed to the same weight reduction program that included calorie intake balance, self-control, and self-monitoring. The self-control treatment group met with the therapist three times and mailed in their monitoring records. The therapist-control treatment group participants were exposed to a financial contingency program (i.e. participants could receive up to two dollars of a deposit back for weight loss). While low self-reinforcing participants did moderately well in either treatment condition, high self-reinforcing participants lost significantly more weight in the self-control condition, compared with the therapist contingency condition. Additionally, the high self-reinforcers in the therapist contingency condition lost less weight than the control group (Rozensky & Bellack 1976). This pattern of results suggests that the match between self-reinforcement style and treatment focus is an important determinant of health behavior change effectiveness. Other research involving weight reduction programs has reported similar interactions between treatment approach and individual differences (Carroll et al 1980).

CONCLUSIONS AND IMPLICATIONS

In summary, it seems that the study of individual differences as moderators for health behavior change has produced some modest results. While some studies fail to find a significant interaction between aptitude and treatment, others studies, such as those examining the interaction of locus of control and focus of control in the treatment context (Best & Steffy 1971), seem to produce fairly consistent results and provide a promising starting point for future research. Future research should include broader conceptualizations of aptitude, such as the categorization of participants based on the Five Factor Model of personality. For example, neuroticism and conscientiousness may play key roles in moderating health behavior change. Along these lines, Gupta (1990) found that individuals high in trait anxiety (a construct closely related to neuroticism) show greater health behavior change in response to a positive punishment reinforcement compared with low-anxiety individuals. Individuals high on neuroticism may also have better success in treatments that include cognitive anxiety management rather than just behavioral techniques. In addition, individuals high in impulsivity do better with positive reinforcement (i.e. a reward), compared with individuals low in impulsivity. Individuals high on conscientiousness may have better success with more highly self-directed or self-controlled intervention approaches than those individuals low on conscientiousness.

The importance of personality or dispositional factors continues to be increasingly recognized by health behavior change researchers. As this chapter has shown, a broad range of individual difference factors play a key role in shaping the patterns of health-related behavior observed across the population. While some of these factors are immutable to modification (e.g. gender, ethnicity), other characteristics (e.g. locus of control, certain personality traits) have themselves been shown to be potentially important moderators or behavior change techniques. By bringing broader theory and research regarding personality and individual difference attributes to bear on the issue of health behavior change, significant advances in our ability to promote health behavior and outcomes are likely to follow.

References

Aharonovich E, Hasin D, Rahav G et al 2001 Differences in drinking patterns among Ashkenazic and Sephardic Israeli adults. Journal of Studies on Alcohol 62:301-305

Amir D 1987 Preventive behaviour and health status among the elderly. Psychology and Health 1:353-377

Best J A 1975 Tailoring smoking withdrawal procedures to personality and motivational differences. Journal of Consulting and Clinical Psychology 43:1-8

Best J A, Steffy R A 1971 Smoking modification procedure tailored to subject characteristics. Behavior Therapy 2:177-191

Booth-Kewley S, Vickers R R 1994 Associations between major domains of personality and health behavior. Journal of Personality 62:281-298

Burton L C, Shapiro S, German P S 1999 Determinants of physical activity initiation and maintenance among community-dwelling older persons. Preventive Medicine 29:422-430

Bush J, White M, Kai J et al 2003 Understanding influences on smoking in Bangladeshi and Pakistani adults: community based, qualitative study. British Medical Journal 326:962-967

Carroll L J, Yates B T, Gray J J 1980 Predicting obesity reduction in behavioral and nonbehavioral therapy from client characteristics: the self-evaluation measure. Behavior Therapy 11:189-197

Centers for Disease Control and Prevention (CDC) 2002 Trends in cigarette smoking among high school students: United States 1991–2001. Morbidity and Mortality Weekly Report 51:409-411

Cockerham W C 1997 Lifestyles, social class, demographic characteristics, and health behavior. In: Gochman D S (ed) Handbook of health behavior research I: personal and social determinants. Plenum Press, New York

Cohn L D, Macfarlane S, Yanez C 1995 Risk-perception: differences between adolescents and adults. Health Psychology 14:217-222

Cook W W, Medley D M 1954 Proposed Hostility and Pharisaic-Virtue scales for the MMPI. Journal of Applied Psychology 38:414-418

Costa P T Jr, McCrae R R 1985 The NEO Personality Inventory manual. Psychological Assessment Resources, Odessa

Costa P T Jr, McCrae R R 1992 Revised NEO Personality Inventory (NEO-PI-R) and NEO Five-Factor Inventory (NEO-FFI) professional manual. Psychological Assessment Resources, Odessa

Dance K A, Neufeld R W J 1988 Aptitude-treatment interaction research in the clinical setting: a review of attempts to dispel the 'patient uniformity' myth. Psychological Bulletin 104:192-213

Dowda M, Ainsworth B E, Addy C L et al 2003 Correlates of physical activity among U.S. young adults, 18 to 30 years of age, from NHANES III. Annals of Behavioral Medicine 26:15-23

Fardy P S, Azzollini A, Magel J R et al 2000 Gender and ethnic differences in health behaviors and risk factors for coronary disease among urban teenagers: the PATH program. Journal of Gender-Specific Medicine 3:59-68

Friedman M, Rosenman R H 1974 Type A behavior and your heart. Knopf, New York

Gough H G 1957 Manual for the California Psychological Inventory. Consulting Psychologists Press, Palo Alto

Gupta S 1990 Personality and reinforcement in verbal operant conditioning: a test of Gray's theory. Psychological Studies 35:157-162

Hampson S E, Andrews J A, Barckley M et al 2000 Conscientiousness, perceived risk, and risk-reduction behaviors: a preliminary study. Health Psychology 19:496-500

James A S, Hudson M A, Campbell M K 2003 Demographic and psychosocial correlates of physical activity among African Americans. American Journal of Health Behavior 27:421-431

Jensen J, Coune M A, Glandon G L 1992 Elderly health beliefs, attitudes, and maintenance. Preventive Medicine 21:483-497

Kemppainen U, Tossavainen K, Vartianinen E 2002 Smoking patterns among ninth-grade adolescents in the Pitkaranta district (Russia) and in eastern Finland. Public Health Nursing 19:30-39

Lemos-Giraldez S, Fidalgo-Aliste A M 1997 Personality dispositions and health-related habits and attitudes: a cross-sectional study. European Journal of Personality 11:197-209

Marshall G N, Wortman C B, Vickers R R et al 1994 The Five-Factor Model of personality as a framework for personality-health research. Journal of Personality and Social Psychology 67:278-286

McCrae R R, Costa P T Jr 1997 Personality trait structure as a human universal. American Psychologist 52:509-516

McDonough P, Walters V 2001 Gender and health: reassessing patterns and explanations. Social Science and Medicine 52:547-559

Mulkana S S, Hailey B J 2001 The role of optimism in health-enhancing behavior. American Journal of Health Behavior 25:388-395

Ouellette S C, DiPlacido J 2001 Personality's role in the protection and enhancement of health: where the research has been, where it is stuck, how it might move. In: Baum A, Revenson T A, Singer J E (eds) Handbook of health psychology. Lawrence Erlbaum Associates, Mahwah, pp 175-193

Penn N E, Kramer J, Skinner J F et al 2000 Health practices and health-care systems among cultural groups. In: Eisler R M, Hersen M (eds) Handbook of gender, culture, and health. Lawrence Erlbaum Associates, Mahwah, pp 105-137

Ross C E, Bird C E 1994 Sex stratification and health lifestyle: consequences for men's and women's perceived health. Journal of Health and Social Behavior 35:161-178

Rotter J B 1966 Generalized expectancies for internal versus external control of reinforcement. Psychological Monographs 80:1, Whole No. 6

Rozensky R H, Bellack A S 1974 Behavior change and individual differences in self-control. Behaviour Research and Therapy 12:267-268

Rozensky R H, Bellack A S 1976 Individual differences in self-reinforcement style and performance in self- and therapist-controlled weight reduction programs. Behaviour Research and Therapy 14:357-364

Scheier M F, Carver C S 1987 Dispositional optimism and physical well-being: the influence of generalized outcome expectancies on health. Journal of Personality 55:169-210

Scheier M F, Carver C S 1992 Effects of optimism on psychological and physical well-being: theoretical overview and empirical update. Cognitive Therapy and Research 16:201-228

Sharkey J R, Haines P S 2001 Black/white differences in nutritional risk among rural older adults: the home-delivered meals program. Journal of Nutrition for the Elderly 20:13-27

Sheppard J A, Maroto J J, Pbert L A 1996 Dispositional optimism as a predictor of health changes among cardiac patients. Journal of Research in Personality 30:517-534

Smith T W 1992 Hostility and health: current status of a psychosomatic hypothesis. Health Psychology 11:139-150

Stronegger W J, Freidl W, Rasky E 1997 Health behaviour and risk behaviour: socioeconomic differences in an Australian rural county. Social Science and Medicine 44:423-426

US Department of Health and Human Services (US DHHS) 2001 Women and smoking: a report of the Surgeon General. US Department of Health and Human Services, Office of Assistant Secretary for Health, Office on Smoking and Health, Atlanta

Vingerhoets A J, Croon M, Jeninga A J et al 1990 Personality and health habits. Psychology and Health 4:333-342

Vollrath M, Knoch D, Cassano L 1998 Personality, risky health behavior, and perceived susceptibility to health risks. European Journal of Personality 13:39-50

Waldron I 1997 Changing gender roles and gender differences in health behavior. In: Gochman D S (ed) Handbook of health behavior research I: personal and social determinants. Plenum Press, New York

Wallston B S, Wallston K A 1978 Locus of control and health: a review of the literature. Health Education Monographs Spring:107-117

Wiebe D J, Smith T W 1997 Personality and health: progress and problems in psychosomatics. In: Hogan R, Johnson J, Briggs S (eds) Handbook of personality psychology. Academic Press, San Diego, pp 891-918

Wood F G 2002 Ethnic differences in exercise among adults with diabetes. Western Journal of Nursing Research 24:502-515

Yen I H, Kaplan G A 1998 Poverty area residence and changes in physical activity level: evidence from the Alameda County study. American Journal of Public Health 88:1709-1712

Attitudes and expectations

Aleksandra Luszczynska and Stephen Sutton

INTRODUCTION

This chapter will be organized around relevant theories of health behavior that incorporate the constructs of 'attitude' and 'expectations' or related concepts. We will discuss the Theory of Reasoned Action (TRA: Ajzen & Fishbein 1980), the Theory of Planned Behavior (TPB: Ajzen 1991, 2002a), Social Cognitive Theory (SCT: Bandura 1997, 2000), and the Health Action Process Approach (HAPA: Schwarzer 2001). Each theory will be outlined in turn, the recommended operationalizations of the components will be described and the extent of empirical support for the theory will be reviewed, drawing where available on evidence from metaanalyses and systematic reviews. The aim is to foster an understanding of how to use the theories in practice to predict relevant target health behaviors.

Using a theory to predict a particular health behavior is an important step towards developing effective interventions to change that behavior. If one or more components of a theory are consistently found to predict a given target behavior in a given target population, then this is consistent with the assumption that these components *influence* the target behavior in this population (although alternative interpretations are always possible). Interventions can then be designed to try to modify these components. Intervention studies may throw further light on whether the predictors of the behavior are truly causal factors.

i see D3

For consistency we will use a single target behavior as an example throughout the chapter: eating at least five portions of fruit and vegetables every day for the next 30 days.

THE THEORIES OF REASONED ACTION AND PLANNED BEHAVIOR

These theories are closely related to each other and are widely used to study health behaviors (Godin & Kok 1996). For an example of the application of the TPB to predicting consumption of a low-fat diet, see Armitage & Conner (1999).

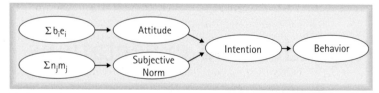

Fig B2.1   The Theory of Reasoned Action. Note: $\Sigma b_i e_i$ refers to behavioral beliefs (belief strength multiplied by outcome evaluation, summed over beliefs); $\Sigma n_j m_j$ refers to normative beliefs (belief strength multiplied by motivation to comply, summed over beliefs)

Figure B2.1 shows the TRA. Intention is the central component. According to the TRA, behavior is determined by the intention to perform that behavior (e.g. the stronger a person's intention to eat at least five portions of fruit and vegetables every day, the more likely they are to do this). Intention, then, is the most proximal determinant and the single best predictor of behavior. The strength of a person's intention is determined by two factors: their *attitude toward the behavior*, that is, their overall evaluation of performing the behavior; and their *subjective norm*, that is, the extent to which they think that important others would want them to perform it. The relative importance of these two components may vary for different behaviors and different populations. Attitude toward the behavior is determined by the total set of *salient* (or *accessible*) *behavioral beliefs* about the personal consequences of performing the behavior. Specifically, the strength of each belief is weighted by the evaluation of the outcome and the products combined additively. ($\Sigma b_i e_i$, where b is belief strength and e is outcome evaluation.) Similarly, subjective norm is determined by the total set of salient *normative beliefs*, that is, beliefs about the views of important others such as parents or friends. Specifically, the strength of each normative belief is weighted by motivation to comply with the referent in question, and the products combined additively. ($\Sigma n_j m_j$, where n is belief strength and m is motivation to comply.) According to the theory, changing behavior requires changing these underlying beliefs (Ajzen & Fishbein 1980, Sutton 2002a).

The TRA does not rule out other causes of behavior. Many other factors such as sociodemographic, cultural, and personality factors may influence behavior, but these are assumed to be distal factors; in other words, to be farther removed from the behavior than the proximal factors specified by the model. The TRA is assumed to be *sufficient*. Distal factors are assumed to influence intention only via their effects on attitude and subjective norm. Similarly, assuming that intentions are stable and that the behavior is completely under volitional control, the effects of distal factors on behavior are assumed to be entirely mediated by attitude, subjective norm, and intention. These assumptions are testable, at least in principle. For example, there may be ethnic differences in the extent to which people eat at least five portions of fruit and vegetables

i see B1, C1

a day. This would be entirely consistent with the TRA. The theory would explain this in terms of different ethnic groups having different attitudes or subjective norms, and hence different intentions, with respect to eating fruit and vegetables. Thus, the TRA divides the determinants of behavior into two classes: a small number of proximal determinants, which are specified by the theory; and all other causes, which are left unspecified but which are assumed to be distal and to influence behavior only via their effects on the proximal determinants.

Behavioral beliefs in the TRA are similar in some respects to the *pros and cons* in the Transtheoretical Model, the most widely used stage theory of health behavior (Prochaska & Velicer 1997). Pros and cons refer to the perceived advantages and disadvantages of performing the target behavior. Behavioral beliefs differ from pros and cons in that they are based theoretically on the expectancy–value principle and they distinguish between expectancy (belief strength) and value (outcome evaluation).

The TRA applies to behaviors that are completely under volitional control, that is, behaviors that can be performed at will. Many behaviors, including most health-related behaviors, are more complex, requiring skills, resources, opportunities, or cooperation of other people for their successful performance.

The TPB is an extension of the TRA that attempts to account for behaviors that are not completely under the individual's control. The theory is shown in Figure B2.2. The additional components are *control beliefs* and *perceived behavioral control*. Perceived behavioral control refers to people's perceptions of their ability to perform a given behavior. It is similar to Bandura's (1997) construct of self-efficacy (see next part of this chapter); indeed, Ajzen (1991) states that the two constructs are synonymous. The theory assumes that perceived behavioral control is determined by salient control beliefs; that is, beliefs about the presence of factors that

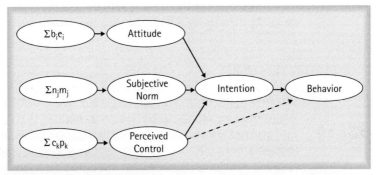

Fig B2.2 The Theory of Planned Behavior. Note: $\Sigma b_i e_i$ refers to behavioral beliefs (belief strength multiplied by outcome evaluation, summed over beliefs); $\Sigma n_j m_j$ refers to normative beliefs (belief strength multiplied by motivation to comply, summed over beliefs); and $\Sigma c_k p_k$ refers to control beliefs (belief strength multiplied by perceived power, summed over beliefs)

i see B5

may facilitate or impede performance of the behavior. Specifically, the strength of each control belief (the perceived likelihood that a given control factor will be present) is weighted by the perceived power of the control factor (the extent to which the control factor will make it easier or more difficult to perform the behavior), and the products combined additively. ($\Sigma c_k p_k$, where c is belief strength and p is perceived power.) Perceived behavioral control is assumed to influence intention and, to the extent that it is an accurate reflection of *actual behavioral control*, perceived behavioral control can, together with intention, be used to predict behavior (see Sutton 2002b for discussion of this point).

Actual behavioral control refers to the extent to which a person has the skills, resources and other prerequisites needed to perform a given behavior. Actual control is difficult to measure and applications of the TPB typically measure perceived control as a proxy of actual control.

Operationalizations

Box B2.1 gives recommended operationalizations of the TRA and TPB variables, based closely on Ajzen (2002b), but using our example of eating at least five portions of fruit and vegetables every day for the next 30 days. All behaviors can be defined in terms of four components: action, target, time, and context. In this example, 'eating ... every day' is the action, 'at least five portions of fruit and vegetables' is the target, and 'the next 30 days' is the time. No context is specified in this example. Using some or all of these four components, the investigator can define the behavior as specifically or as generally as required. Having defined the behavior, the measures of all the TPB components should refer to this definition. This reflects the *principle of correspondence or compatibility*. Measuring all the variables at the same level of specificity or generality maximizes predictive power. This principle is not restricted to the TRA and the TPB; it could be employed with any of the other theories used to predict health behaviors.

NOTE ON SCORING SCHEMES

Measures of intention, attitude, subjective norm, and perceived behavioral control are usually scored 1 to 7 or −3 to +3 (see Box B2.1, points 1–5). It actually makes no difference to the correlations with other variables whether a unipolar or bipolar scoring scheme is used. By contrast, measures of behavioral, normative, and control beliefs are used to create multiplicative composites and in this case, different scoring schemes may yield different correlations with other variables (see Box B2.1, points 6–8). Ajzen (2002b) recommends that investigators compare the results of unipolar and bipolar scoring for the belief measures and use the scores that produce the stronger correlations.

> **Box B2.1** Recommended operationalizations of the Theory of Planned Behavior constructs

1 Behavior

On how many days in the past 30 days have you eaten at least five portions of fruit and vegetables?

2 Intention

I intend to eat at least five portions of fruit and vegetables every day in the next 30 days

extremely unlikely :__:__:__:__:__:__:__: extremely likely

3 Attitude toward the behavior

For me to eat at least five portions of fruit and vegetables every day in the next 30 days would be

good :__:__:__:__:__:__:__: bad

4 Subjective norm

Most people who are important to me think that

I should :__:__:__:__:__:__:__: I should not

eat at least five portions of fruit and vegetables every day in the next 30 days

5 Perceived behavioral control

For me to eat at least five portions of fruit and vegetables every day in the next 30 days would be

impossible :__:__:__:__:__:__:__: possible

6 Behavioral beliefs

Belief strength

My eating at least five portions of fruit and vegetables every day in the next 30 days would increase my food bill

extremely unlikely :__:__:__:__:__:__:__: extremely likely

Outcome evaluation

Increasing my food bill would be

extremely bad :__:__:__:__:__:__:__: extremely good

Continued

Box B2.1   Recommended operationalizations of the Theory of Planned Behavior constructs—(*continued*)

7 Normative beliefs

Belief strength

My family thinks that

I should :___:___:___:___:___:___:___: I should not

eat at least five portions of fruit and vegetables every day in the next 30 days

Motivation to comply

Generally speaking, how much do you want to do what your family thinks you should do?

not at all :___:___:___:___:___:___:___: very much

8 Control beliefs

Belief strength

I will have guests staying in my house in the next 30 days

extremely unlikely :___:___:___:___:___:___:___: extremely likely

Perceived power

Having guests staying in my house in the next 30 days would make it

much more difficult :___:___:___:___:___:___:___: much easier

for me to eat at least five portions of fruit and vegetables every day in the next 30 days

---

For brevity, only one example measure of each component is given in Box B2.1. In practice, it is advisable to use more than one measure of each component, to increase reliability and to ensure that different facets of each component are covered. See Ajzen (2002b) for further examples of measures. Participants may need to be given an explanation of the target behavior, in this case what counts as a portion of fruit and vegetables.

Particularly when the TRA or the TPB is applied to a new behavior or in a new population, it is also advisable to conduct a pilot study to inform the development of the measures. Such a study should always be carried out when the researcher wishes to develop measures of the beliefs that are assumed to underlie attitude, subjective norm, and perceived behavioral control, because these may be unique to a given behavior in a given population (Fishbein 2000). In this case an *elicitation study* should be conducted in a sample of people drawn from the target population, to identify relevant beliefs. Those beliefs that are elicited first, in response to open-ended questions such as 'What do you think would be the advantages for you of eating at least five portions of fruit and vegetables every day?', are assumed to be salient for the individual. Those elicited most frequently in the sample are designated the *modal salient beliefs*. For an example of an elicitation study, see Sutton et al (2003). Closed-ended questions such as those shown in Box B2.1 can then be developed.

The TRA and the TPB have been applied in literally hundreds of studies to predict a wide range of behaviors, including many health-related behaviors. Metaanalyses show that the theories explain on average between 40% and 50% of the variance in intention and between 19% and 38% of the variance in behavior. There are a number of methodological and measurement reasons why the theories do not predict as well as we would like them to (Sutton 1998). Nevertheless, it can be argued that this represents a useful degree of prediction, suggesting that the theories may be capturing important influences on intention and behavior. (For a different view see Sutton 2002b.)

SOCIAL COGNITIVE THEORY

According to Social Cognitive Theory (see Fig B2.3), health behaviors are regulated by cognitions, such as *self-efficacy* and *outcome expectancies* (Bandura 1997, 2000). Self-efficacy is concerned with people's belief in their ability to perform a specific action that is required to attain an expected outcome. According to SCT, behavior is directly influenced by

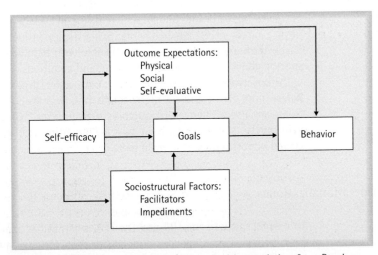

Fig B2.3   Social Cognitive Theory (adapted with permission from Bandura 2000, pp. 120–136)

self-efficacy beliefs (e.g. the stronger a person's self-efficacy to eat at least five portions of fruit and vegetables every day, the more likely the person is to do this). Additionally, these optimistic self-beliefs determine other factors that influence a given behavior. Perceived self-efficacy affects behavior partly through its impact on outcome expectancies. An individual with high optimistic self-beliefs with regard to eating more healthily is likely to believe that adoption of this behavior will lead to a higher number of positive outcomes and a lower number of negative ones.

While perceived self-efficacy refers to personal action control, outcome expectancies pertain to the perception of possible consequences of one's action (Bandura 1997). Physical and social outcome expectancies, such as expectations of discomfort or social reward respectively, refer to the anticipation of what will be experienced after behavior change. Self-evaluative outcome expectancies refer to the anticipation of experiences, such as being ashamed or satisfied, due to internal standards. For example, a person might expect that eating at least five portions of fruit and vegetables every day will result in:

- weight reduction
- approval from their family
- a feeling of pride in having adopted a more healthy lifestyle.

Most of the studies on SCT include only self-efficacy and expectancies about outcomes as predictors of a health behavior. However, SCT includes other factors that determine health behavior change. These are *perceived opportunities and impediments,* as well as *goals* (Bandura 2000). Self-beliefs about personal efficacy determine how people perceive opportunities and impediments. Self-efficacy influences whether individuals pay more attention to opportunities or barriers in their life circumstances. People with strong self-efficacy focus on opportunities. Perceived opportunities and impediments predict goals, but they do not have a direct effect on behaviors. Self-efficacy influences behaviors partly through its impact on goals. People with high self-efficacy in a specific domain select more challenging and ambitious goals. Compared with those with low optimistic self-beliefs, self-efficacious individuals invest more effort and set higher goals (see DeVellis & DeVellis 2000). Goals are also influenced by outcome expectancies. SCT does not provide precise suggestions about how to operationalize goals and perceived opportunities or impediments.

Operationalizations

In a similar way to the TRA and the TPB, when SCT is applied to a specific behavior in a specific population, it is recommended that the investigator develop a new set of measures. These measures should capture the age and culture specificity of the studied population (Resnicow et al 2000). Because both self-efficacy and outcome expectancies are proximal to behaviors, measures usually refer to specific behaviors. Studied behaviors can be defined in general terms (e.g. healthy nutrition) or more specifically (e.g. eating at least five portions of fruit and vegetables every day).

Outcome expectancies are usually worded as 'if–then' statements and self-efficacy items as 'confidence' statements. The usual structure of an outcome expectancy item is: 'If ... (a behavior), then ... (consequences)'. For example, 'If I eat at least five portions of fruit and vegetables every day, then I will lose weight'. Both positive and negative outcomes should be included. For example, a measure of social outcome expectancies should refer to positive and negative reactions of the person's social network to frequent consumption of fruit and vegetables. For self-efficacy, the usual wording is: 'I am confident that I can ... (perform an action), even if ... (a barrier)'; for example, 'I am confident that I can eat at least five portions of fruit and vegetables every day, even if I would prefer to eat something else'. It is necessary to assess a variety of barriers that might arise if an individual tries to adopt or maintain a health behavior.

A number of recent studies have applied SCT to predicting and explaining nutrition behaviors. US national representative surveys on consumption of fruits and vegetables showed that self-efficacy is among the factors most consistently and strongly associated with higher consumption of vegetables and fruits (Van Duyn et al 2001). Resnicow et al (2000) found that self-efficacy to eat more fruits and vegetables, as well as outcome expectancies with respect to fruit and vegetable intake, predicted 24-hour recall of actual fruit and vegetable intake. The use of self-report measures of behavior may introduce bias and inflate the correlations between behavior and measures of the SCT constructs. Some recent studies have attempted to reduce the possibility of bias by employing objective measures of behavior. For example, Anderson et al (2000) derived measures of nutrition behavior from grocery receipts for food items and showed that the effect of self-efficacy on fat, fiber, and fruit and vegetable intake is mediated by physical outcome expectancies. Self-efficacy was a significant predictor of physical, social, and self-evaluative outcome expectancies regarding healthy nutrition.

The constructs included in SCT belong to those most often analyzed or measured in order to test the effectiveness of interventions aimed at health behavior change. In 265 nutrition interventions published in the 1980s and 1990s, outcome expectancies or self-efficacy were used in about 90% of the studies (Contento et al 2002). Manipulations aimed at increasing self-efficacy were found to affect health behaviors. For example, Baranowski et al (2003) used a multimedia game, based on SCT, to try to increase children's preferences for healthy food consumption. Using multiple exposures, this approach increased mastery in asking for fruit and vegetables at home and when eating out.

Compared to controls, preadolescents in the intervention group increased their self-efficacy beliefs and healthy food consumption.

Along with the TRA and the TPB, SCT is one of the most influential theories for predicting and explaining health behavior. Some researchers test the role of different constructs from different theories, combining these constructs within one study. Such an approach provided strong support for SCT and the TPB (see Motl et al 2002). Some constructs within the TRA, the TPB, and SCT, in particular self-efficacy and perceived behavioral control, are defined and operationalized in a similar way. Therefore, if these constructs are examined in the same study, it is necessary to provide evidence for discriminant validity (in other words, evidence that measures of self-efficacy and measures of perceived behavioral control are tapping different underlying constructs).

THE HEALTH ACTION PROCESS APPROACH

The Health Action Process Approach (Schwarzer 2001; see Fig B2.4) suggests a distinction between:

- preintentional motivation processes that lead to the development of a behavioral intention, and
- postintentional processes that lead to actual health behavior.

This model applies to all health-compromising and health-enhancing behaviors and pays attention to post-intentional mechanisms. Different attitudes and expectations are seen to play a role within these two phases.

In the initial *motivation phase*, a person develops an intention to act (Schwarzer 2001), for example to start consuming at least five portions of fruit and vegetables every day. *Risk perception* ('Compared with others of my age and gender, my risk of having colon cancer is extremely unlikely') is seen as a distal antecedent within the motivation phase.

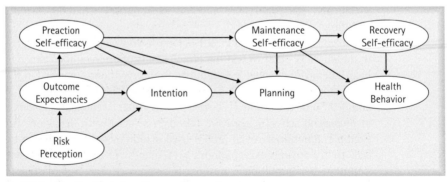

Fig B2.4   The Health Action Process Approach

Risk perception in itself is not enough to enable a person to form an intention. *Outcome expectancies* ('If I eat five portions of fruit and vegetables every day, I will reduce my weight') are important determinants of intention ('I intend to eat five portions of fruit and vegetables every day for the next 30 days'). To develop an intention a person balances the pros and cons of the consequences of the given behavior. The stronger the perceived pros and the weaker the perceived cons, the stronger the intention. Further, a person needs to believe in their capability to initiate a desired action. *Preaction self-efficacy* is an optimistic belief that refers to the first phase of the behavior change process in which an individual does not yet act, but develops a motivation to do so (Luszczynska & Schwarzer 2003). Individuals high in preaction self-efficacy imagine success and anticipate potential positive outcomes of diverse strategies ('I am confident that I can start to eat five portions of fruit and vegetables every day, even if I have to make a detailed plan describing how to remember to do so'). Preaction self-efficacy predicts intention to change a behavior.

The subsequent *adherence phase* is initiated when the intention is transformed into detailed instructions on when, where, and how to perform the desired behavior; that is, when, where, and how to initiate and maintain regular consumption of at least five portions of fruit and vegetables per day. *Plans* may be operationalized as mental representations of suitable situations in which a behavior is performed (see Gollwitzer 1999). Action plans contain algorithms of action sequences (e.g. 'I have my own plan regarding the time of the day when to eat fruit and vegetables'). The number and quality of plans depend on one's perceived competence to initiate the action; that is, on self-efficacy (Schwarzer 2001). In the HAPA model, intention does not affect the behavior directly, but is fully mediated by plans. The most proximal predictors of a behavior are action plans and self-efficacy, specific to the adherence phase.

i see B4

Maintenance of an adopted behavior and recovery from lapses are influenced by self-efficacy. *Maintenance self-efficacy* describes optimistic beliefs about one's capability to deal with barriers that arise during the maintenance period ('I am confident that I can eat five portions of fruit and vegetables per day, even if I have to reschedule and reorganize my meals'). *Recovery self-efficacy* pertains to one's determination to get back to a healthy habit after a lapse or a relapse (see Marlatt et al 1995). The person believes in their own ability to regain control after a setback or failure ('I am confident that I can return to consumption of five portions of fruit and vegetables per day even if I happened to give it up for a week').

As a stage model, the HAPA provides a concise description of the process of behavior change. The expectations, attitudes, or cognitions that play a role in the motivation phase become non-significant as an individual moves to the adherence phase. According to the HAPA, the influence of the variables for the stage progression is likely to be dependent on the

i see B5

stage. Compared to other stage models of health behavior change, the HAPA is simpler, which facilitates its application.

Despite its advantages, the HAPA has been applied in only a few studies to date (Luszczynska 2004, Luszczynska & Schwarzer 2003, Schwarzer & Renner 2000). So far, it has been found to explain between 31% and 48% of the variance in current behavior and 15% and 30% of the variance in behavior change. In a similar way to the TRA and the TPB, the HAPA might serve as a useful heuristic to design interventions aimed at increasing motivation. Additionally, the HAPA emphasizes a role for other factors that help to maintain a behavior, such as plans or phase-specific self-efficacy. An intervention aimed at increasing phase-specific self-efficacy has been shown to promote an increase in breast self-examination (Luszczynska 2004).

CONCLUSION

In this chapter, we have discussed four theories that have been used to predict and explain health behaviors, such as eating more fruit and vegetables. There is substantial overlap between the theories; some of the constructs are similar or identical. Nevertheless, there are also important differences between the theories. For example, the HAPA incorporates the idea that behavior change occurs in two stages, whereas the other theories do not. In deciding which theory to use in a given application, the researcher or practitioner should take a number of factors into consideration, including the strength of empirical evidence for a theory (relatively strong for the TRA, the TPB, and SCT, relatively weak for the HAPA because it has been used in only a few studies to date). Whichever theory is used, we recommend that investigators use a complete version of the theory rather than 'mixing and matching' different constructs from different theories. It may be possible in some cases to use two complete theories in a given study, which would allow a direct comparison between them. Regardless of which theory is selected, researchers and practitioners should give careful consideration to the definition of the target behavior and the measures used to assess behavior and the theoretical constructs.

References

Ajzen I 1991 The theory of planned behavior. Organizational Behavior and Human Decision Processes 50:179-211

Ajzen I 2002a TpB. Available online at: www.people.umass.edu/aizen/

Ajzen I 2002b Constructing a TpB questionnaire: conceptual and methodological considerations. Available online at: www.people.umass.edu/aizen/

Ajzen I, Fishbein M 1980 Understanding attitudes and predicting social behavior. Prentice-Hall, Englewood Cliffs

Anderson E S, Winett R A, Wojcik J R 2000 Social-cognitive determinants of nutrition behavior among supermarket food shoppers: a structural equation analysis. Health Psychology 19:479-486

Armitage C J, Conner M 1999 Distinguishing perceptions of control from self-efficacy: predicting consumption of a low-fat diet using the theory of planned behavior. Journal of Applied Social Psychology 29:72-90

Bandura A 1997 Self-efficacy: the exercise of control. Freeman, New York

Bandura A 2000 Cultivate self-efficacy for personal and organizational effectiveness. In: Locke E A (ed) The Blackwell handbook of principles of organizational behavior. Blackwell, Oxford, pp 120-136

Baranowski T, Baranowski J, Cullen K W et al 2003 Squire's Quest: dietary outcome evaluation of a multimedia game. American Journal of Preventive Medicine 24:52-61

Contento I R, Randell J S, Basch C E 2002 Review and analysis of education measures used in nutrition education intervention research. Journal of Nutrition Education and Behavior 34:2-25

DeVellis B M, DeVellis R F 2000 Self efficacy and health. In: Baum A, Revenson T R, Singer J E (eds) Handbook of health psychology. Lawrence Erlbaum Associates, Mahwah, pp 235-247

Fishbein M 2000 The role of theory in HIV prevention. AIDS Care 12:273-278

Godin G, Kok G 1996 The theory of planned behavior: a review of its application to health-related behaviors. American Journal of Health Promotion 11:87-98

Gollwitzer P M 1999 Implementation intentions. Strong effects of simple plans. American Psychologist 54:493-503

Luszczynska A 2004 Change in breast self-examination behavior: Effects of intervention on enhancing self-efficacy. International Journal of Behavioral Medicine 11(2)

Luszczynska A, Schwarzer R 2003 Planning and self-efficacy in the adoption and maintenance of breast self-examination: a longitudinal study on self-regulatory cognitions. Psychology and Health 18:93-108

Marlatt G A, Baer J S, Quigley L A 1995 Self-efficacy and addictive behavior. In: Bandura A (ed) Self-efficacy in changing societies. Cambridge University Press, New York, pp 289-315

Motl R W, Dishman R K, Saunders R P et al 2002 Examining social-cognitive determinants of intention and physical activity among Black and White adolescent girls using structural equation modelling. Health Psychology 21:459-467

Prochaska J O, Velicer W F 1997 The transtheoretical model of health behavior change. American Journal of Health Promotion 12:38-48

Resnicow K, Wallace D S, Jackson A et al 2000 Dietary change through African American churches: baseline results and program description of the Eat for Life trial. Journal of Cancer Education 15:156-163

Schwarzer R 2001 Social-cognitive factors in changing health-related behavior. Current Directions in Psychological Science 10:47-51

Schwarzer R, Renner B 2000 Social-cognitive predictors of health behavior: action self-efficacy and coping self-efficacy. Health Psychology 19:487-495

Sutton S 1998 Predicting and explaining intentions and behavior: how well are we doing? Journal of Applied Social Psychology 28:1317-1338

Sutton S 2002a Using social cognition models to develop health behaviour interventions: problems and assumptions. In: Rutter D, Quine L (eds) Changing health behaviour: intervention and research with social cognition models. Open University Press, Buckingham, pp 193-208

Sutton S 2002b Testing attitude-behaviour theories using non-experimental data: an examination of some hidden assumptions. European Review of Social Psychology 13:293-323

Sutton S, French D P, Hennings S J et al 2003 Eliciting salient beliefs in research on the theory of planned behaviour: the effect of question wording. Current Psychology 22:229-246

Van Duyn M A, Kristal A R, Dodd K et al 2001 Association of awareness, intrapersonal and interpersonal factors, and stage of dietary change with fruit and vegetable consumption: a national survey. American Journal of Health Promotion 16:69-78

Perceptions, cognitions, and decisions

B3

Jochen Haisch and Rainer Hornung

There are many situations in life where, in retrospect, it seems incomprehensible that we did not recognize a looming danger accurately or in time. When the dangerous event occurs, we ask ourselves why we failed to respond in time to avert the danger. But prior to the event, we often assess the threat as irrelevant and, through delaying action, we in fact inadvertently increase the danger. Ignorant risk evaluations of this kind are very common for many different types of risk. We typically expect that the threatening events are things that happen to other people and that we ourselves will remain unscathed. Presuming it will not happen to us also protects our self-esteem when risks are outcomes of our own personal behavior (Weinstein 1984). In the following chapter, we will examine the Health Belief Model (HBM) which, among other well-developed models and theoretical frameworks, describes possible ways to influence people's perceptions of risk.

 see B2, B5

THE HEALTH BELIEF MODEL

The HBM (Rosenstock 1974) assumes that people will take preventive action for their health and engage in health-promoting behaviors if they believe that they are at personal risk of contracting an illness (perceived susceptibility), perceive the potential seriousness of the illness and its sequelae (perceived severity), are convinced that the recommended measures are effective in reducing the risk or seriousness of impact (perceived benefits), and are not (overly) hindered from engaging in preventive actions by costs, difficulties, or obstacles (perceived barriers). Further, the model assumes that the decision to take health-promoting action is prompted by triggers to behave or 'cues to action'. Cues to action can be internal (experiencing symptoms, for example) or external (health messages in the mass media, for example). According to the model, people will take action to prevent cancer (such as having screening tests or quitting smoking) if they believe that they could be in jeopardy of contracting cancer, believe in the potential seriousness of the condition, believe that recommended preventive measures will be beneficial or effective,

85

and if there are few barriers to overcome in order to perform the action (for example, extremely time-consuming efforts are not required). The cue to action to seek early recognition of cancer might be prompted by experiencing physical symptoms, such as pain (internal), or a health education campaign in the mass media (external) encouraging people to have screening tests, such as mammograms.

Perceived severity and perceived susceptibility determine the strength of an individual's belief that their own health is in jeopardy. Whether or not a person believes in the effectiveness of the healthy behavior to eliminate the threat depends on how specific and accessible the behavior is and the relative weight of the costs and benefits. Perceived susceptibility and perceived severity, which are influenced by health communication and experiences of effective measures, determine how specific action against a threat will be evaluated and the costs and benefits calculated (Stroebe & Stroebe 1995).

The health communication approach in the HBM is often directive and authoritarian, as the sender of a health-related message attempts to motivate the recipient to perceive the health threat more accurately and to appraise and undertake appropriate preventive health actions. Practical interventions, based on the HBM, consist mainly of the right communicator (a highly credible one, for example) designing a message that is likely to persuade individuals to make healthy decisions. The message should produce accurate perceptions of the threat of illness, as well as provide indications of the efficaciousness of preventive measures.

Successful health communication

Successful health communication must present a health threat as a great, personally relevant risk. However, and this is critical for the HBM, threats may trigger cognitive mechanisms in the recipient, which affect the strength and relevance of the threat. One of these cognitive distortions, that can minimize a threat, is an individual's unrealistic belief that they are in a better position than others (positive illusions; Taylor 1989). The majority of people surveyed estimate their own personal health risk as lower than the average risk for others (optimistic bias; Weinstein 1984), thus 'protecting' themselves from threats to their health and an associated possible loss of self-esteem. This form of protection against illness, of course, verges on the irrational and is very fragile, for reality can quickly and irrevocably prove otherwise. By examining 'rational' and 'irrational' protection strategies, Taylor et al (2003) demonstrate, however, that illusionary strategies and interpretations of reality in mentally healthy people do have advantageous functions and benefits, compared with solely rational strategies.

In summary, the health communication aspect of the HBM highlights the importance of positive biases and illusions. Decisions regarding health risks are uncertain; the alternatives are numerous, seldom completely known, and they often entail both health advantages and disadvantages. The consequences associated with the alternatives are, especially in the long-term, unclear. With all of this, illusions are very welcome as an aid to provide some structure and are helpful when solving threatening health problems (Gheorghiu et al 2004). It is essential, therefore, for the health risk communicator to have an understanding of the illusion processes that are a part of coping with threatening health information. Illusion processes both reduce (in an illusionary way only) the complexity of the decision problem and lead the person involved to health alternatives (whether health-promoting or not).

The theory of cognitive dissonance (Festinger 1957) provides a general explanation of the role of illusions in the cognitive processing of threatening health communications. According to the theory, people cannot bear inner contradictions and discrepancies and therefore try to resolve this uncomfortable state of dissonance. Dissonance arises when a person has two or more cognitions at the same time that are not in agreement (such as 'I smoke' and 'Smoking is dangerous to your health'). Eliminating or modifying cognitive elements, or adding new ones, can alleviate cognitive dissonance. Some ways to achieve dissonance reduction are, for instance, to restrict the area to which the threatening communication applies ('Smoking endangers your health only if you smoke more than a certain number of cigarettes a day'), or to emphasize that the connection between smoking and disease is a probability ('Your risk is higher, but health impairment is not certain'), or to hold the illusion of personal invulnerability ('My grandfather lived to smoke into old age').

One way for a health communicator to prevent undesirable dissonance reduction (a devaluation of the communication, for instance) is to use a dissonance shaping strategy. This consists in initially presenting low dissonance communications followed by subsequent dissonance reduction through more accepting attitudes towards the health threat. The assumption is that the lower the dissonance produced, the easier it is for the person to adapt attitudes to the communication and the less important illusion strategies will be in coping with threatening health communications. The health communicator can then develop stronger statements of the health threat that target greater attitude change (Brehm 1976). This message content procedure, involving a multiphase progression of increasing intensity, is necessary to make the threat embodied in the health communication more bearable to the recipient, to protect the recipient's self-esteem, and to increase the effectiveness of the communication.

In addition, for effective health communication, social comparison also plays a significant role. It can further reduce the complexity of the decision problem already outlined. Other people who are in a similar situation play a central, normative, and orientating role with respect to both an individual's estimate of the actual health risk and how they deal with the possible risk (Wood 1989). On the one hand, this social factor can impede the success of information transmitted by the communicator as an authority, forcing the communicator to take on a role as a mediator among psychosocial peers to increase the success of the health communication. On the other hand, fellow patients with similar health problems can be very effective in sharing complex strategies for coping with health risks. This phenomenon may be useful for interventions among lower income groups where health communication campaigns have had limited success. It provides affected individuals with examples of better health behaviors in a relevant social context.

i see D6, D7

For successful health communication, it is very important to resist presenting population risks and to emphasize individual or subgroup risks (Leppin 2001). It has long been known that the high percentage of smokers with smoking-related illnesses in the population (population attributable risk) makes little impression on smokers. Only the smoker's own personal risk plays a role in their perceived threat to health, particularly if the threat is immediate. Only individual risk leads to a relevant reference point for estimating one's own risk. Personal risk, however, is often very small (Jeffery 1989). Health communication that overemphasizes the relative risk, that is, the risk of a person with risky health behaviors as compared to a person who does not engage in the risk behavior, can undermine the credibility of the communication, for the people involved seem to have an intuitive sense of their low personal risk.

Physicians are frequently considered credible health communicators (Stroebe & Stroebe 1995). When patients develop growing trust in their doctors, especially their primary care physicians, they are said to be more willing to modify their health-related behaviors. In the case of chronic illnesses, behavior modifications are required urgently. However, it is here that doctors' health communications are frequently not very successful. For example, in a study that we conducted, at best, only 10% of long-diagnosed diabetics heeded their doctors' advice to attend a short and no-cost diabetes training course. This course often not only makes coping with diabetes easier, but also eliminates the need for medication (for example, type 2 diabetics often require no medication at all as soon as they lose weight). However, participants in training courses led by their physicians profited medically only in the short-term; their blood sugar levels improved only for a short period of time. From a psychological perspective, course participants actually felt worse; they reported worse quality of life after training than at their assessment prior to the training. In other words, the credibility of the communicator per se may not lead to more effective health communication, and certainly not when it comes to repeated training courses that require patients to invest a lot of time.

Positive efficacy experiences

Positive efficacy experiences can make measures to counteract a risk appear effective and not too difficult to perform (Strecher et al 1986).

Information about health risks can serve to highlight effective ways to hinder or cope with the health threat. For example, everyone has experienced the efficacy (high or low) of medications. Ineffective medications can lead to hopelessness and to a total loss of interest in one's own health; on the other hand, effective medications do not inevitably lead to their use, as many patients fear possible side effects. It is important for health information to stress the proven effectiveness of the medication; poor experience of effectiveness should be replaced or complemented by providing additional aids, such as simpler regimens for taking complex medications. This type of information has to present the effectiveness of medications with reference to the particular condition or illness. Some consumer guides to medications do this. If a person has no experience of effectiveness, and effectiveness cannot be transmitted directly, patients with similar health conditions are well suited to communicating credible information on efficacy. This is probably the reason for the favorable effect on health of illness support groups (Davison et al 2000). People coping with similar conditions and illnesses can often transmit health-promoting knowledge and behaviors just as effectively as health professionals do. In addition, simply providing cues that point to appropriate health behaviors can make such behaviors more probable. The cues can be part of a well-designed health communication or a person may take impairment of their physical well-being as grounds for engaging in some new health-promoting action (Rosenstock 1974).

However, even if a particular health measure is highly effective in reducing the threat to health, it will not be employed if the benefit does not appear rationally related to the effort that the individual must expend. Chronic pain patients, for example, may refuse to participate in back strength training if the effort required by regular strength training sessions seems too high in view of the amount of pain, which they believe might just go away without any effort on their part. It is possible to reduce the amount of relative effort required by first giving individuals training that will make it easier for them to engage in the efficacious measure (Bandura 1986). For strength training to alleviate chronic back pain, for example, this may mean helping patients to lose weight first so that strength training will be easier.

i see B2

Efficacy experiences are necessary if people are to take on personal responsibility, which is a decisive variable in preventing and coping with chronic illness. People behave self-responsibly when they believe in the efficacy of the available measure and believe that they have the abilities required to perform the action. As self-responsible health behaviors require effort, however, lack of effective measures or lack of personal ability often serve as grounds for refusal to behave self-responsibly (and for dissonance reduction). As long as we can say that suitable measures against a health risk are not available ('Smoking is an addiction, so of course nothing can be done') or that we lack the personal competency to carry out the health-promoting behavior ('I just don't have the willpower'), then we do not have to take personal responsibility for our own health. Health communicators, to contradict such deluding arguments of the communication recipients, should emphasize efficacy experiences and abilities. Communicators facing these challenges require additional strategic methods in their health communication efforts if they are to succeed (some examples are shown in the next part of this chapter).

SOME SELECTED EMPIRICAL FINDINGS

The HBM has proven useful in the planning and evaluation of public health interventions. A detailed overview is provided by Kirscht (1988). Janz & Becker (1984), from their review of 46 studies of prevention programs based on the HBM, concluded that there is considerable empirical support for the practical significance of the factors in the model. In contrast, a number of studies show only a weak relation between the model variables and behavioral intentions. For example, Abraham et al (1992) found only a very weak association between the intention to use condoms and the variables in the HBM; in fact, these results suggest the opposite to what the model predicts. It does appear, however, that the predictive power of the model can be improved by considering the required behavior competencies. Only when a perceived threat is countered effectively and suitable procedures that can be performed successfully are available, can the motivation to modify the behavior, which was triggered by the threat, result in new behaviors. For this reason, there have been many calls to replace the HBM with more complex models, such as the Protection Motivation Theory (Rogers 1983).

Some studies provide evidence for parts of the model. For example, Weitkunat et al (2003) confirmed the effect of perceived susceptibility on short-term reduction of beef consumption during the BSE crisis ('mad cow disease') in Germany. A computer-assisted telephone survey of 1000 participants asked people to respond to questions on modifications to diet, attitude towards BSE, self-efficacy, perceived severity, and perceived susceptibility to BSE. The respondents reported reduced consumption of all meats during the BSE crisis; beef consumption in particular was clearly down. About a quarter (26%) of the respondents had become vegetarians in response to BSE. The population had been informed about ways to protect themselves effectively through dietary changes. The health threat produced the motivation to change behavior and people succeeded in implementing that change. However, the change was short-lived, as beef consumption returned to its former level when the BSE crisis ended. Because numerous other influencing factors (demographic, cognitive, and social) also had an influence, the authors concluded that the HBM could not explain the main variance in dietary behavior.

Self-efficacy expectations are also a determining influence on adolescents' contraceptive use (Longmore et al 2003). Self-efficacy for contraceptive use is based on the adolescent's conviction that he/she can control sexual situations and practice contraception successfully. Adolescents with self-efficacy in this area behave, for the most part, accordingly and use contraceptives even in difficult situations. Demographic variables also clearly have an influence on contraceptive self-efficacy: young people's confidence in their ability to successfully control their own sexual behavior is lower if they are younger, are male, or if their mothers have a low level of education. Bliemeister (1991) reported on interventions to strengthen self-efficacy in the use of condoms by adolescents and (HIV) risk groups and highlighted the beneficial effect of practical exercises prior to planned condom use.

The adaptive effect of illusions is evident in risk perception or perceived susceptibility. Health communications trigger cognitive distortions in recipients that have favorable effects on health-related behavior intentions and subsequent behaviors. Although experimental and field research studies have consistently found that participants devalue fear-arousing health communications, they find that participants then go on to show great interest in acquiring more information and learning about diagnostic tests (Croyle et al 1997), even if this requires some effort.

For the credibility of health information and its relevance to one's own behavior, social comparison plays a considerable role. Haisch (2003), for example, uses social comparison to communicate the technique of progressive muscle relaxation to patients who fear dental work. The patients read written reports of other dental patients who coped successfully with fear by applying the relaxation method. The results showed that patients experience less fear if the patient in the report is similar to themselves in terms of social characteristics like age, sex, and status.

HEALTH COMMUNICATION IN THE HBM

The HBM is an appropriate conceptual framework for interventions with short-term goals. The health communication aspect of the model, however, also applies to recurring interventions and long-term change. Approaches stressing health communication move the recipient to a more central position in the model and take recipients' personal responsibility into greater consideration. This means that people's uncertainty when making health decisions (such as between a short-term, useful but health-damaging alternative and a health-promoting alternative that requires time) can be utilized to suggest processes and reduce ambiguity.

Perceived susceptibility and perceived severity

All health risk communications can arouse fear and the effect of fear-inducing messages is often uncertain (Kirscht 1988). For people to be able to accept risk communications, a sense of personal control over the fear-inducing threat seems necessary. It is most important that health messages do not support the target person's beliefs that they are not responsible for their own state of health. Instead, messages should reinforce people's beliefs that they can indeed deal with threatening illnesses and that they have the ability to cope with health threats. The transmission of new experiences through social peers is particularly effective. It is also helpful to stress areas of life in which people feel that they are in control of their health. Taylor (1989) provides an impressive report on patients who, despite repeated blows to their health-related beliefs and despite repeated relapses in cancer, maintain their own health control by focusing on the areas of life that they can indeed control. Health communication can support this process through systematic provision of information about similar experiences from social peers. This can take the form of self-help materials or counseling sessions with the physician. Further (based on attribution theory), health communication can emphasize that there are indeed situations in which people succeed in exercising health control (for example, increase their well-being by changing jobs), that there are persons with the same illness in a similar situation that succeed in maintaining control (for example, by coping better with everyday stress), that there have been times in the past when the patient exercised better control over health than at present (e.g. engaged in more regular physical exercise), and that each person has personal strengths and resources that help them to cope with illness (such as family support). Proceeding in this way provides the target audience with the perspective that, although they may be at risk from a serious health threat, they can act to improve or regain their health.

i see C3

If in addition the health communication is designed to proceed stepwise, and the contents of the messages only gradually magnify the perceived potential health threat, then people will ultimately be able to accept the fear-inducing content as personally relevant for their own health and will be able to make appropriate changes in their behavior.

Perceived benefits and perceived barriers

The recipients of health communications can use inefficacy as a strategy to reduce dissonance between the information and the effort required to perform new actions. This strategy can be countered in a number of ways. One way is to reduce the amount of effort that would be required, by offering recipients low threshold health programs that require little money and time and provide easy access to health professionals. Another way is to enhance people's abilities so that they can cope with the required efforts more easily. Here, the increased experience of self-efficacy is of central importance. For health communication, it is interesting that role models can also support self-efficacy. Health communications should use role models with whom the addressees can readily identify.

i see D5, D6

It is important for people to experience the advantages of health-promoting actions just as immediately as they experience the advantages of health-damaging behavior. It is unfortunately the case that health-damaging behaviors often bring immediate relief (e.g. smoking produces relaxation), while the advantages of health-promoting behaviors are experienced only in the longer term, if at all (for example, lung cancer is avoided). For this reason, health communication should emphasize the immediate potential advantages of health-promoting actions (Perrez & Gebert 1994) and also stress that health-promoting actions have a positive effect on self-esteem ('I did it!').

Cues to action

Health communication in the HBM should consider the recipient of the health messages. This will lead to greater success in the long term. We think the key lies in communicating to recipients their personal responsibility for their own health. This can be achieved at a population level through self-help materials (Haisch 2003), which result in improvements in health-related behavior that are comparable to improvements reached with the aid of professional guidance (for example, with diabetes mellitus patients, treatment of alcohol and nicotine abuse, and lack of physical exercise). In this way, according to the HBM, effective health communication can provide external cues for necessary, new health behaviors as well as eliciting internal cues in the recipient. However, for this to happen, health communicators will have to abandon the idea that comprehensible information on health risks alone produces knowledge in people that will lead them to change their behaviors.

 i see A2

IMPLICATIONS

The HBM addresses complex decision situations in which people must deal with ambiguous information that does not clearly point to any one alternative. In this situation, people are particularly open to illusions and suggestive processes. Working in the framework of the variables in the model, we have shown which suggestions in particular can be implemented in order to increase people's cooperation and their willingness to assume personal responsibility. For health communicators who want to utilize the model, using these suggestions not only leads to increased success by taking the recipients' motivation into consideration, but also allows more extensive application of the model. The model can now be applied to health behavior situations where it has previously been less useful: namely, in cases where long-term behavior change is necessary. And with the increasing prevalence of chronic illnesses, long-term behavior changes are becoming ever more important. Figure B3.1 provides an overview of the relations between the HBM, illusions, and suggestive interventions.

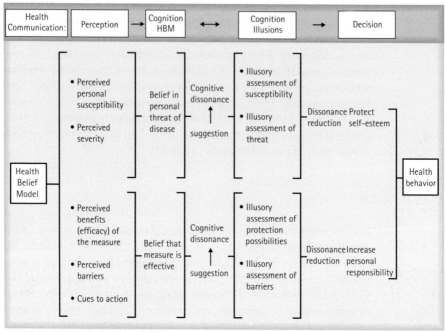

Fig B3.1 Health Belief Model, illusions, and suggestive health communication

At the start of the process there are the person's *perceptions*: perception of chances of contracting the condition; of the severity of the condition and its consequences; of the efficacy of the advised action to reduce risk or seriousness of impact; and of the costs (tangible and psychological) of the advised health-promoting action. These perceptions lead to *cognitions* (beliefs): the person believes that they are susceptible or not and that recommended measures will be effective or not. Health messages can trigger cognitive dissonance in the recipient, which in turn can be resolved through cognitive mechanisms of the recipient, such as suggestions and positive illusions (Taylor 1989). The *decision* phase can be differentiated according to whether protection of self-esteem or enhancement of personal responsibility is the priority.

The health communicator should, of course, utilize all variables in the HBM equally and additively and should not, for example, only seek to provide information about a health risk. The model itself intends all of its components to be applied. Health communicators can work more successfully with the model, however, if they make use of the suggested path that we have outlined and design specific information content in a targeted fashion to be more acceptable to the individual recipient. To do this, it is necessary to select and define the target population. Use of appropriate measurement scales allows the determination of important factors, such as determination of health locus of control (Wallston et al 1978), relevant attributions (Peterson & Villanova 1988, Weiner 1994), or self-efficacy (Schwarzer & Jerusalem 1995). Then, it is crucial to activate the recipients' resources by motivating them to take personal responsibility for health. All of this naturally increases the efforts that are required for health communication, but the advantage is that the target individuals feel that the messages are relevant to them personally. They recognize themselves in the experiences that are communicated to them. They feel that the communication addresses them personally and that they are being taken seriously. As a result, they are more likely to trust the health communication and health communicator (Petermann 1997). If this type of communication, in the framework of the HBM, succeeds in increasing personal responsibility and self-efficacy in the patient, the patient can be expected to comply with health or medical care recommendations even in the long-term. This has been confirmed by health research (see, for example, Haisch 2003). Box B3.1 summarizes the necessary steps for an intervention guided by the HBM.

Box B3.1   Intervention steps in the framework of the HBM

Goal
Appropriate perception of health threat and of the efficacy of the health-promoting measure.

To be achieved
Attitude that supports health-promoting actions.

To be assessed
Perception of personal susceptibility, perception of health threat, perception of benefits of specified measures, perception of barriers to taking recommended action, perception of the extent of improved health outcomes.

1 Define in detail the characteristics of the target population to which the intervention is to be addressed.
2 Determine current magnitudes of these characteristics using suitable test scales (health locus of control, attributions, self-efficacy).
3 Begin health communication with initial, general statements about the threat to health for the target population.
4 Begin with initial, general statements on the significance of personal resources and strengths.
5 Present clearly the short-term benefits of the health-promoting action with regard to the health threat.
6 Stress how difficult the decision to engage in health-promoting behaviors is.
7 Provide consensus information: other people in the target population have responded successfully to the health threat by engaging in health-promoting action.

Continued

Box B3.1 Intervention steps in the framework of the HBM—(*continued*)

8 Describe in detail how other people succeeded in responding to the health threat by engaging in health-promoting action.

9 Describe in detail the personal resources and strengths of these persons.

10 Explain the threat to health in clear detail.

11 Explain the susceptibility of the target population in clear detail.

12 Provide distinct information: describe situations in which persons in the target population, despite the threat to health, engaged in health-promoting action.

13 Provide consistent information: describe past situations in which persons in the target population engaged in health-promoting action.

14 Show the ways in which persons in the target population acquired the necessary resources and strengths.

15 Elaborate further on the threat to health.

16 Elaborate further on the susceptibility of the target population.

References

Abraham S C S, Sheeran P, Spears R et al 1992 Health beliefs and the promotion of HIV-preventive intentions among teenagers: a Scottish perspective. Health Psychology 11:363-370

Bandura A 1986 Social foundations of thought and action: a cognitive social theory. Prentice-Hall, Englewood Cliffs

Bliemeister J 1991 Zur Problematik AIDS-protektiven Verhaltens: Überlegungen aus sozialpsychologischer Sicht zur Steigerung der Effektivität von AIDS-Präventionsstrategien. In: Haisch J, Zeitler H P (eds) Gesundheitspsychologie. Zur Sozialpsychologie der Prävention und Krankheitsbewältigung. Asanger, Heidelberg, pp 123-144

Brehm S S 1976 The application of social psychology to clinical practice. Hemisphere, Washington

Croyle T R, Sun Y C, Hart M 1997 Processing risk factor information: defensive biases in health-related judgments and memory. In: Petrie K J, Weinman J A (eds) Perceptions of health and illness. Harwood, Amsterdam, pp 267-290

Davison K P, Pennebaker J W, Dickerson S S 2000 The social psychology of illness support groups. American Psychologist 55:205-217

Festinger L 1957 A theory of cognitive dissonance. Stanford University Press, Stanford

Gheorghiu V A, Molz G, Pohl R F 2004 Suggestion and illusion. In: Pohl R F (ed) Cognitive illusions: a handbook on fallacies and biases in thinking, judgment, and memory. Psychology Press, Hove

Haisch J 2003 Suggestion in prevention and health promotion. Paper presented at the Fifth Symposium on Suggestion and Suggestibility, July 2003. University of Krakow, Poland

Janz N, Becker M 1984 The HBM: a decade later. Health Education Quarterly 11:1-47

Jeffery R W 1989 Risk behaviors and health: contrasting individual and population perspectives. American Psychologist 44:1194-1202

Kirscht J P 1988 The HBM and predictions of health actions. In: Gochman D S (ed) Health behavior. Emerging research perspectives. Plenum Press, New York, pp 27-41

Leppin A 2001 Informationen über persönliche Gefährdungen als Strategien der Gesundheitskommunikation: Verständigung mit Risiken und Nebenwirkungen. In: Hurrelmann K, Leppin A (eds) Moderne Gesundheitskommunikation. Huber, Bern, pp 107-127

Longmore M A, Manning W D, Giordano P C et al 2003 Contraceptive self-efficacy: does it influence adolescents' contraceptive use? Journal of Health and Social Behavior 44:45-60

Perrez M, Gebert S 1994 Veränderung gesundheitsbezogenen Risikoverhaltens: Primäre und sekundäre Prävention. In: Schwenkmezger P, Schmidt L R (eds) Lehrbuch der Gesundheitspsychologie. Enke, Stuttgart, pp 169-187

Petermann F (ed) 1997 Patientenschulung und Patientenberatung. Hogrefe, Göttingen

Peterson C, Villanova P 1988 An Expanded Attributional Style Questionnaire. Journal of Abnormal Psychology 97:87-89

Rogers R W 1983 Cognitive and physiological processes in fear appeals and attitude change: a revised theory of protection motivation. In: Cacioppo J T, Petty R E (eds) Social psychophysiology: a sourcebook. Guilford Press, New York, pp 153-176

Rosenstock I 1974 The HBM and preventive health behavior. Health Education Monographs 2:354-386

Schwarzer R, Jerusalem M 1995 Generalized Self-Efficacy Scale. In: Weinman J, Wright S, Johnston M (eds) Measures in health psychology: a user's portfolio. Causal and control beliefs. NFER-Nelson, Windsor, pp 35-37

Strecher V, DeVellis B, Becker M et al 1986 The role of self-efficacy in achieving health behavior change. Health Education Quarterly 12:73-92

Stroebe W, Stroebe M S 1995 Social psychology and health. Brooks/Cole, Pacific Grove

Taylor S E 1989 Positive illusions: creative self-deception and the healthy mind. Basic Books, New York

Taylor S E, Lerner J S, Sherman D K et al 2003 Portrait of the self-enhancer: well adjusted and well liked or maladjusted and friendless? Journal of Personality and Social Psychology 84:165-176

Wallston K A, Wallston B S, DeVellis R 1978 Development of the Multidimensional Health Locus of Control (MHLC) scales. Health Education Monographs 6(2):160-170

Weiner B 1994 Sünde versus Krankheit: Die Entstehung einer Theorie wahrgenommener Verantwortlichkeit. In: Försterling F, Stiensmeier-Pelster J (eds) Attributionstheorie. Hogrefe, Göttingen, pp 1-26

Weinstein N D 1984 Why it won't happen to me: perceptions of risk factors and illness susceptibility. Health Psychology 3:431-457

Weitkunat R, Pottgiesser C, Meyer N et al 2003 Perceived risk of bovine spongiform encephalopathy and dietary behavior. Journal of Health Psychology 8:365-373

Wood J V 1989 Theory and research concerning social comparisons of personal attributes. Psychological Bulletin 106:231-248

Habits and implementation intentions

Bas Verplanken

INTRODUCTION

We do not often do things for the first time. Although we forget about most first-time activities, some stick in your memory for life, such as your first day at school, your first kiss, or your first driving lesson. However, the vast majority of everyday activities are behaviors we repeat over and over again. These include many behaviors that social scientists find important to study, such as behaviors that have consequences for health, safety, and the environment. What most of our first-time experiences have in common is that we act in a deliberate and conscious fashion. We may search out information, plan when, where, and how to perform the behavior, be careful when doing it, ask for assistance from other people, and perhaps act clumsily or awkwardly. Afterwards we may think back to what we have done, evaluate the outcome, plan to do it again, or do it differently next time. This process changes dramatically once we start repeating a behavior. After a while we do not plan, think, or evaluate any more. When the time has come to act, we simply act: a *habit* has been born.

Few would dispute the claim that most behaviors are repetitive, yet in spite of a large literature on learning and conditioning, the habit concept has received only minor attention in the social psychological literature. The most widely discussed theme with respect to past behavior is the dictum 'Past behavior is the best predictor of future behavior', which can often be found in writings on attitude–behavior relations. It refers to the frequently reported finding that measures of past behavior significantly contribute to the prediction of future behavior. This effect usually remains significant even when controlling for variables, such as attitudes and intentions, which are considered important antecedents of behavior. In fact, past behavior often appears as the strongest of all predictors. Although there may be other reasons why one would find such a relationship, such as instability of attitudes and intentions (e.g. Ajzen 2002), one reason might be habituation. As behavior is repeated over and over again, the control of behavior shifts

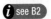 see B2

from being internally guided (attitudes and intentions) to being controlled by environmental cues. Thus, when I move to a new job, I may initially evaluate the pros and cons of taking the bus or going by car to the new place. However, after some bad bus experiences and finding the car more convenient, I typically do not make such an evaluation any more, no matter whether circumstances remain similar or change (e.g. a new bus route). Rather, at 8 a.m. I simply take the car and get to work. The empirically found stronger effect of past behavior compared with attitudes and intentions in the prediction of repeated behavior may thus be a reflection of habituation (Ouellette & Wood 1998).

In this chapter, I want to make a case for habit, not only as an interesting construct in itself but also as a construct that has an impact on attitude–behavior relations and may influence how we think about behavioral change and design interventions. I will first focus in more detail on the habit construct itself, and the question of how to measure habits. I will then focus on habits as obstacles to behavioral change. Next, I address the bright sides of habits. In particular, I will argue that establishing habits may be an important intervention goal. Finally, I will speculate on using so-called implementation intentions as a promising tool to establish new habits.

WHAT ARE HABITS?

Verplanken & Aarts (1999) defined habits as ' . . . learned sequences of acts that have become automatic responses to specific cues, and are functional in obtaining certain goals or end-states' (p. 104). Obviously, many behaviors may fall under this definition, varying from being very simple (e.g. saying 'Hi' to your secretary) to being complex (e.g. dieting). Let us take a closer look at some elements of the definition. Habits are *learned sequences of acts*. Thus, a certain degree of practice is required for a habit to develop. It is difficult to give numbers: how many times do we have to repeat a particular behavior before we can call it a habit? Ronis et al (1989) described a habit as behavior that is repeated at least twice a month and has been performed at least 10 times, but this is probably too general a statement. It may well be that some behaviors take a long time to habituate (e.g. changing eating patterns), whereas other habits may be installed after only a few trials (e.g. going to the canteen at your new workplace). In any case, habits have a history of repetition, whether this history is long and painful or short and easy.

Habits are *automatic responses to specific cues*. At 8 a.m. you walk to your car and go to work; a hunger pang in the afternoon makes you grab that candy bar; you hold the door for the lady who accompanies you. Habitual acts are instigated as immediate responses to specific cues. Such cues can be anything, ranging from physical objects to time, geographical features, people, labels, or internal cues like hunger or pain. Importantly, these responses occur without purposeful thinking or reflection and often without any sense of awareness. Bargh (1994) broke down the concept of automaticity into four possible components, i.e. a process or behavior that:

- occurs outside awareness
- is difficult to control
- is mentally efficient (one can do other things in parallel), and
- is unintentional.

Each of these components may or may not be present, which results in a number of qualitatively different types of automaticity. The habit concept fits three of these components, as a habit most often occurs outside awareness, can be difficult (but not impossible) to control, and is mentally efficient. As for the fourth component, most habits behavioral scientists are interested in may not so much be intentional in the sense of being consciously planned, but rather in the sense of being goal directed (Aarts & Dijksterhuis 2000). This refers to the last part of our habit definition.

Habits are *functional in obtaining certain goals or end-states*. We develop habits because they serve us and make our lives livable. In terms of the behaviorist tradition, in which the establishment and maintenance of behavior was a central theme, habits are created and maintained under the influence of reinforcement. In other words, behavior that has positive consequences is more likely to be repeated, whereas negative consequences make repetition less likely. Habits thus serve *some* goal. For instance, a habit of exercising serves the goal of health maintenance. Eating snack food gives a physical sensation of satisfaction. The habit of taking the car to work may be the most efficient solution to a particular transportation mode choice problem. Sometimes it is difficult to discover the reinforcer or there may be other reinforcers for different persons. For instance, eating candy bars may serve a purely hedonic goal, but may also subdue feelings of failure or personal dissatisfaction. Thus, analyzing which goal is served, and which reinforcers are in the game, is important for understanding a particular habit.

HOW TO MEASURE HABITS

In order to work with the habit construct, one should have a measurement instrument. The measurement of habit is problematic and this may be a reason why the topic has not advanced as much as one would have expected (Eagly & Chaiken 1993). Most researchers use self-reports of past behavioral frequency as a measure of habit. Although repetition of behavior is certainly part of the habituation process, repeated behavior need not be a habit (Ajzen 2002). Some repeated behaviors may be executed deliberately and consciously every single time, for instance cooking a dinner for friends, a doctor examining a patient, or an air traffic controller's decision to clear a plane for take-off. Although these behaviors involve repetition, they do not match our definition given earlier, in particular concerning the aspect of automaticity. Thus, behavioral frequency is not necessarily a valid measure of habit.

Recently, Verplanken & Orbell (2003) developed an alternative measure of habit strength, a 12-item scale called the Self-Report Habit Index (SRHI). This scale breaks down the habit construct into a number of features, i.e. perceptions of frequency, automaticity, and self-identity. Following Bargh's (1994) analysis, automaticity is further broken down into lack of awareness, difficulty to control, and mental efficiency. The 12 items are presented in Box B4.1. Note that the content of the items should be scrutinized and, if necessary, adapted according to the behavior under study.

One of the advantages of the SRHI is that the measure is not based on behavioral frequency estimates and may thus be used to monitor habit strength independently of actual behavioral frequency. For instance, a person who is put on medication may take her medicine every day, but may only gradually develop a habit. Assuming that she takes the medication conscientiously, this cannot be measured by behavioral frequency, but might be revealed by the SRHI. Furthermore, the scale is short and easy to fill out (Verplanken et al 2004). To date, the SRHI has been used in a variety of areas, such as health behavior

---

Box B4.1   The Self-Report Habit Index

(Behavior X) is something:

1 ... I do frequently.
2 ... I do automatically.
3 ... I do without having to consciously remember.
4 ... that makes me feel weird if I do not do it.
5 ... I do without thinking.
6 ... would require effort not to do it.
7 ... that belongs to my (daily, weekly, monthly) routine.
8 ... I start doing before I realize I'm doing it.
9 ... I would find hard not to do.
10 ... I have no need to think about doing.
11 ... that's typically 'me'.
12 ... I have been doing for a long time.

Responses can be given on seven-point scales anchored by *agree – disagree*.
Some items may be adapted according to the nature of the behavior.
Reprinted with permission from Journal of Applied Social Psychology 33(6):1313–1330.
Copyright V H Winston & Son Inc, 360 South Ocean Boulevard, Palm Beach, FL 33480.
All rights reserved.

(e.g. fruit consumption, eating snack food, exercising, teeth brushing), consumer behavior (e.g. impulsive buying, buying candy), leisure behavior (e.g. listening to music, watching television), as well as other behaviors, such as transportation mode choice, chatting at work, and negative thinking. In all studies the SRHI relates to other measured constructs in meaningful ways. The scale also has excellent psychometric properties. For instance, internal reliabilities are around and mostly above 0.90 and a test–retest reliability of 0.91 (over a week) was found for transportation mode choice habit (Verplanken & Orbell 2003).

THE DARK SIDE OF HABITS

In everyday language, 'habit' is sometimes equated with 'bad habit'. Indeed, when we focus on undesirable behaviors, habituation is particularly problematic. One only has to think of potentially problematic behaviors such as unhealthy eating, the use of alcohol and drugs or dangerous driving. If we remember our definition of habit, three aspects make bad habits difficult to cope with. First, bad habits imply relatively frequent occurrence of behavior. Eating an occasional candy bar does not hurt anyone, but turning this into a daily habit does. Second, habit is a form of automaticity. Thus, engaging in undesirable habits occurs without thinking or reflection and is difficult to avoid. Thus, the habitual car driver does not weigh pros and cons of taking the car versus public transport, even if conditions may have changed in favor of an alternative to the habitual choice. Third, habits are sustained by reinforcers. Like any other habit, undesirable behaviors may be functional in the sense of providing something good or pleasurable. In some areas, such as unhealthy eating habits, smoking, or drug use, physical reinforcers are at work, which can be extremely powerful and addictive.

The three features of habits – frequency, automaticity, and functionality – make habits strong and durable structures. If undesirable habits are the target of interventions, one should be aware of these qualities. In an extensive research program on travel mode choices, we showed that habituation has a number of consequences that should be worrying for those who want to change behavior by providing information and changing attitudes (Aarts et al 1998, Verplanken & Aarts 1999). In particular, two findings were relevant. First, we found that those who had developed strong habits were less attentive to information, both when this information concerned travel mode choice options (e.g. costs, efficiency) and features of the choice situation (e.g. distance or weather conditions). In other words, habituation leads to 'tunnel vision'. Second, when we looked at how attitudes and intentions were related to behavior (the use of car versus public transport), we found that these relations were weak among those who had developed strong car use habits. In other words, although the Theory of Planned Behavior suggests that attitudes and intentions predict behavior, our results suggested that these relationships are much weaker under strong habit conditions. This has been confirmed in a metaanalysis of the relations between behavioral intentions, past behavior, and future behavior (Ouellette & Wood 1998).

Applying these findings to a behavior change intervention context, the attention findings suggest that strong habit individuals are less likely to attend to new information. These individuals might thus not even be aware of information campaigns in the first place. The attitude–intention–behavior relation results suggest that *if* attitudes and intentions change on the basis of new information, these are less likely to lead to new behavior. Thus, in light of our findings, the prospects for interventions that consist of providing information and aim at changing attitudes are particularly grim when the target behavior is habitual.

HABIT AS AN INTERVENTION GOAL

If there is a dark side of habits, there must be a bright side too. Actually, there are several. One is that not all behavior is habitual. We perform many acts on the basis of at least some considerations. Behavior may not *yet* be habitual, which provides opportunities to influence it. For example, new car drivers have not yet developed their driving habits, including sloppy or dangerous driving. In particular, people who move from one life phase to another have to adopt new behaviors and routines, such as adolescents, young families, or retiring persons. Such phases are important in terms of establishing new, correct, or desired behaviors. There are also situations where old habits are explicitly broken, for instance when a person switches jobs or moves to another place. Such events are especially interesting if they occur at a relatively large scale or among a distinct group. For instance, when two companies merge, many procedures and behaviors have to change, many of which were old habits and routines. Another example is the building of new residential areas. In these cases, relatively large groups of people will have to establish new behaviors with respect to transportation, energy use, leisure, or shopping within a relatively short time. Situations like these thus provide interesting opportunities for interventions aimed at propagating new and desired behaviors. In designing and planning behavior change programs, it may thus be particularly useful to search for situations where old habits are broken and/or new habits have not (yet) been established.

Perhaps the brightest side of habits is the argument that habit formation itself may become an *intervention goal*. After all, intervention programs designed to establish new behavior aim at behavior that is performed frequently, is stable over time, and is resistant to other influences. The very features that make old, unwanted habits obstacles to change can thus be considered as desirable when it comes to new behavior, which a behavior change program aims to establish. Thus, if individuals adopt the promoted behavior, we would want that behavior to be frequently and automatically executed and to be functional and efficient. The planning of new habits may therefore be explicitly adopted as an intervention goal.

PLANNING NEW HABITS

Texts on persuasion and behavioral change programs mostly focus on information processing, attitude change, and the implementation of behavior. Much less attention has been given to the stability and maintenance of newly adopted behavior. One perspective on maintenance is to focus on embedding the new behavior in the environment (Bartholomew et al 2001). For instance, health promotion programs flourish better when they are institutionalized and made part of an organization, as institutionalization may help an individual to sustain and routinize behavior (Goodman & Steckler 1989). However, here I would like to argue that focusing on habituation itself is important in creating stable future behaviors and might thus be part of an intervention design.

How can new habits be created? First and foremost, individuals who are the target of an intervention should be motivated to change or adopt new behavior. Thus, any intervention program can only expect results if individuals have positive attitudes and strong intentions with respect to the target behavior. This aspect is addressed elsewhere in this volume and is beyond the scope of the present chapter. However, it is important to note that motivation and good intentions are necessary but not sufficient ingredients. Intentions do not necessarily translate into behavior, let alone into habits (Sheeran 2002). There may be many reasons for such an intention–behavior gap, such as the presence of competing intentions, not knowing how to act, being undecided about when to start, or simply forgetting. An intervention aimed at creating new habits should at least focus on the three key elements of habit, i.e. frequency of occurrence, automaticity, and functionality. One helpful way of designing and establishing new habits may be the use of *implementation intentions*.

IMPLEMENTATION INTENTIONS

Implementation intentions are specific plans of action, which specify exactly when, where and how to act in future situations (Gollwitzer & Schaal 1998). For instance, given that a person has a particular and well-formed intention to start exercising, implementation plans specify:

- *when* this person will exercise (every day after work)
- *what* exactly she will do (running), and
- *where* she will do that (around the lake).

The important thing about an implementation plan is the linkage of specific cues (time cues: when; place cues: where) with specific responses (what), such that these connections become strong and lead to the planned actions once the individual encounters the specified cues.

Implementation plans have been found to be impressively effective, both when it comes to the likelihood of enacting intentions, as well as the speed of action initiation (Sheeran 2002). This is even more remarkable considering the simplicity of most implementation intention instructions that have been used. For instance, Orbell and colleagues (1997) demonstrated in a field experiment that 100% of women who intended to perform breast self-examination *and* had furnished these intentions with implementation intentions actually did perform self-examination, compared with only 53% in a control group who had expressed intentions but had not explicitly formed implementation intentions. Implementation intentions have also been found to be effective in establishing complex behavior, such as healthy eating (Verplanken & Faes 1999).

So first of all, an implementation intention seems very useful to bridge the intention–behavior gap discussed in this chapter. More important for the issue of how to create habits, forming implementation intentions may help to establish behavior that has the three key elements of habit, i.e. frequency of occurrence, automaticity, and functionality. First, an implementation plan regulates behavioral frequency which means that behavior will be repeated at the specified times. Following up on the running example, running frequency may be scheduled at a desired frequency, such that it is likely to become habitual (e.g. five times a week after work).

Second, one of the reasons why implementation intentions are so powerful may be that control over behavior is at least partly transferred from the person (i.e. reliance on motivation and willpower) to the situation where behavior should take place (i.e. reliance on cues that automatically initiate responses). An implementation plan thus aims at establishing automatic cue–action links. These (planned) automatic responses thus mimic habitual responses and may in fact turn into genuine habits when practiced sufficiently frequently. Thus, running after work is initially the result of a planned implementation intention, but may gradually develop into a habit and the initially planned cue and response now become the habit.

Implementation plans should also take care of the third habit feature, functionality of behavior. The cues and responses should be selected such that these are optimally functional. For example, the running habit should be well scheduled such that it is convenient and does not interfere with other activities. Furthermore, the running itself may give rewards such as fresh air after a long office day, time to think, and feeling healthy. Implementation plans may also be used to target and kick old, undesirable habits. Thus, by analyzing existing habits in terms of cue–response links and functionality of the habit, one may attempt to replace the original responses to cues by new responses (e.g. running instead of watching television after work). In all, in addition to increasing the likelihood of enacting intentions, which has been the main focus of implementation intentions theory so far, implementation intentions may be very effective in creating behavior that is executed frequently and automatically, and is functional. In other words, implementation intentions may form the cognitive framework for the development of future habits.

CONCLUSION

Box B4.2 summarizes the main points concerning habitual behavior. Habitual behavior is markedly different from reasoned action. Although a habit may start as the result of conscious decision making, a habitual act is typically executed without much thinking and deliberation, occurs mostly beyond our awareness, and may be difficult to control. Research has demonstrated that attitudes and intentions are less predictive of future behavior when this behavior has become habitual. The presence of strong habits also seems to lead to 'tunnel vision',

---

Box B4.2   A summary of habitual behavior

- We seldom do new things; most behaviors are repeated, but researchers and practitioners do not pay much attention to this aspect.
- Repeated behaviors may turn into habits, which are automatic responses to specific cues and are functional in obtaining certain goals or end-states.
- Although repetition is part of the habituation process, repeated behavior is not necessarily a habit. Using past behavioral frequency as a measure of habit is thus problematic. The Self-Report Habit Index provides a better alternative.
- The three core features of habit – frequency, automaticity, and functionality – make undesirable (bad) habits problematic and difficult to change.
- Habituation leads to 'tunnel vision', making people inattentive to new information.
- We may want new and desired behaviors to become habits, which makes them stable and difficult to change. Habituation may thus become an explicit intervention goal.
- Because the basic mechanism of implementation intentions and habits seems very similar – automatic responses to specific cues – planning new behavior by means of implementation intentions may well be an efficient tool to create future habits.
- The habit concept should be included in the toolbox of researchers and practitioners of behavioral change.

---

i.e. relatively little attention paid to and interest in new information. All this is bad news for those who hope to change habits through information campaigns. At the same time, it shows that habit strength is an important criterion to include in the segmentation of target groups when planning interventions. The SRHI may be a useful instrument for this purpose.

i see D2

The other side of the habit coin is that habituation implies behavior being stable and repetitive. If we think of behavioral change programs, these features are exactly what we would like a new behavior to acquire. Thus, habituation may be an important intervention goal. The use of implementation intentions may then be a powerful tool in order to create new habits. The core mechanism by which implementation plans work seems very similar to habits. The initially planned cue-response associations included in an implementation plan may gradually become the habitual cues and responses that we call a habit. In addition to bridging the intention-behavior gap, implementation intentions may therefore be an important self-regulation instrument in order to kick old habits and create new ones. In conclusion, the habit concept should definitely be included in the toolbox of those who work on social engineering and behavioral change.

References

Aarts H, Dijksterhuis A 2000 Habits as knowledge structures: automaticity in goal-directed behavior. Journal of Personality and Social Psychology 78:53-63

Aarts H, Verplanken B, van Knippenberg A 1998 Predicting behavior from actions in the past: repeated decision-making or a matter of habit? Journal of Applied Social Psychology 28:1355-1374

Ajzen I 2002 Residual effects of past on later behavior: habituation and reasoned action perspectives. Personality and Social Psychology Review 6:107-122

Bargh J A 1994 The four horsemen of automaticity: awareness, intention, efficiency, and control in social cognition. In: Wyer R S, Srull T K (eds) Handbook of social cognition, vol 1. Lawrence Earlbaum Associates, Hillsdale, pp 1-40

Bartholomew L K, Parcel G S, Kok G et al 2001 Intervention mapping: designing theory- and evidence-based health promotion programs. Mayfield, Mountain View

Eagly A H, Chaiken S 1993 The psychology of attitudes. Harcourt Brace Jovanovich, Fort Worth

Gollwitzer P M, Schaal B 1998 Metacognition in action: the importance of implementation intentions. Personality and Social Psychology Review 2:124-136

Goodman R M, Steckler A 1989 A model for the institutionalization of health promotion programs. Family and Community Health 11:63-78

Orbell S, Hodgkins S, Sheeran P 1997 Implementation intentions and the theory of planned behavior. Personality and Social Psychology Bulletin 23:945-954

Ouellette J A, Wood W 1998 Habit and intention in everyday life: the multiple processes by which past behavior predicts future behavior. Psychological Bulletin 124:54-74

Ronis D L, Yates J F, Kirscht J P 1989 Attitudes, decisions, and habits as determinants of repeated behavior. In: Pratkanis A R, Breckler S J, Greenwald A G (eds) Attitude structure and function. Lawrence Erlbaum Associates, Hillsdale, pp 213-239

Sheeran P 2002 Intention–behavior relations: a conceptual and empirical review. European Review of Social Psychology 12:1-36

Verplanken B, Aarts H 1999 Habit, attitude, and planned behaviour: is habit an empty construct or an interesting case of goal-directed automaticity? European Review of Social Psychology 10:101-134

Verplanken B, Faes S 1999 Good intentions, bad habits, and effects of forming implementation intentions on healthy eating. European Journal of Social Psychology 29:591-604

Verplanken B, Orbell S 2003 Reflections on past behavior: a self-report index of habit strength. Journal of Applied Social Psychology 33:1313-1330

Verplanken B, Myrbakk V, Rudi E 2004 The measurement of habit. In: Betsch T, Haberstroh S (eds) The routines of decision making. Lawrence Erlbaum Associates, Mahwah

Stages of change, readiness, and motivation

James Prochaska

STAGES OF CHANGE

Historically, behavior change was equivalent to taking action. Patients were assessed as having changed, for example, when they quit abusing substances like alcohol, food, or tobacco. According to the Transtheoretical Model, change is viewed as a process that unfolds over time and involves progress through a series of stages:

- Precontemplation
- Contemplation
- Preparation
- Action
- Maintenance
- Termination.

Precontemplation

Precontemplation is the stage in which people are not intending to take action in the foreseeable future, usually measured as the next 6 months. People may be in this stage because they are uninformed or underinformed about the consequences of their behavior. Or they may have tried to change a number of times and become demoralized about their ability to change. Both groups tend to avoid reading, talking, or thinking about their high-risk behaviors. They are often characterized, in other theories, as resistant or unmotivated clients or as not ready for therapy or health promotion programs. The fact is traditional treatment programs were not ready for such individuals and were not motivated to match their needs.

People in Precontemplation underestimate the benefits of changing and overestimate the costs. But they typically are not aware that they are making such mistakes. If they are not conscious of making such mistakes, it will be difficult for them to change. So, many remain stuck in the Precontemplation stage for years, doing considerable damage to their bodies, their self-esteem, and others. We have found no inherent

i see A3

motivation for people to progress from one stage to the next. These are not like stages of human development, where children have inherent motivation to progress from crawling to walking, even though crawling works very well and learning to walk can be painful and embarrassing.

We have identified two major forces that can move people to progress. The first is developmental events. In our research, the *mean* age of smokers reaching longer term maintenance is 39. Those of us who have gone through age 39 know that it is a mean age! It is an age at which to reevaluate how we have been living and whether we want to die from the way we have been living or whether we want to enhance the quality and quantity of the second half of our lives.

The other naturally occurring force is environmental events. One of my favorite examples is a couple that we followed who were both heavy smokers. Their dog of many years died of lung cancer. This eventually moved the wife to quit smoking. The husband bought a new dog. So even the same events can be processed differently by different people. There has been a common belief that people with addictions must hit bottom before they will be motivated to change so family, friends, and physicians wait helplessly for a crisis to occur. But how often do people turn 39 or have a dog die? When people show the first signs of a serious physical illness, like cancer or cardiovascular disease, others around them can become mobilized to help them seek early intervention. We know that early interventions are often life saving and we wouldn't wait for such patients to hit bottom. We shall see that we have created a third force to help addicted patients in Precontemplation to progress. It is called planned interventions.

Contemplation

Contemplation is the stage in which people are intending to take action in the next 6 months. They are more aware of the pros of changing, but are also acutely aware of the cons. When people begin to seriously contemplate giving up their favorite substances, their awareness of the costs of changing can increase. There is no free change. This balance between the costs and benefits of changing can produce profound ambivalence. This profound ambivalence can reflect a type of love–hate relationship with an addictive substance and it can keep people stuck in this stage for long periods of time. We often characterize this phenomenon as chronic Contemplation or behavioral procrastination. These folks are not ready for traditional action-oriented programs.

Preparation

Preparation is the stage in which people are intending to take action in the immediate future, usually measured as the next month. They have typically taken some significant action in the past year. These individuals have a plan of action, such as going to a recovery group, consulting a counselor, talking to their physician, buying a self-help book, or relying on a self-change approach. These are the people we should recruit for action-oriented programs.

Action

Action is the stage in which people have made specific overt modifications in their lifestyles within the past 6 months. Since Action is observable, behavior change often has been equated with Action. But in the Transtheoretical Model, Action is only one of six stages. Not all modifications of behavior count as Action in this model. People must attain a criterion that scientists and professionals agree is sufficient to reduce risks for disease. In smoking, for example, only total abstinence counts. With alcoholism and alcohol abuse, there are many who believe that only total abstinence can be effective, while others accept controlled drinking as effective Action.

Maintenance

Maintenance is the stage in which people are working to prevent relapse but they do not apply change processes as frequently as do people in Action. They are less tempted to relapse and increasingly more confident that they can continue their changes. Based on temptation and self-efficacy data, we estimated that Maintenance lasts from 6 months to about 5 years.

One of the common reasons why people relapse early in Action is that they are not well prepared for the prolonged effort needed to progress to Maintenance. Many think the worst will be over in a few weeks or a few months. If they ease up on their efforts too early, they are at great risk of relapse.

To prepare people for what is to come, we encourage them to think of overcoming an addiction as like running a marathon rather than a sprint. They may have wanted to enter the 100th running of the Boston Marathon but if they had little or no preparation, they know they would not succeed so would not enter the race. If they had done some preparation, they might make it for several miles before failing to finish the race. Only those well prepared could maintain their efforts mile after mile.

In the Boston Marathon metaphor, people know they have to be well prepared if they are to survive Heartbreak Hill that hits after some 20 miles. What is the behavioral equivalent of Heartbreak Hill? The best evidence we have, across addictions, is that the majority of relapses occur at times of emotional distress. Times of depression, anxiety, anger, boredom, loneliness, stress, and distress are when we are at our emotional and psychological weakest.

How does the average American cope with such troubling times? The average American drinks more, eats more, smokes more, and takes more drugs (Mellinger et al 1978). It is not surprising therefore that people struggling to overcome addictions will be at greatest risk of relapse when they face distress without their substance of choice. We cannot prevent emotional distress from occurring. But we can help prevent relapse if our patients have been prepared for how to cope with distress without falling back on addictive substances.

If so many Americans rely on oral consumptive behavior as a way to manage their emotions, what is the healthiest oral behavior they could use? Talking with others about one's distress is a means of seeking support that can help prevent relapse. Another healthy alternative that can be relied on by large numbers of people is exercise. Not only does such physical activity help manage moods, stress, and distress but for 60 minutes a week a recovering addict can receive over 75 health and mental health benefits (Reed et al 1997). Exercise should be prescribed to all sedentary patients with addictions as the bargain basement of behaviors. A third healthy alternative is some form of deep relaxation, like meditation, yoga, prayer, massage, or deep muscle relaxation. Letting the stress and distress drift away from one's muscles and one's mind helps to keep progressing at the most tempting of times.

Termination

Termination is the stage in which individuals have zero temptation and 100% self-efficacy. No matter whether they are depressed, anxious, bored, lonely, angry, or stressed, they are sure they will not return to their old unhealthy habit as a way of coping. It is as if they never acquired the habit in the first place. In a study of former smokers and alcoholics, we found that less than 20% of each group had reached the criteria of no temptation and total self-efficacy (Snow et al 1992). While our ideal goal is to be cured or totally recovered, we recognize that for many people the best we can achieve is a lifetime of Maintenance.

REACH

Research in the USA comparing stage distributions across populations finds that about 40% of smokers are in Precontemplation, 40% in Contemplation, and less than 20% in Preparation (Velicer et al 1995). These data suggest that action-oriented interventions match the needs of less than 20% of smokers in the USA. In many European and Asian countries, the challenge is even greater, since about 70% of smokers are in the Precontemplation stage and only about 5% are prepared to quit (Etter et al 1997). If prevention practices are to match the needs of entire populations, then interventions are needed for the vast majority who are not prepared to take action.

To reach entire populations requires a shift from a passive-reactive to a proactive approach to practice. Most professionals have been trained to be passive-reactive, to passively wait for clients to seek services and then react. The biggest problem with this approach is that the majority of people with behavior risks never seek services.

Offering stage-matched interventions and applying proactive or outreach recruitment methods, we have been able to motivate 80–90% of smokers to enter our treatment programs in a series of large-scale clinical trials (Prochaska et al 2001a,b, Velicer et al 1999). This is a quantum increase over the 1–4% participation rates found in earlier studies.

What happens if professionals change only one practice and pro-actively recruit entire populations into action-oriented clinics? This experiment has been tried in one of the United States' largest health-care systems (Lichtenstein & Hollis 1992). Physicians spent time with all smokers to recruit them for a state-of-the-art, action-oriented, clinic-based smoking cessation program. If that didn't work, nurses spent up to 10 minutes to get them to sign up, followed by 12 minutes of health education and a counselor call to the home. This intensive recruitment protocol motivated 35% of smokers in the Precontemplation stage to sign up. But only 3% showed up, 2% finished up and 0% ended up better off. Sixty-five percent of individuals in the Contemplation and Preparation stages signed up, 15% showed up, 11% finished up and some percent ended up better off.

RETENTION

What motivates clients to continue with intervention? Or conversely, what moves patients to terminate treatment quickly and prematurely? A metaanalysis of 125 studies found that nearly 50% of clients drop out of behavior change programs (Wierzbicki & Pekarik 1993). These drop-out rates from behavior medicine are remarkably similar to the 50% discontinuation rates found across most categories of biological medicines (Johnson et al 1999).

One excellent predictor of premature drop-out from treatment is the stage of change of the client at intake (Brogan et al 1999). Professionals should not treat patients in the Precontemplation stage as if they were in the Action stage and expect them to continue therapy. Health professionals try to pressure patients to take Action when they're not prepared, driving them away, and then blaming patients for not complying with action-oriented treatments.

With smokers who enter therapy in the Action stage, relapse prevention strategies are appropriate. But would relapse prevention make any sense with the patients in Precontemplation? What might be a good match here? We recommend a drop-out prevention approach, since we know these patients are likely to drop out early if we don't help them to continue.

We now have six studies that examine program retention rates of individuals receiving stage-matched interventions (e.g. Prochaska et al 1993, 2001a,b). What is clear is that when treatment is matched to stage of change, people in Precontemplation complete programs at the same high rates as those who started in the Preparation stage. This result held when participants were recruited proactively (we reached out to them to offer help) and when they were recruited reactively (they called us for help).

PROGRESS

What moves people to progress in therapy and to continue to progress after therapy? The *stage effect* predicts that the amount of successful action taken during treatment and after treatment is directly related to the stage people are in at the start of treatment (Prochaska et al 1992). In one example, interventions with smokers ended at 6 months. The group of smokers who started in the Precontemplation stage showed the least amount of effective action as measured by abstinence at 6, 12 and 18 month assessment points. Those who started in the Contemplation stage made significantly more progress. And those who entered treatment already prepared to take action were most successful at every assessment.

The stage effect has been found across a variety of problems and populations, including rehabilitative success for brain injury and recovery from anxiety and panic disorders following random assignment to placebo or effective medication (Beitman et al 1994, Lam et al 1988). In the latter clinical trial, the psychiatrist leading the trial concluded that patients will need to be assessed for their stage of readiness to benefit from such medication and will need to be helped through the stages so that they are well prepared prior to being placed on the medication.

Here is one strategy for applying the stage effect clinically. We have already seen that if we try to move all people with addictions to immediate action we are likely to have the majority of them not show up for therapy or not finish up. An alternative is to set a realistic goal for brief encounters with clients at each stage of change. A realistic goal is to help clients progress one stage in brief therapy. If clients move relatively quickly then we can help them progress two stages. The results to date indicate that if clients progress one stage in 1 month, they almost double the chances of taking effective action by 6 months. If they progress two stages, they increase their chances of taking effective action by three times (Prochaska et al 2004). Setting such realistic goals can enable many more people to enter therapy, continue in therapy, progress in therapy, and continue to progress after therapy.

PROS AND CONS OF CHANGING

In our original research on decision making we followed the model of Janis & Mann (1977) who identified four types of pros or benefits:

1 instrumental benefits to self
2 instrumental benefits to others
3 approval from self
4 approval from others

and four categories of cons:

1 instrumental costs to self
2 instrumental costs to others
3 disapproval from self
4 disapproval from others.

Across more than 12 behaviors, we always found that measures produced only two principal components for decision making: the pros and cons of changing. These results have been interpreted to mean that, when it comes to motivation for changing, populations do not differentiate between internal (self) and external (other) sources of motivation. This certainly simplifies assessments and interventions when we apply decision-making variables to produce progress.

PROCESS

If health promotion programs are to help individual patients and entire populations progress from one stage to the next, they will need to know how to match particular principles and processes of change to specific stages of change. There are at least 15 such principles and processes of change.

Principle 1

The pros of changing must increase for people to progress from Precontemplation. We found that, in 12 out of 12 studies, the pros were higher in Contemplation than in Precontemplation (Prochaska et al 1994). This pattern held true across 12 problem behaviors: quitting cocaine, smoking, delinquency, obesity, consistent condom use, safer sex, sedentary lifestyles, high-fat diets, sun exposure, radon testing, mammography screening, and physicians practicing behavioral medicine. It also held true for patients' views of psychotherapy. Those in Precontemplation for changing their problems perceived the cons of psychotherapy as outweighing the pros. Those in Contemplation perceived the pros and cons as about equal, reflecting their ambivalence. Those in Action or Maintenance were convinced the pros of therapy clearly outweighed the cons.

Here's a technique we use in our population-based programs. Ask a patient in Precontemplation to tell you all the benefits or pros of changing, such as quitting smoking or starting to exercise. They typically can list four or five. Let them know there are 8–10 times that amount. Challenge them to double or triple their list for your next meeting. If their list of pros for exercising starts to indicate many more motives, like a healthier heart, healthier lungs, more energy, healthier immune system, better moods, less stress, better sex life, and enhanced self-esteem, they will be more motivated to begin to seriously contemplate changing.

Principle 2

The cons of changing must decrease for people to progress from Contemplation to Action. In 12 out of 12 studies, we found that the cons of changing were lower in Action than in Contemplation (Prochaska et al 1994).

Principle 3

The pros and cons must cross over for people to be prepared to take Action. In 12 out of 12 studies, the cons of changing were higher than the pros in Precontemplation but, in 11 out of 12, the pros were higher than the cons in the Action stage. The one exception was with quitting cocaine, which was the only population where we had a large percentage of people as inpatients. We interpret this exception to mean that with these addicts, their action may have been more under social controls of residential care than under self-control.

Principle 4

The strong principle of progress holds that to progress from Precontemplation to effective Action, the pros of changing must increase one standard deviation (Prochaska 1994).

Principle 5

The weak principle of progress holds that to progress from Contemplation to effective Action, the cons of changing must decrease one half standard deviation. Since the pros of changing must increase twice as much as the cons decrease, we place twice as much emphasis on the benefits of changing than on the costs.

Principle 6

We need to match particular processes of change to specific stages of change. Figure B5.1 presents the empirical integration that we have found between processes and stages of change.

Processes

CONSCIOUSNESS RAISING

Involves increased awareness about the causes, consequences, and cures for a particular problem. Interventions that can increase awareness include observations, confrontations, interpretations, feedback, and education. Some techniques are high risk in terms of retention and are not recommended as much as motivational enhancement methods, like

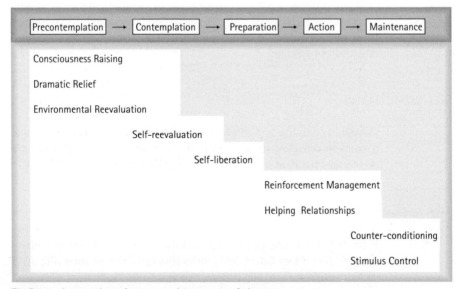

Fig B5.1   Integration of stages and processes of change

personal feedback about the current and long-term consequences of continuing with the problem. Increasing the cons of not changing is the corollary of raising the pros of changing. So clearly, part of applying consciousness raising is designed to increase the pros of changing.

DRAMATIC RELIEF

Involves emotional arousal about one's current behavior and relief that can come from changing. Fear, inspiration, guilt, and hope are some of the emotions that can move people to contemplate changing. Journals, role playing, grieving, and personal testimonies are examples of techniques that can move people emotionally.

ENVIRONMENTAL REEVALUATION

Combines affective and cognitive assessments of how a behavior affects one's social environment and how changing would impact on that environment. Empathy training, value clarification, and family or network interventions can facilitate such reevaluation.

Here is a brief media intervention aimed at smokers in Precontemplation. A man clearly in grief says, 'I always feared that my smoking would lead to an early death. I always worried that my smoking would cause lung cancer. But I never imagined it would happen to my wife'. Beneath his grieving face appears this statistic: 50 000 deaths per year are caused by passive smoking – the California Department of Health.

In 30 seconds, we have consciousness raising, dramatic relief, and environmental reevaluation. No wonder such media interventions have been evaluated to be an important part of California's successful reduction of smoking.

SELF-REEVALUATION

Combines cognitive and affective assessments of one's image free from a problem. Imagery, healthier role models, and value clarification are techniques that can move people evaluatively.

SELF-LIBERATION

Is the belief that one can change and the commitment and recommitment to act on that belief. Techniques that can enhance such willpower include public rather than private commitments. Motivational research also suggests that if people only have one choice they are not as motivated as if they have two choices. Three is better, but four does not enhance motivation. We try to provide people with three of the best choices for applying each process.

REINFORCEMENT MANAGEMENT

Involves the systematic use of reinforcements for taking steps in the right direction. Contingency contracts, overt and covert reinforcements, and group recognition are procedures for increasing reinforcement and incentives that increase the probability that healthier responses will be repeated.

    To prepare people for the longer term, we teach them to rely more on self-reinforcements than social reinforcements. We find clinically that many clients expect much more reinforcement and recognition from others than what others actually provide. Too many relatives and friends can take Action for granted too quickly. Average acquaintances typically generate only a couple of positive consequences early in Action. Self-reinforcements are obviously much more under self-control and can be given more quickly and consistently when temptations to lapse or relapse are resisted.

HELPING RELATIONSHIPS

Combines caring, openness, trust, and acceptance, as well as support for changing. Rapport building, a therapeutic alliance, counselor calls, buddy systems, sponsors, and self-help groups can be excellent resources for social support.

COUNTERCONDITIONING

Requires the learning of healthier behaviors that can substitute for unhealthy behaviors. Counterconditioning techniques tend to be quite specific to a particular behavior and include desensitization, assertion, and cognitive counters to irrational self-statements that can elicit distress.

STIMULUS CONTROL

Involves modifying the environment to increase cues that prompt healthier responses and decrease cues that are tempting. Avoidance, environmental reengineering, like removing addictive substances and paraphernalia, and attending self-help groups can provide stimuli that elicit healthier responses and reduce risks for relapse.

CONCLUSION

What this chapter should make clear is that the full benefits of a stage approach to behavior change cannot be derived from treating stage of change as just a single factor or variable. A stage approach, like that applied by the Transtheoretical Model, provides an alternative paradigm from traditional action approaches to behavior change. A stage approach provides an alternative paradigm for reaching entire populations with health promotion programs, retaining people in the program until they complete it, and helping people progress by particular principles and processes of change, applied to specific stages of change. In brief, stage is best understood not as a single factor or variable, but as an alternative scientific and professional paradigm for maximizing population impacts of health promotion programs.

References

Beitman B D, Beck N C, Deuser W et al 1994 Patient stages of change predicts outcome in a panic disorder medication trial. Anxiety 1:64-69

Brogan M M, Prochaska J O, Prochaska J M 1999 Predicting termination and continuation status in psychotherapy by using the Transtheoretical Model. Psychotherapy 36:105-113

Etter J F, Perneger T V, Ronchi A 1997 Distributions of smokers by stage: international comparison and association with smoking prevalence. Preventive Medicine 26:580-585

Janis I L, Mann L 1977 Decision making. Free Press, New York

Johnson S S, Grimley D M, Prochaska J O 1999 Prediction of adherence using the Transtheoretical Model: implications for pharmacy care practice. Journal of Social and Administrative Pharmacy 15(3):135-148

Lam C S, McMahon B T, Priddy D A et al 1988 Deficit awareness and treatment performance among traumatic head injury adults. Brain Injury 2:235-242

Lichtenstein E, Hollis J 1992 Patient referral to smoking cessation programs: who follows through? Journal of Family Practice 34:739-744

Mellinger G D, Balter M B, Uhlenhuth E H et al 1978 Psychic distress, life crisis, and use of psychotherapeutic medicines: National Household Survey Data. Archives of General Psychiatry 35:1045-1052

Prochaska J O 1994 Strong and weak principles for progressing from Precontemplation to Action based on twelve problem behaviors. Health Psychology 13:47-51

Prochaska J O, DiClemente C C, Norcross J C 1992 In search of how people change: applications to the addictive behaviors. American Psychologist 47:1102-1114

Prochaska J O, DiClemente C C, Velicer W F et al 1993 Standardized, individualized, interactive and personalized self-help programs for smoking cessation. Health Psychology 12:399-405

Prochaska J O, Velicer W F, Rossi J S et al 1994 Stages of change and decisional balance for 12 problem behaviors. Health Psychology 13:39-46

Prochaska J O, Velicer W F, Fava J L et al 2001a Evaluating a population-based recruitment approach and a stage-based expert system intervention for smoking cessation. Addictive Behaviors 26:583-602

Prochaska J O, Velicer W F, Fava J L et al 2001b Counselor and stimulus control enhancements of a stage matched expert system for smokers in a managed care setting. Preventive Medicine 32:23-32

Prochaska J O, Velicer W F, Prochaska J M et al 2004 Size, consistency and stability of stage effects for smoking cessation. Addictive Behaviors 29:207-213

Reed G R, Velicer W F, Prochaska J O et al 1997 What makes a good staging algorithm: examples from regular exercise. American Journal of Health Promotion 12:57-67

Snow M G, Prochaska J O, Rossi J S 1992 Stages of change for smoking cessation among former problem drinkers: a cross-sectional analysis. Journal of Substance Abuse 4:107-116

Velicer W F, Fava J L, Prochaska J O et al 1995 Distribution of smokers by stage in three representative samples. Preventive Medicine 24:401-411

Velicer W F, Prochaska J O, Fava J et al 1999 Interactive versus non-interactive and dose response relationships for stage matched smoking cessation programs in a managed care setting. Health Psychology 18:21-28

Wierzbicki M, Pekarik G 1993 A meta-analysis of psychotherapy dropout. Professional Psychology: Research and Practice 29:190-195

External Factors

Socio-economic environments

Mel Bartley

INTRODUCTION

Since the time of *The Black Report*, the ground-breaking official British government report on health inequality, both individual research reports and official surveys have repeatedly documented persistent differences between social groups in various types of consumption and leisure activities that are related to health. Most prominent among these are, of course, smoking, leisure-time exercise, and the amount of fats, sugars, and salt in the diet.

Table C1.1 shows the differences in the rates of cigarette smoking for men and women from the *Health Survey for England 2000*. The measure of socio-economic position was the one most frequently used in British official health reports at that time: the Registrar-General's social classification.

Smoking displays a clear 'social gradient': the less advantaged the social class position, the more likely it is that a man or woman will smoke. A large number of different 'risky behaviors' show similar social gradients. The social gradients are visible when using various different measures of social position and circumstances, such as income or status (Lynch et al 1997). The lower the income or status, the more likely it is that a person will engage in 'riskier' forms of behavior, such as smoking, consumption of refined white bread and high-fat meat, and the less likely it is that they will engage in 'health-promoting' behaviors, such as leisure-time exercise (Blane et al 1996) or eating adequate amounts of fruit and vegetables (Johansson et al 1999).

The Black Report and a large number of subsequent studies use the term 'behavioral/cultural explanation' to refer to the role played by smoking, eating, alcohol, and exercise in eventually producing social inequality in disease. The purpose of this chapter, however, is to ask how much we know about the relationship of socio-economic context to health behaviors. This task is less frequently undertaken than the examination of health behaviors themselves as causes of socio-economic differences in health.

Table C1.1   Cigarette smoking in England in 2000 by Registrar-General's social class (Health Survey for England 2000, author's analysis): ages 20–74 years

Registrar General's social class	% Men	% Women
Professional	12.3	7.3
Managerial	25.1	18.2
Other non-manual	33.5	24.5
Skilled manual	33.6	35.8
Semi-skilled manual	32.5	33.9
Unskilled manual	45.1	38.9
Number of respondents	2433	2905

Studies have identified three different types of features of the socio-economic environment as likely to influence health. These are: material factors such as income (Williams 2002), wealth (Duncan et al 2002), and the quality of the physical environment (housing quality, pollution, hazardous employment) (Blane et al 2000); psychosocial factors, such as social support, social cohesion, autonomy, and control over work and life circumstances (Hemingway & Marmot 1999); and cultural factors, such as beliefs and norms of behavior (Landman & Cruickshank 2001).

i see C2, C3, C5 The relationships of cultural norms and beliefs to behaviors may be most easily understood. Individuals engage in or refrain from a given practice because the communities to which they belong, and wish to continue belonging, encourage or forbid it. Of course, things are never as simple as this and any parent will be well aware of the difficulties involved in enforcing certain norms of behavior! So we still need to look more deeply, perhaps, into what it is that makes the cultural environment more or less powerful in different cases.

The commonly presented statistics on social variation in health behaviors do not generally give us a great deal of help in deciding what is most important about the social environment for health behavior. A table such as Table C1.1 shows a sharp difference in smoking rates according to a measure of 'social class' used in British official statistics. There are limits to how enlightening such data may be. An undefined measure of socio-economic position, such as this one, can be taken as an indicator for a wide range of possible causal influences. Is it the fact that those in higher social classes have generally a better material environment that is important or the fact that they generally have higher income, higher prestige, or more favorable and secure working conditions? What about the influence of education? In order to attain a professional or technical occupation, further or higher education is usually necessary. And although many managers may have risen through their work experience rather than because of specific qualifications, the majority of them do have at least the equivalent of a high school graduation. Could it be that the more education a person has, the better they may understand health education messages? The important influences could be any or all of these and this list is just a beginning. The problem here, for those who must deal with practical efforts to improve health, is that our understanding is not sufficient as a guide to action.

INTERNATIONAL AND CULTURAL DIFFERENCES

As an example of the problems that exist in interpretation of social gradients in health behaviors, let us look at some international differences. The kinds of strong relationships between socio-economic circumstances and unhealthy behaviors, which have been described in this chapter, are found in the Nordic nations, the USA, and the UK. The international patterns offer something of a puzzle to those who believe that material inequality influences differences in health behaviors between social groups. In nations such as Sweden, where income inequality is relatively low, differences between social classes in diseases linked to unhealthy behaviors, such as heart disease, are quite large. In the Mediterranean nations and in Japan, these patterns are far less clear. There is a group of southern European nations where income inequalities are quite large, implying that the difference in the material environments of those at the extremes of the income distribution will be great, but where inequalities in life expectancy are relatively modest. One of the most important differences between the Nordic and Mediterranean nations is that, in the latter nations, the diet followed by the majority of people seems to be rather healthier than the average diet of citizens of northern Europe and the USA (Kunst 1997, p. 206).

These observations give us a good example of the importance of the cultural environment. In Mediterranean countries, eating fruit, salads, and olive oil is a normal part of everyday life, not seen as a 'lifestyle' choice associated with social advantage or disadvantage. The middle-class obsession with healthy lifestyle is not yet as widely adopted in France, Spain, Italy, Greece, or Switzerland as it has been in Sweden, Norway, or Britain. The kind of social variation in smoking seen in Table C1.1 has been typical of the USA, UK, and much of northern Europe for many decades now but it is only just beginning to emerge in southern Europe. In Italy or Spain, we may see many people (men in particular) from all social backgrounds whose diet is 'healthy' but who also smoke. The 'causal force' of social advantage or education in producing different kinds of health behaviors therefore depends on the cultural meanings of these behaviors in different societies.

In northern Europe and the USA, non-smoking, low-fat food, and leisure exercise have been adopted as a way of expressing superior social status, a 'lifestyle choice'. This is not yet the case in Spanish, Italian, or

Greek society. If everyone eats olive oil and sun-dried tomatoes, these are useless as a way of displaying one's high status. However, the differences in the relationship of socio-economic position to health behaviors may also be, in part, a result of the material realities of local existence. In countries where fruit and vegetables (and perhaps wine in moderate quantities) are cheap and plentiful, they form part of everyone's diet and are affordable to all. One does not need to have intelligence, coping skills, self-control, etc. to decide to eat tomatoes, citrus fruit, garlic, and olive oil in Spain or Italy. Nor is such a lifestyle a signal of wealth. But these climatic factors are not able to explain why it is that, in southern European nations, smoking is not strongly related to socio-economic position (although this is changing). Nor is there a plausible economic explanation. In most countries of northern Europe, the cost of cigarettes is far higher.

For the practical purposes of understanding health behaviors, we might think of cultural explanations as those that relate behavior to symbolically valued social statuses. If the status of masculinity is, in a given social context, signaled by partaking in dangerous sports, then those who aspire to the status will tend to engage in the activities. It could even be surmised that dangerous sports may be more important, relatively speaking, to those who lack other forms of access to this valued social status.

A similar point might be made for *social* status. The work of Pierre Bourdieu shows the importance of social status for choices of reading, music, and other leisure activities. He also remarks on the ways in which 'taste' is conditioned by childhood experiences. In French, as in English, the word for 'taste' (*le gout*) has the same ambivalence. It is used to signify both the taste of food and preferences for such things as types of clothing, literature, and music. Bourdieu believed that tastes, in both these senses, were powerful discriminators of social class and social status, far more than, for example, political ideas (Bourdieu 1984). People use their consumption choices as a way of displaying their social status (Wilkinson 1996). Changes in consumption choices are, therefore, necessary in order to pursue membership of, and achieve acceptance by, higher status social groups. In the everyday experience of a British or American middle-class person, it is known that smoking in another person's house is likely to be frowned upon and that overweight in oneself or one's children is a major cause for embarrassment. Many forms of leisure-time exercise are costly and, even when this is not the case, seen as middle-class activities. The importance of both money and cultural meanings, in limiting access of the less advantaged to the more pleasant forms of exercise, has not been very widely researched.

MATERIAL ENVIRONMENT AND HEALTH BEHAVIOR

The material environment is generally thought of as exerting an effect on health that is direct and independent of behavior. It is far from clear why there should be any relation between the material environment and health *behaviors*, despite the fact that many studies report that those living in poorer environments have higher rates of smoking and lower rates of fruit and vegetable consumption and leisure exercise (Ecob & Macintyre 2000, Twigg et al 2000). In some cases, such as mesothelioma, it is even more important for those living in polluted environments to refrain from some unhealthy practice (smoking in this case) than for more privileged persons.

The relationship of poverty and social exclusion to smoking is one of the most consistent observations in the whole of social epidemiology (Jarvis 1997) but it is poorly understood. Nor do we well understand the reasons for the intercorrelations between health behaviors and other forms of socio-economic disadvantage, such as hazardous work conditions, poor housing, or weak social networks. These may be no more than statistical artefacts of the ways in which income and wealth are themselves related (in some cases causally) to other forms of social and economic advantage and disadvantage.

However, statistical artefact or not, there is a powerful relationship between the material environment and health behaviors. Since 1991, as part of the effort to monitor the effectiveness of government policies designed to reduce health inequality, an annual Health Survey has been carried out in England (a similar survey was later instituted in Scotland). This large data set contains great detail on both health behaviors and a wide range of possible causal factors. Topics have varied over the years and the Health Survey for England of 1993 is unique in its coverage of psychosocial as well as material and cultural topics. The 1993 survey did not ask directly about income. As in many other nations, direct questions on income are not always regarded as acceptable by survey respondents. Two widely accepted measures of the material circumstances of the household are home ownership (whether the home is rented or is being or has been purchased) and ownership of a car. In a dedicated analysis of the 1993 Health Survey for England, I found that a variable combining home and car ownership was very strongly related to smoking (odds ratio: 3.6) and that this relationship was not explained away by social class or by measures of social relationships such as marital status and social support (odds ratio after adjustment: 2.9).

The relative importance of material living standards and cultural or psychosocial environment for health-related behaviors is a topic that is only just beginning to be understood. One plausible explanation might be that those with fewer material resources place less value on 'future years of life'. In order to give up a present pleasure, on the promise that life will be extended later on, it is presumably necessary to place a higher value on future life than present 'indulgence'. It would make perfect sense if this kind of mental valuation exercise resulted in a different decision according to how the individual envisaged the enjoyment of future life years. If the prospect is one of experiencing a few more years of poverty, there is no great surprise in the different outcome of health education messages in those with different living standards.

see A2

PSYCHOSOCIAL ENVIRONMENT AND HEALTH BEHAVIOR

The relationship of the psychosocial environment to health behaviors may be rather less difficult to understand. Here the relationship is less direct than is the case for the cultural environment: the psychosocial environment does not in itself offer norms or guidelines to acceptable or correct behaviors. So we need to be aware that the types of behavior that are prescribed or proscribed depend on culture. As it often seems to be the case that recipes for healthy behavior entail either the performance of some difficult set of tasks or the forgoing of an addictive substance, norms are not enough. The ability to fulfill the norms of behavior often seems to depend either on personality or on support from the social environment over and above cultural sanction. As a result, it would not be surprising to find that those with stronger social networks (Ford et al 2000), more social support, and more opportunity for self-actualization, through the use of skills and work autonomy, engaged in healthier behaviors (Martikainen et al 1999).

i see C3

It is possible to examine, in a simple way, the likely mediating roles of psychosocial employment conditions and social support in the relationship between social class and one health-related behavior, smoking, using data from a large cross-sectional health study in England (the Health Survey for England 1993). My logistic regression analysis focused on the familiar social gradient in smoking, this time according to a measure of social class based explicitly on employment relations and conditions. In comparison with the social class reference category 'higher professional and managerial', the relative risk of current smoking in the other social groups – 'lower professional and managerial (odds ratio: 1.4), 'routine non-manual' (odds ratio: 1.7), 'small employers and self-employed (odds ratio: 2.0), 'lower technical and skilled manual' (odds ratio: 2.2), and 'semi- and unskilled manual' (odds ratio: 2.5) – did not change after adjustment for control at work and variety in working life. Work control and variety have no independent relationship to smoking and do not help to explain the differences in rates between the social classes.

Most research that has been interpreted as showing a relationship of psychosocial conditions to health behaviors has assumed that social class or social status gradients in behavior exist because of some unmeasured psychosocial exposure. This assumption perhaps needs to be questioned. Landsbergis et al (1998) report weak or non-existent effects of changes in work control and autonomy on changes in health behaviors over a 3-year study. It would, of course, be far more convincing to show that changes in psychosocial conditions were followed by changes in behavior than merely to demonstrate cross-sectional associations. There may be all kinds of reasons why people with different patterns of health behaviors may be attracted to, or selected into, different kinds of occupation or have different earning power in the labor market. But these 'selection' effects, if they exist, are not relevant to the topic of this chapter, which is the *effect* of social environmental factors on health behaviors.

HEALTH BEHAVIORS, SELF-REGULATION, AND PSYCHOLOGICAL REWARD

One promising way to look at the relationship of social position to health behaviors has recently emerged from the psychological and neu-rological literature. It centers on the concept of 'self-regulation'. The work has begun to be assimilated into social epidemiology by Siegrist (1998, 2000) who regards the fulfillment of central social roles (worker, family or intimate group member, active citizen) as supportive of what he calls personal self-regulation. The concept of self-regulation encom-passes a notion of 'positive feedback' to the individual about their acceptance and esteem within their immediate social context, and by society more widely. Self-regulation thereby creates a stable contact between the individual and society which also gives signals about desir-able behavior, by rewarding actions that are valued. These positive sig-nals appear to actually influence certain chemicals inside the brain. In their absence, tensions are experienced which can be to some extent alleviated by means of substances including sweet and carbohydrate-rich foods, alcohol, and nicotine, as well as certain 'hard' drugs.

Siegrist argues that when deprived of access to central social roles, as when a close relationship breaks down or a job is lost, a source of self-regulation is removed from the individual. We could go on to see the ways in which socio-economic position and circumstances are related to the risk of such adverse events. Those in less advantaged social positions, in terms of income, are often also found in less secure jobs. In this light, it would not be surprising if people with lower incomes were found to be more likely to smoke or to have less healthy diets. Couples with low income, or living on state benefits, are known to be more likely to expe-rience separation and divorce, putting them at high risk of this kind of 'role loss'. Social differences in active citizenship, in the form of partici-pation in voluntary organizations, churches, political parties, and simi-lar activities, are less well researched and understood (Veenstra 2000). However, there is some evidence that 'social capital' in an area, defined in terms of how many people belong to local organizations, may be related to health (Whitehead & Diderichsen 2001).

A LIFE-COURSE PERSPECTIVE

One sociodemographic variable that is consistently found to be related to health behaviors, at least in the northern European nations and the USA, is education. Those with more years of schooling, and with more qualifications, are found to have healthier diets, to smoke less, and to do more exercise in the great majority of studies (Irbarren et al 1997). It is important to note here that perhaps the most popular explanation for this relationship has nothing to do with 'the role of the social environment in health behavior', which is the topic of this chapter. This explanation holds that individuals who, as children, do better in education also gravitate towards the higher end of the social spectrum as adults and are best able to evaluate and follow health education advice. The reasons for this may be to do with various psychological characteristics such as intelligence, coping abilities, future orientation, and so on. Thus, the apparent relationship of education to health behavior tells us no more than that people with greater psychological resources are better able to attain privileged social positions and to adopt healthier lifestyles. Likewise, the relationship of social class or social status to health behaviors would just confirm that it is the most able who attain the highest social status.

In this argument, the relationship of the social environment to health behavior is 'confounded' by psychological characteristics. This is quite a seductive argument, although it has seldom been directly tested. Empirical tests are difficult. If intelligence were hypothesized to be the relevant variable, a study would require data on intelligence very early in life, before the influence of family environment became predominant, and then, much later in life, evidence on health behaviors and social mobility. Stronks et al (1997) reported that citizens of The Netherlands with lower levels of education were likely to smoke and have a poor diet. This study did not pretend to measure 'intelligence', but rather focused on relevant psychological characteristics, such as coping abilities and locus of control. It found that, although those with less education did have lower coping abilities and a more external locus of control, this was only partly responsible for the relationship between education and behavior. The less successful had more risky behaviors in part because they were psychologically different from the more successful ones, but it was even more important that they had lower incomes (Stronks et al 1997). In policy terms, to improve the health behaviors of those with less education, it would have been more effective to increase their incomes than to attempt to change their psychological traits.

Perhaps the best way to consider the relationship of health behaviors to the social environment is to look across longer periods of the life course (Kuh et al 1997, Osler et al 2000). Maybe in the culture of more advantaged social groups, both education and health are given more priority than they are in those with a harsher socio-economic environment. As children grow up, they may acquire a certain disposition towards a set of behaviors (a 'habitus' in Bourdieu's terms). Those in a materially and culturally favorable environment achieve more highly at school, in part because material security at home enables them to study, in part because of the value their families place on education. As a consequence, they are more likely to stay in the same culturally and economically advantaged social positions as their parents were in and the habitus of these groups includes 'healthier' lifestyles (Lynch

see B4

et al 1997). Any relationship between social position and smoking, for example, would in this perspective not depend on attitudes, but rather on a set of habits acquired over time.

POLICY IMPLICATIONS

The relationship of the socio-economic environment to health behavior remains at present largely as a description of observed regularities. There is a need for theory to guide researchers through the complex data relating health behaviors to the socio-economic environment. Only in this way will studies be able to improve their relevance to policy and practice.

At the present time, the best evidence we have points to the importance of material living standards (including expectations of future living standards) and secure social roles. Insecurity of social bonds is associated with risky behaviors in all cultures. A person whose life is devoid of sources of security and esteem within their social environment is unlikely to care as much about how long that life may last. There are different ways in which this insecurity may come about. In some cases chronic poverty or unemployment is the main cause, in others it may be the breakdown of social relationships due to economic and political crises.

For those in clinical practice, the evidence points to the importance of awareness of the material circumstances of each service user, and of life changes that affect them. Declines in living standards, disappointments over rewards for work, and the breakdown of relationships all seem to increase the risk of deterioration in health behaviors.

From what we know already about the relationship of income, social support, and employment security to health behaviors, it would even be possible to predict the effects on health behaviors of proposed economic and social policies, a 'health behavior impact statement'. Enacting economic policies that reduce employment security and increase income inequality have long been believed to increase the 'flexibility' of national economies. These may not appear to be connected to population health in any very obvious way. By increasing national economic output, such policies may even appear likely to improve health. Evidence-based impact assessments could well show that there are hidden health costs, however. By carrying out this kind of exercise, policy makers may even manage to avoid promoting the very risks that they attempt to diminish by health education campaigns.

References

Blane D, Hart C L, Smith G D et al 1996 Association of cardiovascular disease risk factors with socioeconomic position during childhood and during adulthood. British Medical Journal 313:1434-1438

Blane D, Mitchell R, Bartley M 2000 The inverse housing law and respiratory health. Journal of Epidemiology and Community Health 54:745-749

Bourdieu P 1984 Comment peut-on etre sportif? In: Bourdieu P (ed) Questions de sociologie. Editions de Minuit, Paris

Duncan G J, Daly M C, McDonough P et al 2002 Optimal indicators of socioeconomic status for health research. American Journal of Public Health 92:1151-1157

Ecob R, Macintyre S 2000 Small area variations in health behaviours: do these depend on the behaviour itself, its measurement, or on personal characteristics? Health and Place 6:261-274

Ford E S, Ahluwalia I B, Galuska D A 2000 Social relationships and cardiovascular disease risk factors: findings from the Third National Health and Nutrition Examination Survey. Preventive Medicine 30:83-92

Hemingway H, Marmot M 1999 Psychosocial factors in the aetiology and prognosis of coronary heart disease: systematic review of prospective cohort studies. British Medical Journal 318:1460-1467

Irbarren C, Luepker R V, McGovern P G et al 1997 Twelve-year trends in cardiovascular disease risk factors in the Minnesota Heart Survey. Are socioeconomic differences widening? Archives of Internal Medicine 157:873-881

Jarvis M 1997 Patterns and predictors of smoking cessation in the general population. In: Bolliger C, Fagerstrom K (eds) Progress in respiratory research: the tobacco epidemic. Karger, Basel

Johansson L, Thelle D S, Solvoll K et al 1999 Healthy dietary habits in relation to social determinants and lifestyle factors. British Journal of Nutrition 81:211-220

Kuh D, Power C, Blane D et al 1997 Social pathways between childhood and adult health. In: Kuh D, Ben-Shlomo Y (eds) A life course approach to chronic disease epidemiology. Oxford University Press, Oxford, pp 169-200

Kunst A 1997 Cross-national comparisons of socio-economic differences in mortality. CIP-Gegevens Koninklijke Bibliotheek, Den Haag

Landman J, Cruickshank J K 2001 A review of ethnicity, health and nutrition-related diseases in relation to migration in the United Kingdom. Public Health and Nutrition 4:647-657

Landsbergis P A, Schnall P L, Deitz D K et al 1998 Job strain and health behaviors: results of a prospective study. American Journal of Health Promotion 12:237-245

Lynch J W, Kaplan G A, Salonen J T 1997 Why do poor people behave poorly? Variation in adult health behaviours and psychosocial characteristics by stages of the socioeconomic lifecourse. Social Science and Medicine 44:809-819

Martikainen P, Stansfeld S, Hemingway H et al 1999 Determinants of socioeconomic differences in change in physical and mental functioning. Social Science and Medicine 49:499-507

Osler M, Gerdes L U, Davidsen M et al 2000 Socioeconomic status and trends in risk factors for cardiovascular diseases in the Danish MONICA population, 1982–1992. Journal of Epidemiology and Community Health 54:108-113

Siegrist J 1998 Reciprocity in basic social exchange and health: can we reconcile person-based with population-based psychosomatic research? Journal of Psychosomatic Research 45:99-105

Siegrist J 2000 Place, social exchange and health: proposed sociological framework. Social Science and Medicine 51:1283-1293

Stronks K, vandeMheen H D, Looman C W N et al 1997 Cultural, material, and psychosocial correlates of the socioeconomic gradient in smoking behavior among adults. Preventive Medicine 26:754-766

Twigg L, Moon G, Jones K 2000 Predicting small-area health-related behaviour: a comparison of smoking and drinking indicators. Social Science and Medicine 50:1109-1120

Veenstra G 2000 Social capital, SES, and health: an individual-level analysis. Social Science and Medicine 50:619-629

Whitehead M, Diderichsen F 2001 Social capital and health: tip-toeing through the minefield of evidence. Lancet 358:165-166

Wilkinson R G 1996 Unhealthy societies: the afflictions of inequality. Routledge, London

Williams D R 2002 Racial/ethnic variations in women's health: the social embeddedness of health. American Journal of Public Health 92:588-597

Physical environments

Ben Smith and Adrian Bauman

INTRODUCTION

Among the range of environmental factors that promote and enable health behaviors, the physical features of the environment are potentially the most pervasive and important. The physical environment exerts an influence upon the behaviors of individuals within the immediate surrounds of their homes, schools, and workplaces and through the wider characteristics of the neighborhoods, cities, and natural environments in which they live. Environmental change strategies have the potential to reach people with varying levels of knowledge and readiness for behavior change, as well as those from diverse locations and socio-economic and cultural backgrounds.

While the discourse on health promotion has given a central place to the role of supportive environments, it has been recognized that health promotion efforts have tended to focus upon intrapersonal determinants of behavior and this has limited the scale and duration of their impact (O'Donnell 2003). The upward trends in obesity in many nations are a demonstration of the ineffectiveness of individually oriented strategies to influence dietary and physical activity habits in the face of opposing pressures in the physical and social environment (Nestle & Jacobsen 2000). There is a need to address this shortcoming in health promotion efforts, particularly in light of the growing global importance of non-communicable diseases and injuries which are heavily influenced by interactions between human behaviors and physical environments.

This chapter examines the role that the physical environment plays in relation to health behaviors. To begin, theories are canvassed which describe various patterns of interaction between the physical environment and behaviors. Evidence about the relationships between features of the environment and several important behaviors is considered and implications for health promotion interventions and research are highlighted.

THEORETICAL PERSPECTIVES

The physical environment incorporates all of the physical elements within the surroundings of humans and other organisms, including air, water, land, flora, fauna, manufactured products, and built structures. The multifaceted nature of the physical environment, with its different degrees of proximity to individuals and direct or indirect influences upon behaviors, indicates that, while this is a promising arena for health promotion, it is also a complex area of study. Theoretical models about the environment–behavior relationship, therefore, provide an important foundation for knowledge development and interventions.

Several theories concerned with the impact of the physical environment upon behaviors could be grouped under a heading of stimulus response theories. Arousal theories address the psychophysiological response caused by environmental factors, such as heat and noise, and the impact that this has on behavioral performance (Sundstrom et al 1996). Conditions of moderate arousal are said to lead to optimal performance. Stress and adaptation theories are concerned with human reactions to elements in the environment which evoke a stress response and the behaviors which are undertaken to cope with environmental stressors (Bonnes & Secchiaroli 1995). Similar to these are environmental load theories (Cohen 1978), which address the way in which individuals deal with an excess of inputs from the environment. These highlight the selective attention strategy that humans employ in situations of overload and explain poor behavioral performance in terms of an attention deficit arising from excessive stimulation.

Social cognitive theory, developed by Bandura (1986), states that the environment, as with other behavioral influences, rarely exerts unidirectional control over the actions that people take. Instead, behavior is said to be a product of reciprocal relationships between cognitive and personal characteristics, the environment (both physical and social), and the action itself. The relative influence of the three interacting factors is said to vary according to individual characteristics, the nature of the activity, and environmental circumstances. Environmental conditions may exert overriding restraints upon behavior in some situations, but in others these constraints may be weak or personal beliefs may be so strong that an action is taken irrespective of environmental influences.

Ecological approaches have been an important development in understanding relationships between the physical environment and human behaviors. Barker's (1968) behavior setting theory, as a leading example of these, states that the behaviors of individuals are determined by the physical objects in their environment and the 'setting program', which sets down the nature and sequence of actions that are appropriate in that context. Examples of behavior settings include schools and churches, both of which include the essential elements of people (students, worshippers), physical factors (buildings, doorways, furniture, equipment, etc.), and programs for behavior (sitting, reading, listening, singing, etc.).

Individuals with a greater 'level of penetration' into a setting, due possibly to their responsibilities within it, are considered subject to more direct behavioral pressures, and settings which are 'undermanned' are considered to exert greater influence upon their members.

Social ecological models (Stokols 1992) adopt a systems theoretical position which holds that the physical, social, and cultural dimensions of the environment are interrelated and cumulatively influence behaviors. Environmental domains at different levels (home, neighborhood, and city) are considered to be interdependent; therefore, both immediate and more distant environments have an influence upon health-related behaviors and present opportunities for intervention. Because the utility of the social ecological perspective is threatened by its inclusiveness of many determinants, 'middle range' models have been developed to identify ecological variables that can be addressed in health promotion. For instance, Cohen et al's (2000) structural model of health behavior identifies four levels of health promotion action:

- the availability of health-related products
- the structure of the physical environment
- social structures that regulate behaviors
- cultural and media messages.

RESEARCH ADDRESSING
THE PHYSICAL ENVIRONMENT AND BEHAVIOR

There is evidence to show that the physical environment can influence the ease with which behaviors that have long-term health benefits (e.g. physical activity, healthy eating) can be performed and whether routine activities (e.g. driving, performing work duties) can be carried out without risk of injury. Elements of the environment which have an influence upon behaviors in a way that enhances or threatens health can be identified in homes, schools and workplaces, neighborhoods, cities, and the natural environment.

Homes

Hazards in the home environment, including slippery walking surfaces, obstacles in hallways, inadequate lighting, deficient stairways, uneven ground, and loose floor coverings, influence whether the elderly can mobilize and perform their daily activities without the risk of falling. Studies reveal that home hazards increase the risk of falls among older people who are not independent in self-care (Cesari et al 2002) and those who are vigorously active (Northridge 1995). Interventions by occupational therapists to identify and remove environmental hazards in the homes of older people who are considered at risk (due to past

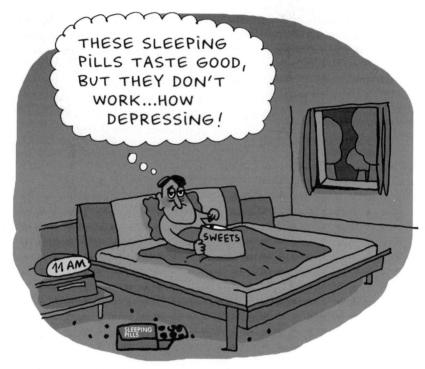

WINTER IN SWEDEN

falls) have been found to reduce falls (Cumming et al 1999). Among general community living older people, home hazard modification has been found to add to the benefits of group-based exercise in falls prevention (Day et al 2002).

The safety of children is affected by whether or not safeguards are present in the home, including pool fencing to prevent submersions and drowning (Thompson & Rivara 2003), hot water thermostat controls to prevent scalds (NHS CRD 1996), and window barriers to prevent falls (Cummins & Jackson 2001). For each of these types of injury, longitudinal data are available to show that an increase in the prevalence of the respective safety device in the child's environment, due to legislation and/or awareness campaigns, has reduced the population incidence of the related injury.

Schools and workplaces

The provision of shade structures in child-care centers and schools is a widely adopted sun protection strategy, although research about the impact that this has upon sun protection behaviors is limited. Milne et al (1999) investigated the relationship between the amount of shade cover of playgrounds upon children's sun exposure as part of the evaluation of a primary school sun protection intervention. They found that the amount of shade available was not related to sun exposure, although it was noted that shade provision was measured throughout the school and not specifically in play areas used by the study group. Experience in other settings indicates that for maximum impact shade structures need to be provided as part of multifaceted interventions that incorporate education, role modeling, and policy development (Glanz et al 2002).

Evidence about the impact of the physical characteristics of playground equipment upon child injury identifies factors that can be readily addressed in interventions, namely hard undersurfaces (e.g. concrete), inadequate guardrails, and equipment with a height of greater than 150 centimeters (Mott et al 1997). The most effective injury prevention strategies for children are those that combine proper installation and maintenance of equipment with playground safety policies and adequate adult supervision (Purvis & Hirsch 2003).

Physical risk factors in workplaces, in addition to the organizational and psychosocial characteristics of the work environment, are a significant cause of injury in this setting. Musculoskeletal injuries and disorders among nurses have been found to be higher when adjustable beds and transfer sheets are used and to be reduced by access to mechanical lifting devices (Trinkoff et al 2003). Melamed et al (1999) reported that active hazards (e.g. exposed sharp angles, protruding parts), overcrowding, excessive noise, climate discomfort (e.g. uncomfortable temperature or air currents), and vibration caused by machinery were environmental factors that predicted injuries in a range of industries in Israel. Research in Sweden has found that defective equipment (e.g. broken ladders) and slippery surfaces (due to spillages or snow and ice) are contributing factors in a substantial proportion of slip, trip, and falls injuries in workplaces (Kemmlert & Lundholm 2001).

Neighborhood facilities

Neighborhood characteristics that have been found to be positively associated with physical activity participation include self-reported access to exercise facilities and parks, pleasant scenery, and sidewalks (Brownson et al 2001). Booth et al (2000) found perceived accessibility to facilities to be related to leisure-time activity among older adults. In a study where objective distance between residences and exercise facilities was measured, Sallis et al (1990) reported that proximity to pay facilities (e.g. gymnasiums) and not free facilities (e.g. parks, sports fields) was inversely related to levels of activity. Another study using objective measures found that proximity to recreation and exercise facilities was associated with their use and that an overall rating of the physical environment (access to facilities, appeal, availability of footpaths and shops) had a significant, albeit weak, relationship with activity participation (Giles-Corti & Donovan 2002). The presence of signs encouraging people to use the stairs instead of elevators or lifts in venues such as shopping centers and train stations has been found in several studies to be an environmental influence upon the number of people who choose this option (Kerr et al 2001).

The contribution that fast-food consumption appears to be making to the rising prevalence of obesity (Binkley et al 2000) suggests that the proliferation of fast-food outlets is having a harmful effect upon dietary habits. Evidence is not yet available to substantiate this, although cross-sectional research has found that having supermarkets in the local area is associated with a greater likelihood of meeting recommendations for fruit and vegetable and fat intake (Morland et al 2002). In the same study, fast-food outlets were evenly distributed across the neighborhoods studied so there was little basis for examining dietary differences in relation to this factor. Research showing a trend of increased fast-food portion sizes indicates that this is one characteristic of these outlets which is contributing to increased dietary fat consumption (Nielsen & Popkin 2003).

Environmental strategies to control fast-food outlets are being considered a necessary part of the response to the obesity epidemic in many countries and these may include limiting the number of fast-food outlets not meeting nutritional standards per capita in a community, setting a minimum distance between these outlets and youth facilities, and prohibiting drive-through services (Ashe et al 2003).

Cities

Aspects of road transport routes and their surrounds that affect driving safety and motor vehicle accidents include road and shoulder width, curves, separation of carriageways, the presence of traffic controls, and road surfaces (Waller 1985). Enhancements of these factors, together with improved motor vehicle design, seatbelt legislation, and enforcement of drink driving and speeding laws, have led to substantial reductions in rates of vehicle crashes and fatalities (Wintemute 1992). Furthermore, there is good evidence that the use of traffic calming measures within urban precincts, such as street closures, street narrowing, staggered one-way regulations, and speed humps, are an effective environmental strategy for reducing speeding, unsafe driving, and traffic accidents (Elvik 2001).

Research in the fields of urban design and transportation has identified a cluster of land use characteristics that are associated with levels of walking or cycling. The proximity of residences to shopping areas and other regular destinations (e.g. schools, recreation facilities) has been found to have a significant effect upon walking participation (Greenwald & Boarnet 2002). Underlying land use patterns identified as influences upon physical activity participation are:

- residential density, which is positively correlated with the use of non-motorized transport
- a mixture of residential, commercial, and recreational zones, which is associated with greater walking
- high connectivity of streets, characterized by a grid rather than a cul-de-sac pattern, enabling greater use of walking for transportation (Handy et al 2002).

Geographical information system (GIS) software has been an important tool in studies about the relationship between residential location, land use structure, and participation in physical activity.

Natural environment

Dietary practices among people in developing countries living on low incomes are often dependent on the quality of forests and other ecosystems in their vicinity. The Food and Agriculture Organization (FAO) of the United Nations (1996) has described the contribution of 'wild foods' to nutrition, both as primary sources of food and as safety net provisions when food stocks are low. The range of indirect contributions made by forests to household nutrition is also described, including providing fuels so that food can be properly prepared, supplying products that can generate income for food purchases, and enhancing soil quality which enables the growth of a wider range of food plants. A wider dimension of the natural environment which has implications for food availability in developing countries is global climate change due to greenhouse gases. Based upon modeling of the impact of climate change upon yields of major grain cereals and soybean, Parry et al (1999) estimate that an additional 80 million people will be at risk of hunger in 2080, with Africa the most severely affected.

ENVIRONMENTAL STRATEGIES TO PROMOTE HEALTH

The evidence about the range of factors in the physical environment that impact upon behaviors indicates that there is much scope to give these greater attention in health promotion. Table C2.1 presents examples of strategies to modify and control elements of the physical environment in the various contexts examined already.

The behavior change strategies listed in the table have important implications for the way in which health promotion is practiced. The need for multisectoral collaboration is apparent in many of the strategies. For instance, the introduction of equipment and safety standards to reduce injury risk in workplaces will require collaboration with government occupational health and safety agencies, employers, and unions in various industries. Political advocacy will be required to bring about

Table C2.1 Strategies to facilitate behavior change through the physical environment

Context	Health-related behavior	Environment feature	Behavior change strategies
Home	Falls in the elderly	Slippery surfaces Obstructed doors and passageways Uneven floors and pathways Loose rugs	Home safety audits Subsidized home modification services
	Submersion, exposure to hot substances and falls in children	Pool fencing Hot water thermostats Window barriers	Legislation on pool fences Industry standards requiring thermostat controls on hot water heaters Building regulations requiring window barriers
Schools and workplaces	Falls in children	Hardness of surfaces under play equipment Guardrails on equipment Height of play equipment	Equipment standards and insurance requirements governing undersurfacing, guardrails, and height of play equipment
	Child sun protection	Availability of shade structures	School policies about playground shade coverage
	Occupational accidents	Availability of mechanical lifting devices Protective guards on machinery Overcrowding Excessive noise Climatic discomfort Defective equipment Slippery surfaces	Industry-specific standards governing equipment safety, minimum work space, noise levels, and climate Safety standards included in industrial agreements Regular workplace safety audits

Neighborhoods	Physical activity	Availability of parks and recreation venues Availability of pay facilities for exercise Aesthetic quality of parks and streets Quality of sidewalks	Local government development plans to enhance parks, recreation areas, sidewalks, and lighting Waiving of local government levies for exercise facilities Signs to prompt use of stairs
	Dietary fat consumption	Availability of fast-food outlets Fast-food portion size and fat content	Planning controls over number of fast-food outlets and proximity to youth facilities Standards governing portion size and fat content of foods
Cities	Speeding and unsafe driving	Width and quality of roads Traffic signals Traffic calming devices	Advocacy for road improvements through motorists' lobby groups Government standards for roads with various traffic volumes Traffic calming plans to meet accident reduction targets
	Physical activity	Proximity of residential areas to shops, schools, and other facilities Availability of public transport	Planning policies to locate residential areas within walkable distance of shops and schools Integrating walking and cycling paths with public transport
Natural environment	Nutrition in developing countries	Forest conservation Soil quality and erosion Availability of natural fuels Average air temperatures	Advocacy for forest conservation National policies concerning greenhouse gas emissions

legislation and regulatory controls over potentially harmful influences in the physical environment. An example is advocacy for regulation of the location of fast-food outlets and the size and fat content of the food portions that they sell, which is likely to be strenuously opposed by commercial interest groups. The strategies listed in the table also highlight the need for the budget and duration of health promotion interventions to be reconsidered and, in many cases, increased. For instance, working with local government authorities to enhance the amenity of neighborhood environments for physical activity is likely to require 5 years or more to implement and large investments of public funds.

FUTURE DIRECTIONS

One explanation for the overemphasis upon individual determinants of behavior in health promotion is that evidence about the contribution of these factors is more easily collected and consequently abundant. Another is that interventions at this level are less complex to manage, given that they require less involvement in multisectoral collaboration, advocacy, and policy change. Building the knowledge base about the role played by the physical environment in relation to behavior and the environmental interventions that have a beneficial impact upon behaviors will help to redress this unfavorable trend.

The development of accurate measures of exposure to elements of the physical environment is fundamental to understanding environment and behavior relationships. As already mentioned, a positive development in physical activity research has been the use of GIS software that enables accurate, unobtrusive measurement of land use patterns, transport routes, and distances between points of interest. In the area of sun protection, solar light meters have been used to objectively measure shade coverage (Parsons et al 1998). Audit tools provide a more labor-intensive but potentially more detailed method of collecting environmental data. Pikora et al (2002) have developed a Systematic Pedestrian and Cycling Environmental Scan (SPACES) for the assessment of aspects of residential environments that are relevant to physical activity and have reported this to have good interrater reliability. There are also examples of tools that have been found to be reliable in the assessment of home hazards for falls among older people (Mackenzie et al 2002). Measurement of environmental characteristics by self-report represents another option, but experience in physical activity research indicates that assessments by survey respondents may have little agreement with objective measurements (Kirtland et al 2003). There is a need to continue to develop detailed measures of environmental variables specific to a range of health-related behaviors (e.g. child injury, sun protection) and to ascertain their reliability and validity in different geographical locations.

Disentangling the effects of the physical environment upon behaviors from those caused by socio-economic status, social norms and support structures, and intrapersonal factors is an area that clearly deserves attention. There is ample evidence that poor environmental conditions are associated with low socio-economic status and it is likely that environmental conditions are a major cause of the social gradient in health (Evans & Kantrowitz 2002). What is required is determination of the extent to which modifiable features of the physical environment exert an independent influence. Given that intrapersonal and interpersonal factors can moderate the way in which individuals respond to their physical environment, there is also a need to understand the combinations of physical, social, and psychological factors that influence behaviors in particular ways. This knowledge could then be used in strategies to enhance the behavioral impact of environmental modifications.

Because elements of the physical environment are usually fixed, much of the research about environment–behavior relationships is cross-sectional. Natural experiments, where individuals or communities are exposed to major changes in their physical surroundings so that effects of these can be measured, are rare. In spite of this, it is necessary to recognize that knowledge about the effects of the physical environment upon behaviors will improve most rapidly through longitudinal and intervention research, particularly using designs that can control for the social and psychological influences upon behaviors discussed in this chapter. The research conducted so far, in regard to home hazard reduction for children and older people, the sun protection effects of shade structures and, to a lesser extent, the effects of modifying physical activity environments, indicates that this is possible, at least at the level of homes, schools and workplaces, and neighborhoods.

Environmental variables have the potential to reach large proportions of populations and to have an impact that is sustained beyond the life of funded programs. In fact, many behaviors can only be influenced at the population level when strategies directed towards individuals are complemented by those that address barriers and opportunities for the behavior in the physical and social environment. A good foundation of research about the impact of the environment upon a number of behaviors has been built. Important next steps are to undertake more sophisticated modeling of the relative impact of variables in the physical environment compared with other factors identified by ecological models, and to test the impact that environmental change strategies can have in addressing specific health needs.

References

Ashe M, Jernigan D, Kilne R et al 2003 Land use planning and the control of alcohol, tobacco, firearms, and fast food restaurants. American Journal of Public Health 93:1404–1408

Bandura A 1986 Social foundations of thought and action: a social cognitive theory. Prentice-Hall, Englewood Cliffs, New Jersey

Barker R G 1968 Ecological psychology: concepts and methods for studying the environment of human behavior. Stanford University Press, Stanford

Binkley J K, Eales J, Jekanowski M 2000 The relation between dietary change and rising US obesity. International Journal of Obesity and Related Metabolic Disorders 24:1032-1039

Bonnes M, Secchiaroli G 1995 Environmental psychology: a psycho-social introduction. Sage, London

Booth M L, Owen N, Bauman A et al 2000 Social-cognitive and perceived environmental influences associated with physical activity in older Australians. Preventive Medicine 31:15-22

Brownson R C, Baker E A, Housemann R A et al 2001 Environmental and policy determinants of physical activity in the United States. American Journal of Public Health 91(12):1995-2002

Cesari M, Landi F, Torre S et al 2002 Prevalence and risk factors for falls in an older community-dwelling population. Journals of Gerontology Series A – Biological Sciences and Medical Sciences 57(11):M722-726

Cohen D A, Scribner R A, Farley T A 2000 A structural model of health behavior: a pragmatic approach to explain and influence health behaviors at the population level. Preventive Medicine 30(2):146-154

Cohen S 1978 Environmental load and the allocation of attention. In: Baum A, Singer J E, Valins S (eds) Advances in environmental psychology, vol 1. Lawrence Erlbaum Associates, Hillsdale, New Jersey

Cumming R G, Thomas M, Szonyi G 1999 Home visits by an occupational therapist for assessment and modification of environmental hazards: a randomized trial of falls prevention. Journal of the American Geriatrics Society 47(12):1397-1402

Cummins S K, Jackson R J 2001 The built environment and children's health. Pediatric Clinics of North America 48(5):1241-1252

Day L, Fildes B, Gordon I et al 2002 Randomised factorial trial of falls prevention among older people living in their own homes. British Medical Journal 325:128-133

Elvik R 2001 Area-wide traffic calming schemes: a meta-analysis of safety effects. Accident Analysis and Prevention 22:327-336

Evans G W, Kantrowitz E 2002 Socioeconomic status and health: the potential role of environmental risk exposure. Annual Review of Public Health 23:303-331

Food and Agriculture Organization of the United Nations 1996 Considering nutrition in national forestry programmes. Food and Nutrition Division, Nutrition and Programmes Service, FAO, Rome

Giles-Corti B, Donovan R J 2002 The relative influence of individual, social and physical environment determinants of physical activity. Social Science and Medicine 54:1793-1812

Glanz K, Geller A C, Shigaki D et al 2002 A randomized trial of skin cancer prevention in aquatics settings: the Pool Cool program. Health Psychology 21:579-587

Greenwald M, Boarnet M G 2002 The built environment as a determinant of walking behavior: analyzing non-work pedestrian travel in Portland, Oregon. Transportation Research Record 1780:33-42

Handy S L, Boarnet M G, Ewing R et al 2002 How the built environment affects physical activity: views from urban planning. American Journal of Preventive Medicine 23(2S):64-73

Kemmlert K, Lundholm L 2001 Slips, trips and falls in different work groups – with reference to age and from a preventive perspective. Applied Ergonomics 32:149-153

Kerr J, Eves F, Carroll D 2001 Six-month observational study of prompted stair climbing. Preventive Medicine 33:422-427

Kirtland K A, Porter D E, Addy C L et al 2003 Environmental measures of physical activity supports: perception versus reality. American Journal of Preventive Medicine 24:323-331

Mackenzie L, Byles J, Higginbotham N 2002 Reliability of the Home Falls and Accidents Screening Tool (HOME FAST) for identifying older people at increased risk of falls. Disability and Rehabilitation 24(5):266-274

Melamed S, Yekutieli D, Froom P et al 1999 Adverse work and environmental conditions predict occupational injuries. The Israeli Cardiovascular Occupational Risk factors Determination in Israel (CORDIS) study. American Journal of Epidemiology 150:18-26

Milne E, English D R, Corti B 1999 Direct measurement of sun protection in primary schools. Preventive Medicine 29:45-52

Morland K, Wing S, Diez-Roux A 2002 The contextual effect of the local food environment on residents' diets: the Atherosclerosis Risk in Communities Study. American Journal of Public Health 92:1761-1767

Mott A, Rolfe K, James R et al 1997 Safety of surfaces and equipment for children in playgrounds. Lancet 349:1874-1876

Nestle M, Jacobsen M F 2000 Halting the obesity epidemic: a public health policy approach. Public Health Reports 115:12-24

NHS Centre for Reviews and Dissemination (NHS CRB) 1996 Preventing unintentional injuries in children and young people. Effective Health Care 2(5):1-16

Nielsen S J, Popkin B M 2003 Patterns and trends in food portion sizes, 1977–1998. Journal of the American Medical Association 289:450-453

Northridge M E, Nevitt M C, Kelsey J L et al 1995 Home hazards and falls in the elderly: the role of health and functional status. American Journal of Public Health 85(4):509-515

O'Donnell M P 2003 Health promoting community design. American Journal of Health Promotion, Editor's Notes Sept/Oct 2003. Available online at: www.healthpromotionjournal.com/publications/journal/en2003-09.htm

Parry M, Rosenzweig C, Iglesias A et al 1999 Climate change and world food security: a new assessment. Global Environmental Change 9:S51-S67

Parsons P G, Neale R, Wolski P 1998 The shady side of solar protection. Medical Journal of Australia 168:327-330

Pikora T J, Bull F C L, Jamrozik K et al 2002 Developing a reliable audit instrument to measure the physical environment for physical activity. American Journal of Preventive Medicine 23:187-194

Purvis J M, Hirsch S A 2003 Playground injury prevention. Clinical Orthopaedics and Related Research 409:11-19

Sallis J F, Hovell M F, Hofstetter C R et al 1990 Distance between homes and exercise related facilities related to frequency of exercise among San Diego residents. Public Health Reports 105:179-185

Stokols D 1992 Establishing and maintaining healthy environments: toward a social ecology of health promotion. American Psychologist 47(1):6-22

Sundstrom E, Bell P A, Busby P L et al 1996 Environmental psychology 1989-94. Annual Review of Psychology 47:485-512

Thompson D C, Rivara F P 2003 Pool fencing for preventing drowning in children. Cochrane Database of Systematic Reviews 1

Trinkoff A M, Brady B, Nielsen K 2003 Workplace prevention and musculoskeletal injuries in nurses. Journal of Nursing Administration 33:153-158

Waller J A 1985 Injury control: a guide to the causes and prevention of trauma. Lexington Books, Massachusetts

Wintemute G J 1992 From research to public policy: the prevention of motor vehicle injuries, childhood drownings, and firearm violence. American Journal of Health Promotion 6:451-464

Psychosocial environments

Christian Janßen and Holger Pfaff

INTRODUCTION

How can we maintain our health? What can we do to avoid illness? Since disease prevention and progression have many causes, the answer to these questions may depend on how you approach it scientifically. The causes will vary, therefore, depending on whether you investigate it from a biological, chemical, physical, psychological, or social point of view. Taking a psychosocial perspective of health and population-level behavior change, we hope to demonstrate the most important social factors that influence psychological states and possibly cause good health and illness.

Social stratification by profession, education and income, social networks through friends and organizations and social subsystems, such as the labor market or educational system, contribute to our behavioral skills and psychological resources, which can help to sustain health and prevent disease. For example, people from higher social classes who have a larger number of social contacts have healthier living conditions, can handle adverse life events, and can cope with disease better than those in lower social classes (Marmot & Wilkinson 1999). They can achieve this because they have behavioral skills and psychological resources, such as knowledge, money, respect, and social support, which empower them to cope with stress better.

Social structures, such as social class, social networks, the labor market, and the educational system, as well as preventing disease, can promote disease if their design engenders social disadvantage. Unemployment and effort–reward imbalance (e.g. high work demand accompanied by low pay and recognition), as well as social isolation, can increase an individual's stress levels and lead to distress. This distress can provoke disease.

Thus social health and disease factors can be summarized as the result of social structures and opportunities. In the last few decades, specific sociological health and disease models have been developed to explain the mechanisms of these social factors. These models will be described in detail in this chapter.

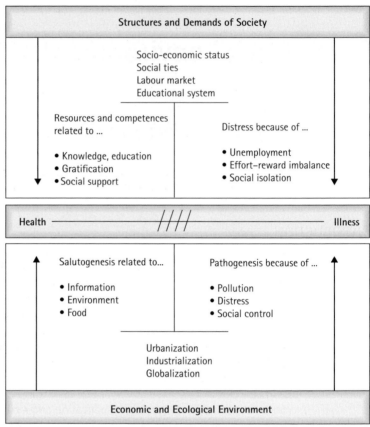

Fig C3.1 Sociological factors of health and illness (Adapted with permission from von Troschke et al 1998)

Figure C3.1 shows the determinants and effects of social, economic, and ecological factors on health. Economic and ecological environmental influences on health have evolved through three important social economic developments: urbanization, industrialization, and globalization. The process of modernization, which is reflected in these developments, was determined essentially by progress in the natural sciences, for example disinfectants, automation, and immunization. Today, it is commonly agreed that this progress improves the living conditions of society in general, as well as particular working, transport, living, and nutrition conditions. This in turn affects population morbidity and mortality rates (von Troschke et al 1998). Accordingly, life expectancy has improved in line with progress. This health-promoting effect of social economic change is, however, accompanied by risks, which can have pathological consequences. During the course of industrialization and urbanization, chronic diseases, such as coronary heart disease, have increased. The spectrum of morbidity has also changed. As a consequence of industrialization, the increase in traffic, for example, has led to new problems such as traffic accidents, environmental pollution, and noise. Industrial pollution, for example, has been accompanied by an increase in daily stressors, which have become a part of modern life (intensification of work stress due to noise, for example).

Health-related effects of social economic change are evident in the current heath status of eastern European states. The difference in life expectancy between Organization for Economic Cooperation and Development (OECD) countries and central and eastern European countries has continuously increased. Insufficient health behavior, malnutrition, alcohol consumption, and, in particular, smoking are the most important causes of higher mortality in eastern Europe. Medical services and environmental pollution seem to play a smaller role (Bobak & Marmot 1996).

Assuming that basic systems influence our lives, scientists have gradually developed a sophisticated division of labor: biological organisms, mental systems, social systems, and machines. Medicine deals with the human organisms, psychology with mental systems, engineering focuses on technical systems, and sociology on social systems, such as society, organizations, groups, and the social interactions and behavior which take place within these systems (Luhmann 1995). Thus, a psychosocial model of health promotion and disease progression tries to identify causal factors, located at the interface between social and psychological systems. As a result, there are two basic psychosocial approaches to explain health and disease: one concentrates on systems and their states while another focuses on psychological factors, i.e. the individual. The former are called system-related models, the latter individual-centered models (Table C3.1). System-centered models, in particular, assume causal relationships between social, economic, and cultural system-states, on the one hand, and health-related system-states on the other; for example, life expectancy of a population. These models can be subdivided into materialistic and non-materialistic models. The latter concentrate on social and cultural social factors instead of economic ones.

Table C3.1 System- versus individual-related psychosocial models of health and illness

Approach	Model
System	Social Capital
	Social Cohesion
Individual	Social Support
	Effort–Reward Imbalance
	Demand–Control
	Stress-Process

SOCIAL CAPITAL MODEL

The Social Capital Model was originally based on a model of social cohesion. The term 'social cohesion' describes the degree of bonding and solidarity in social groups (Pfaff 1989). Cohesive societies, organizations and groups have strong interrelated bonds and a high degree of integration. In sociology, it is assumed that networks with high cohesion have sustainable and amenable effects on health. Durkheim (1997), for example, showed in an early study that in the 19th century suicide rates were higher among Protestants than Catholics. He explains that the tendency for suicide is lower in societies with a combination of high normative regulation, strong inner cohesion, and strong involvement of individuals in the group. According to his view, this combination was present more in Catholic religious groups than Protestant ones. The mechanisms by which a cohesive social system influences health are multiple. Not only do cohesive systems satisfy our need for involvement in strong social groups, but they also help and support us to cope with crises and keep control of our lives.

Cohesive societies have a large amount of social capital. Social capital comprises those structures of a society which are resources for individuals and support collective behavior (Berkman & Kawachi 2000). These resources include the degree of trust in a social group (e.g. neighborhoods), the relevance of norms (e.g. generally accepted rules of interaction), as well as the degree of solidarity within a social system. If societies are built on reliable structures and relationships, they may accumulate social capital, which can be used in multiple ways. Social capital is a feature of social systems and therefore a so-called 'ecological variable'. According to this concept, an individual cannot have social capital. Social capital belongs instead to the society in which we live. It is therefore possible for an individual with a large social network to live in a society with little social capital. Societies with high social capital due to strong internal connectedness (friends and clubs) have the ability to exert effective social control, as well as the ability to motivate collective actions.

The social capital of society can promote health through more than one pathway:

- by influencing health-related behavior
- by influencing access to helpful community services (e.g. public transport, hospitals)
- through psychosocial processes (e.g. society as a source of emotional support and a means of protecting self-esteem).

A US study showed that the degree of mistrust within certain states was strongly correlated with age-adjusted mortality rates in these states (Kawachi et al 1997). The same was true for the number of memberships in self-selected associations (e.g. church groups, sport clubs, hobby groups, unions). Another study showed that individuals living in states with low trust capacity reported worse health compared with individuals in states with high interpersonal trust (Kawachi et al 1999).

SOCIAL SUPPORT MODEL

The roots of the interdisciplinary model of social support can be traced back to the 1897 suicide study mentioned previously (Durkheim 1997). In its modern form, the concept was developed and empirically tested by psychiatrists, epidemiologists, psychologists, and sociologists. The Social Support Model comprises three dimensions of social relationships:

- presence (i.e. social integration)
- structure (i.e. social networks)
- content (i.e. extent of support).

The social integration of an individual includes such aspects as the availability of relationships, the number of possible relationships, and contact frequency. The level of contact in social networks, for example, can differ by size, density, duration, intensity, structure, and reciprocity (Macinko & Starfield 2001). The content of social relationships can vary and include the following types of support: love/affection, trust, inclusion/belonging, caution, esteem, confirmation, advice, information, care, material help, common sense, and solidarity. These supportive behaviors can be divided into two categories: emotional support (e.g. affection) and instrumental support (e.g. information). Existing objective support is separated conceptually from perceived subjective support. Receivers of perceived and actual support assess the availability and potential for support. Potential sources of support are, for example, friends, relatives, partners and colleagues, social workers, doctors, and nurses (Levy & Pescosolido 2002).

What is the effect of social support? The Social Support Model consists of four principles (see Fig C3.2):

1 stress affects health
2 support prevents stress build-up and mitigates existing stress
3 support reduces the negative consequences of stress and deflects these consequences before they take effect
4 support directly fosters health and wellness.

The strongest empirical evidence is that stress and support affect health. The principle that stress and its consequences can be prevented still requires more research (Pfaff 1989). Many cohort studies show that social isolation, the opposite of social integration, is a risk factor for mortality. After a heart attack, for example, individuals who are socially isolated, lack emotional support, or a trusted companion have an increased mortality risk (Badura et al 1987). Another important health factor is whether you believe you would have sufficient support in a

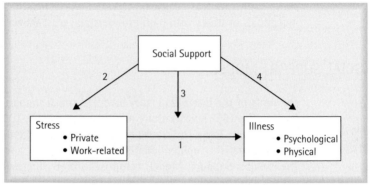

Fig C3.2   The Social Support Model (e.g. Pfaff 1989). (1) Stress affects health. (2) Support prevents stress build-up and mitigates existing stress. (3) Support reduces the negative consequences of stress and deflects these consequences before they take effect. (4) Support directly fosters health and wellness

serious situation. Perceived potential support promotes and protects health. The positive effects of social integration and perceived support are based, among other things, on social relationships which:

- positively regulate thinking, feeling, and behavior
- strengthen the feeling of meaning and cohesion
- support health-promoting behavior
- support coping with stress
- increase self-esteem
- strengthen the feeling of control (health locus of control; Wallston et al 1978) or sense of coherence (Antonovsky 1987)
- influence the immune system
- by their mere presence emotionally and physically stabilize the individual (Berkman 1995).

EFFORT–REWARD IMBALANCE (ERI) MODEL

The ERI Model was developed by the sociologist Johannes Siegrist (Siegrist & Peter 2000) to explain work-related mortality due to coronary heart disease. In its original form it was mainly concerned with occupational health. Two central dimensions characterize the model: effort and reward. Occupational over demand consists of work-related strain and duties (external demands) and an exaggerated desire for job control (internal demands). The reward can be material or immaterial and includes three aspects of control: income, recognition, and status. The model's central premise is that an imbalance between high job strain and low reward results in an imbalance of effort and reward,

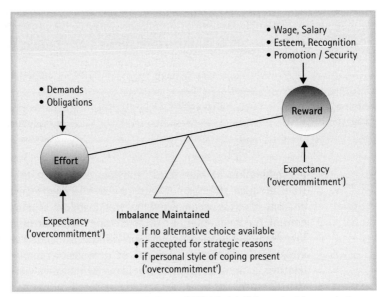

Fig C3.3   Effort–Reward Imbalance (ERI) Model (Adapted with permission from Siegrist 2000)

which may result in impaired health. This imbalance is demonstrated in Figure C3.3.

High job strain is not problematic if there is appropriate reward for the effort involved. If, in contrast, the employee feels that he is receiving insufficient monetary reward and recognition for the effort he has exerted and that despite his hard work his career progression is not guaranteed nor his job secure, then a kind of crisis may occur. In summary, the ERI Model sets its focus on the non-reciprocity of efforts and rewards which is partly fixed in the employment contract. The model has been well supported in both national and international studies (Siegrist 2002).

DEMAND–CONTROL (DC) MODEL

The Demand–Control Model was conceived by the sociologist Robert Karasek (Karasek & Theorell 1990). It was developed to analyze the correlation between work and health but, unlike the ERI Model, it was aimed at occupational tasks with high demand and low control. There are two central dimensions: stress and control. Stress concerns the amount of work performed by an employee (quantitative workload). The control dimension describes how far an employee has decisional power in his work and how far he can employ his personal skills.

According to the DC Model, health risks are anticipated when there is an imbalance between stress and control. If both stress and control are dichotomized into high and low levels, then ill health results from

Table C3.2 The Demand–Control (DC) Model (Reprinted with permission from Karasek & Theorell 1990)		
	Low demand	**High demand**
High control	Low stress	Active work
Low control	Passive work	High stress

a combination of high stress and low control. In this case, distress from the high strain is not mitigated by sufficient control. The lowest amount of stress occurs when low workloads are accompanied by high control. A combination of high strain and high control (active work) or low strain and low control (passive work) is associated with intermediate stress levels. Active work can be described as managerial tasks. In contrast, a night receptionist would perform passive work, for example. The DC Model has been well tested empirically in national and international studies. Further, there are studies which show that employees with a negative stress–control work environment have a two- to fourfold greater risk of heart attack compared with individuals with a favorable stress–control balance (Badura et al 1987). This effect is independent of genetic and coronary risk factors.

STRESS-PROCESS MODEL

The Stress-Process Model is based on sociological and psychosocial findings from interdisciplinary stress research. The main founder of this model is, among others, the American sociologist and social epidemiologist Leonard Pearlin (Pearlin et al 1981). The model is supported by several American and German studies which have investigated the health consequences of losing a job, the death of a spouse, and suffering a heart attack (Badura et al 1987). According to the model, the variables can be divided into five categories:

1 social background
2 stressors
3 self-esteem
4 mediator/moderators
5 stress outcomes.

The social background of an individual contributes to the nature of the stress response. Important social background factors include the social conditions within a society and the position of the individual within society. Belonging to a certain social class, your professional status, sex, age, involvement in social networks, and your roles in different institutions also have an influence on the stress situation. Individuals' health and stress-related attitudes and behaviors also partially determine access to and ability to use social resources.

Stressors are defined as all external conditions which influence an individual and are potentially dangerous, for example conflicts, time pressures, loss, and insecurity. Depending on an individual's social background, the effect of the stressors varies. Stressors in the Stress-Process Model, in contrast to the Life-Event Model (Geyer 1999), are not understood as single events but as situations that result from other social conditions and are therefore part of a stress process. To clarify this, primary and secondary stressors have been identified. Primary stressors are potentially dangerous external conditions which can initiate the stress process, for example a heart attack or adverse life event. Secondary stressors develop from primary stressors, for example altered occupational status after a heart attack. According to the Stress-Process Model, life events (e.g. job loss) can be considered as primary stressors, which in turn can induce secondary stressors (e.g. reduced income). The power of secondary stressors to cause ill health may be stronger than that of primary stressors. Thus, in this model, life events may also be considered as secondary stressors (e.g. job loss) arising from a primary stressor (e.g. conflict with a work manager). Further, in the Stress-Process Model, it is possible that interactions between various stressors (e.g. work and family) occur. The main assumption of this model is the dynamic nature of the stress process, which goes beyond the notion of stressors as stationary isolated events.

In the Stress-Process Model, stress includes all the consequences of stress for the individual. According to this model, stress is strongly influenced by self-esteem. A positive self-image (i.e. self-esteem) means that an individual is convinced that they can handle the demands of the environment (e.g. high sense of control and self-efficacy) and can help an individual to resist negative stress effects. Self-confidence and self-reliance can also be damaged by the stress process itself; for example, persistent failure and pressure to succeed can lead to doubts about one's capabilities and skills. Other individuals, however, can help to stabilize self-confidence.

The term 'mediator' (sometimes moderator) covers all personal and social resources which have the potential to compensate for and control the effects of stressors. The Stress-Process Model focuses on the mediators of coping and social support. In combination with social esteem, they contribute to an individual being a victim of stress or, at the other end of the spectrum, they can protect an individual from the health-threatening consequences of stress. Social support has already been fully addressed in this chapter. Coping, on the other hand, relates to all behaviors and cognitions (e.g. attitudes and assessments) that help individuals to avoid or minimize dangerous developments. Coping has four main aims: to avoid stress, to minimize existing stress (e.g. problem solving), to reframe stressful situations (rather than try to change them), for example to perceive them as less threatening, and to control the consequences of stress (e.g. reduce stress symptoms by relaxation exercises). The sociological Stress-Process Model in this context presumes that such individual coping techniques are likely to have only limited success. They are more likely to be effective, however, for interpersonal stress situations than for stress in an organizational context (e.g. job strain or role conflict). To solve such problems, collective forms of coping are more appropriate (e.g. self-help groups).

In the Stress-Process Model, multiple stress consequences are considered. It assumes principally that stress consequences are manifest at very different levels (physiological, psychological, and behavioral) but not necessarily at all these levels simultaneously. The particular form that stress outcomes take depends on both background factors (e.g. gender) and stress mediators.

CONCLUSION AND IMPLICATIONS

The psychosocial health environment and health behavior involve social factors which can influence our psychological processing and may be related to or cause health and illness. There are two distinct principles that separate health and disease models. Either models focus on social systems and their states (e.g. the Social Capital or Social Cohesion Models) or they focus on individuals and their relationships with the social environment (e.g. the Social Support Model, the Effort–Reward Imbalance Model, the Demand–Control Model, or the Stress-Process Model). An overview of the different models and their variables has been provided in this chapter and is summarized in Table C3.3.

The synopsis of these models indicates that multiple and varied factors can damage an individual's health or, equally, protect and promote positive health. Future prevention programs should therefore intervene at two levels: the individual and the social system. The aim of preventive medicine should be to implement a comprehensive biopsychosocial strategy of health promotion. As the examples given show, there is plenty of support for the notion that social structures and psychosocial factors can influence health. Finally, having considered the consequences of preventive medicine programs, which include these factors, we can suggest some recommendations for best practice.

Health practitioners should attempt to promote adequate individual health and disease preventive behavior in large parts of the population. At the same time, however, social environments should be designed to promote health. At the core of modern disease prevention and health promotion lie workplace, community, and state-level health policies which strengthen potential health and disease outcomes. Medical prevention and health promotion should therefore target several social determinants of health and disease. The most important target is changing health behavior because the practitioner can directly influence this, in terms of health education for example. For some other

Table C3.3 Dependent and independent variables of psychosocial models related to health and illness

Model	Independent variables	Dependent variables
Social Capital	Trust and reciprocity Participation in (voluntary) groups	Mortality, morbidity, and health indicators
Social Support	Number and frequencies of social relationships/ties Content of social relationships/ties Emotional support (e.g. affection, empathy) and instrumental support (advice, information, material help) Sources of support, e.g. friends, relatives, partners, colleagues, superiors, physicians, and nurses Objective vs subjective support	Mortality, morbidity, and health indicators Health-related behavior Self-esteem Sense of coherence Health locus of control
Effort–Reward Imbalance	Demands, obligations, expectancy, wage/salary, esteem/recognition, promotion/security	Indicators of mortality and morbidity
Demand–Control	Amount/kind of work, control over amount/kind of work	Indicators of morbidity (heart attack)
Stress-Process	Primary stressors: critical life events, temporary events, chronic burden, burden resulting from social roles, burden resulting from environment Secondary stressors: continuing problems of critical life events and burden Mediators: coping and social support Self-perception	Indicators of mortality and morbidity Emotional distress and disturbances

social determinants, the practitioner can exert additional indirect pressure (e.g. decisions concerning return to work after a heart attack). In medical practice it is important that doctors employ both their direct and indirect spheres of influence.

Other important targets for health promotion in the community are workplace prevention and community administration interventions. Nowadays, there are plenty of examples of this not only in the USA but also in Europe (Naidoo & Wills 2000). Health promotion measures in workplaces, to a large degree, still focus on individual employee health behavior. Results of several studies indicate that behavioral interventions are more successful when senior managers support the measures, employees participate in the planning process, and the intervention does not focus on medical risk factors (e.g. interventions that simply address 'back care' or 'skin care' rather than skin cancer) (Breucker et al 1998). Selecting a target group and directly addressing them during the intervention has also proved successful in order to implement routine evaluation and to account for the self-determining nature of decentralized organizations.

In addition, modern health promotion projects should focus on the organization's structures and processes. It is preferable to modify these than to try to change individual behavior. Ideally, health promotion should be implemented in a sustainable way as part of an organization's development and as an integral part of good business and management. Integrating health promotion into daily routine in this way enables health to be considered as an important part of the organization's culture. An organization's structures and processes should be changed, following the principles outlined in this chapter, by reducing the stress–resource gap, strengthening psychological resources, and avoiding psychosocial stressors.

References

Antonovsky A 1987 Unraveling the mystery of health: how people manage stress and stay well. Jossey-Bass, San Francisco

Badura B, Kaufhold G, Lehmann H et al 1987 Leben mit dem Herzinfarkt. Eine sozialepidemiologische Studie. Privately published, Berlin

Berkman L F 1995 The role of social relations in health promotion. Psychosomatic Medicine 57:245-254

Berkman L F, Kawachi I (eds) 2000 Social epidemiology. Oxford University Press, New York

Bobak M, Marmot M 1996 East-West mortality divide and its potential explanations: proposed research agenda. British Medical Journal 312:421-425

Breucker G, Kloppenburg H, Menckel E et al 1998 Success factors of workplace health promotion. BKK, Bremerhaven

Durkheim E 1997 Suicide: a study in sociology. Free Press, New York

Geyer S 1999 Macht Unglück krank? Lebenskrisen und die Entwicklung von Krankheiten. Juventa, Weinheim

Karasek R, Theorell T 1990 Healthy work. Stress, productivity, and the reconstruction of working life. Basic Books, New York

Kawachi I, Kennedy B P, Lochner K et al 1997 Social capital, income inequality, and mortality. American Journal of Public Health 87:1491-1498

Kawachi I, Kennedy B P, Lochner K 1999 Social capital and self-rated health. A contextual analysis. American Journal of Public Health 89:1187-1193

Levy J A, Pescosolido B A 2002 Social networks and health. Elsevier, Oxford

Luhmann N 1995 Social systems. Stanford University Press, Stanford

Macinko J, Starfield B 2001 The utility of social capital in research on health determinants. Milbank Quarterly 79:387-427

Marmot M, Wilkinson R G 1999 Social determinants of health. Oxford University Press, Oxford

Naidoo J, Wills J (eds) 2000 Health promotion: foundations for practice. Baillière Tindall, London

Pearlin L I, Menaghan E G, Lieberman M A et al 1981 The stress process. Journal of Health and Social Behavior 22:337-356

Pfaff H 1989 Stressbewältigung und soziale Unterstützung. Zur sozialen Regulierung individuellen Wohlbefindens. Juventa, Weinheim

Siegrist J 2002 Effort–reward imbalance at work and health. In: Perrewe P, Ganster D (eds) Research in occupational stress and well-being: historical and current perspectives on stress and health. Elsevier, New York, pp 261-291

Siegrist J, Peter R 2000 The effort–reward imbalance model. In: Schnall P (ed) Stressors at the workplace: theoretical models. Hanley and Belfus, Philadelphia, p 264

von Troschke J, Herrmann M, Stössel U 1998 Fortschritt und Gesundheit. In: Schwartz F W, Badura B, Leidl R et al (eds) Das Public-Health-Buch: Gesundheit und Gesundheitswesen. Urban and Fischer, München, pp 81-93

Wallston K A, Wallston B S, DeVellis R 1978 Development of the Multidimensional Health Locus of Control (MHLC) scales. Health Education Monographs 6:101-105

Political and legal environments

Tim Barnett

INTRODUCTION

This chapter will illustrate how people and agencies strategize to generate change and then review how important such pressure for change is for a health-promoting political and legal environment. It will then, in the light of that, discuss how people can best empower themselves and how campaigns can be structured to become a successful catalyst for improvement. Lastly, it will review the impact of law and policy on behavior and behavior modification.

A friend of mine recently celebrated his 90th birthday. His family, fellow retirement village residents, and a wide variety of companions gathered for what was to be a sparkling evening. Three of us had been chosen to make eulogy speeches. And through them emerged a story of which, until that evening, only the birthday boy knew all the elements.

He had moved into the retirement village 5 years before. Every aspect of it either delighted or satisfied him, except for its ban on residents owning cats or dogs. He had a lifetime desire to own a cat, frustrated by his wife (who had died just before he moved there) being allergic to them. He proceeded to engage in what (knowing him well) I am certain was a deliberate and superb lobbying strategy. Stage 1 was to *raise awareness* of the issue. So he acquired a very life-like toy cat, which was placed prominently in his downstairs lounge window, so every other resident could not fail to see it when they passed. Stage 2 was to *communicate confidence that things could change* – and to expose how silly the status quo was, compared to the desirability of change. So he installed a cat door in the most prominent of his unit's external doors. The rules may have banned cats but were silent on cat doors. Stage 3 was to *bring others on board* – a form of partnership creation. So he called in on every resident in his part of the village and (with their agreement, which was, naturally, always forthcoming) he appointed them honorary aunts and uncles of the cat, which he still did not own. Again the naivety of those rules was exposed! Stage 4 was to *create a catalyst for action.* He voiced urgent concern to neighbors that he had seen mice in the village. (Some even claim that he introduced a couple of very live mice to embellish the argument. His denials of this at the birthday party left lingering doubts.) And that brought it all to a peak, at Stage 5: *delivery.* He simply acquired a cat and moved it in. And waited for something to happen. Of course, nothing did. Not even cat-haters dared, because their position had been so marginalized. The aunts and uncles met and welcomed their new niece. My friend had his cat, in his flat. The lobby aim was achieved.

LOBBYING FOR PUBLIC HEALTH POLICIES

New Zealand has developed a proud policy of active opposition to smoking, most recently through a ban on smoking in eating places and bars. This sea change in attitude has been evidenced in law reform, arriving in waves over the last 15 years, depending on the bravery of the Minister of Health and/or the wider government of the time, on public policy, and on the statistics of smoking. In a less tangible sense, it has been evidenced in the marginalization of the pro-smoking lobby. Big tobacco interests have very limited opportunity to flaunt their oceans of cash and even the comparatively powerful free-market libertarian lobby does not seek to highlight the arguments of those opposing restrictions on smoking.

This position has been reached through a coordinated lobby process. It first saw success in 1998, through having *friends in high places* (notably the then Health Minister who in a subsequent government became Prime Minister), through creation of a *coherent public health policy* in which harm minimization played a central role and which was compatible with significant moves to dissuade tobacco use, and through the *need to change* becoming increasingly evident through health statistics. It has succeeded in delivering lobbying through a *partnership approach*, straddling the divide between the health voluntary sector and the range of ministry and locally based public health services and (at least from the outside) being *unified*. (Political parties which present an externally united face and manage to handle internal debate and criticism in a way which does not cause ongoing disaffection seem to be winners publicly. This is equally true of lobbies.) The other key factor is *sustainability*. The lobby has delivered a stream of successes through the past 15 years and so is associated with *getting things done*.

These two examples, contrasting starkly the personal and the political but commonly illustrating some of the essential elements of lobby success, both achieved apparently sustainable change. But why do we need to do it in the first place? Why do we not have systems which deliver fair outcomes without the need for vast resources to be devoted to the process of persuasion?

POLITICAL SYSTEMS

In short, lobbying exists because we are only human. It is we who create our government systems. We, as human beings, naturally and passionately disagree on many things. And because the system itself (be it a retirement village management committee or public health law and policy) is not neutral. Bureaucracies have a dynamic all of their own. By necessity they are governed by rules and all too easily become obsessive about secrecy in order to protect them from outside influence. That secrecy stunts openness to change and to new ideas. When the body governing the development of policy is not debate focused, the emerging policy will fail to be as good as it could be. Reluctant consultation, with only part of the story being told and only part of the response being heard, can generate even more harm since it can give false validation to apparent truths. When the political element is added to this equation, public officials are given a common target or even an enemy, namely the minister.

Politicians have a natural desire to make laws. Government policy advisers are wary about that, because at both the stage of authorship and then in the passage through Parliament, politicians can do astonishing things to proposed legislation, damaging or even rendering unrecognizable the best conceived words and concepts of officials. Those officials much prefer policies, over which they can exert much firmer control and which – if they go wrong or are not what the official wanted in the first place – can be reversed more easily than laws, given a change of government. Many of the general public are vague about the difference between laws, regulations, and policies, but just expect the government to 'do something' about a problem.

Things are changing. Policy developers are challenged as never before. For example, in Western Europe, North America, Australasia, and South Africa, we live in societies which are increasingly multiracial, where minorities and the female majority are determined and entitled to achieve fair treatment, and where the additional layer of cultural appropriateness is quite properly being applied to laws and policies. The traditional public sector cannot cope with this, because of its composition and strong internal culture. It can maintain a successful resistance for years but not for ever, since those population-driven pressures are insistent and growing. So, unless the 'system' is designed in extraordinarily sensitive ways, public input to counteract or complement the views of public officials becomes not a luxury but an absolute necessity, if the system is to preserve its integrity. Western democracy, given its limited range of governance models, requires lobbying and advocacy for maturity and public credibility. It is not an exaggeration, in our increasingly diverse and complex societies, to suggest that the survival of a functioning democracy relies on good, accountable lobbying sensitive to its contemporary culture.

So lobbying has an ever more essential function. Without it, the ability of politicians to promote and deliver new ideas, and the ability of government and other officials to come up with options for action and consult on those options, is extraordinarily limited. Take me as an example. In my split life of 3 or 4 days in Parliament in New Zealand's capital city of Wellington and 3 or 4 days in my South Island electorate/constituency of Christchurch Central, I touch on many things but delve deeply into few. Even grassroots contact with people who understand specific issues and solutions in my own city can be measured in minutes rather than hours each week, in spite of the fact that I represent fewer people than most Western politicians and manage to spend more time than most in my own area. I rely heavily and extensively on voluntary organizations and highly motivated individuals to analyze their own experiences and reflect them back to me in meaningful and quality ways. To present the problem and at least start to shape the solution. And I regularly expect too much, sending groups back to improve their explanations and justifications of what they are seeking before approaching me again.

SUCCESSFUL LOBBYING

Lobbies often, in my experience, fall at the first hurdle. They know the outcome they desire, but fail to identify the vehicle required. They understand their own issue very well, but too often that understanding is on their own terms, from their own viewpoint. That view is insufficiently dispassionate to generate realistic strategic thinking on how to achieve their goal. They have a misty and often severely warped idea of how successful lobbies have achieved their success or of the intimate and creative nature of great relationships between lobbies and politicians, which have molded our contemporary democratic system. Without that, they stand little chance of understanding how to use the system to demolish the barriers and rebuild in a more sensible way. They are so driven by the injustice they see in the current arrangements that they fail to understand alternative points of view, the balance of powerful forces which have molded public policy, the sensible considerations which have quashed their ideas until now, or even the possibility that thoroughly sensible people may be able to mount a powerful and sustained argument against them for genuine reasons.

The choice of vehicle for achieving the change required is at the very core of every successful campaign. It is the key strategic decision. My friend knew that the retirement village committee could have vetoed his desires at any stage, ultimately through expelling him for breaking the contract between them and him. But he also knew that they were sensitive enough to public (i.e. village resident) and potentially media opinion not to take such a ridiculous stand. The Smoke Free Coalition knew that they would need a combination of laws to restrict cumulatively the environments in which smoking was allowed, economic interventions to increase the price of tobacco, and public education, including minimization of exposure to the messages from the tobacco industry.

Before going any further, it is necessary to establish a few definitions. I tend to use the term *'lobby'* as a generic one to apply to the wide range of persuasion-focused pressure exerted to achieve one's established aim. Others, particularly in my experience those from the health sector, prefer the word *'advocate'*. I am relaxed about that alternative – I don't really think there is a material difference. However, there is a difference between either of those terms and *'campaign'*. I regard campaigning as the generic term, including not only lobbying and advocacy but also more direct action. A demonstration outside the office of a Member of Parliament is a valid part of a campaign, but could not be described as lobbying. (Indeed, it is a dramatic statement of a lobby having failed or of the people involved understanding confrontation better than engagement.)

Within the range of lobby options, described by me above as 'persuasion-focused pressure', I would include personal letter and email writing, personal visits, phone calls, and the sending (and possible subsequent presentation) of submissions. They are all constructive in that arguments are presented and the opportunity for response and engagement is allowed for.

Having established some of the terminology and elements of a successful lobby and enquired into why lobbying is not just an option but is an essential part of democratic life-blood, we now need to consider how best to strategize to achieve the aim, to guide how the part of the lobby which seeks a specific outcome is to be shaped.

LOBBYING STRATEGIES

The choice of appropriate delivery mechanism for any particular lobby aim is heavily influenced by five key factors.

The first factor is the *nature of the aim*. If what is sought is a comparatively modest policy change in the direction of the government's value base or a specific action to deter high risk, a friendly chat with a minister or even a relevant adviser could conceivably be enough. If it requires some sense of permanence and is of sufficient scale, law change may be required. This could (depending on the jurisdiction) be primary or secondary legislation, the former needing a law change through the Parliament, the latter being delivered through resolution of a group of ministers or the Cabinet (in Westminster and most other European systems). There are of course degrees of law change, ranging from the non-controversial to high profile and intensely controversial.

The second factor is *timing*. Organizations have significant control over the timing of their lobbies, but events can rapidly take over. For example, a campaign for tougher laws controlling the behavior of pet dogs can work and talk for years without noticeable success. Their point of take-off could well be a particularly nasty attack by a dog (preferably owned by people who generate minimal public sympathy) on a young (and attractive) child whose parents are prepared to see them exposed to media attention. A lobby for significant law change cannot always rely on fortuitous tragedy. The key work is done with the people developing policy manifestos for the next election. Ideally, especially if the cause is not particularly politically ideological, a number of parties can be persuaded to back the cause.

Time scales are immensely variable. In general, legislation is taking longer to pass through Parliaments as electoral systems give greater emphasis to representation, as the Parliaments become more diverse, as the public consultation process attracts more and more expert interest. For example, New Zealand's Parliament agreed a new Prostitution Reform Bill in 2003. The possibility of such legislation had first been mooted in 1987. Ministers of Health were advocating it from 1990 onwards. The Bill was drafted in 1997 and introduced to Parliament (as a Private Members' Bill) in 2000. The Select Committee process took nearly 2 years. Once back in Parliament, it took 9 months to pass. Throughout the process, given the nature of such an issue, the lobby had to regroup and reinvent itself to face the new reality, including that resulting from an average 33% turnover in Members of Parliament after each general election (held every 3 years). This is the necessary price of diversity and the development of deeper forms of democracy.

The third factor is the *scale of the challenge*. Tough aims take longer to achieve (unless luck is on the side of the lobbyist) and may involve a more circuitous route. Complex challenges will involve many lobby tools at different stages. Assuming that legislation is an eventual aim of the campaign, the initial challenge is to get the item on the agenda of both politicians and key potential partner lobby groups. This is likely to involve media work, research, maybe even very public and persuasive expressions of the lack of sustainability, or other unfairness of the current situation. As the item creeps on to the agenda of parties well-placed on the political spectrum to be of some influence, so the process becomes more legally exacting and is subject to more rigorous (and thus high-risk) monitoring by the media and public. Some issues, notably environmental ones, can generate sufficient public excitement to stimulate the sending of postcards and emails or even mass lobbying of politicians, either in their offices or through select committee submissions in those countries which have significant public involvement in select committees. Other issues (e.g. euthanasia, prostitution) are harder to explain to the public and are best communicated by those directly affected (e.g. a sex worker, the relative of someone who has died a very painful death).

The fourth factor is the *nature of the person or agency driving the lobby*. One person, who may be a figurehead or may be the effective driver, embodies some lobbies. This depends on the complexity of the issue under discussion, the size and culture of the country or jurisdiction where the lobby is being attempted, and the length of time which the campaign is likely to take. It is clearly good for a campaign to be linked to an identifiable person, since media usually respond well to that and personalization of a difficult cause can help to give it coherency, while validating others supporting it. The risk is that the person may turn out to be autocratic in their management of the campaign or they may turn out to be profoundly flawed (and that, rather than their cause, becomes the story).

The fifth factor is the reputation, notably the *level of unity*, of the lobby. Perhaps the most effective deterrent to politicians, media, and the general public in relation to a lobby is the perception that it is internally divided, in terms of either method or desired outcome. That acts as a strident and insistent warning signal that effort could be wasted, that both warring sides in the lobby will focus on the lobby target, and that independent research (expensive and difficult to organize) may be required. Disunity also acts as an emotional lightning rod for the people who feel ownership over the lobby and much energy is wasted on usually sterile disputes. Many perfectly worthy and necessary causes have been delayed and polluted by disputation.

POLITICAL AND LEGAL ENVIRONMENTS

The final topic I will address is the broader context of much lobbying, the political decision-making environment and the associated legal environment. It is the shape of and the degree of dynamism within that environment which determine political receptiveness to lobbying and serves to channel lobbies towards achievable solutions. The previous section identified the five key factors which a lobby can influence in its approach. Clearly much remains beyond its direct control and yet careful observation of it can help mold a winning strategy.

In 'Western' democracies, a variety of democratic forms can be observed. Not wishing to launch into a lecture on constitutional forms, suffice it to say that there are four broad but different models which a lobby might be faced with. They are:

1 parliamentary
2 presidential (European-type)
3 presidential (United States-type)
4 supra national (e.g. European Union).

Any of these institutions may also have subsidiary bodies (e.g. local councils, state governments) serving particular regions or population groups.

Legal systems also vary and the constitution of each country (written in all countries except Britain, Israel, and New Zealand) determines the relationship between presidency or monarchy, Parliament, and the courts. Generalizations are difficult, since these systemic devices are overlain with the particular culture or cultures of all or part of the nation state. I venture to suggest that beyond superficially dramatic differences (for example, the ability of the courts in some countries to overturn laws; delegation or centralization of power), debates about and exploration of solutions in these various jurisdictions follow comparable and predictable courses and are capable of being broadly described.

The late 20th century saw the rise of the lobby, as a response to the limitations of traditional political and governmental decision-making processes. The longer that coherent and increasingly well-funded lobbies have existed, the more sophisticated their methods have become. Cautious approaches to the outer edges of the political system have been replaced by bold moves focused on the centre. Rebuttal was initially met with resignation. Now it is much more likely to be met with a more determined second approach. A sterile response from the politicians once meant that lobbyists had to wait for the next generation of politicians – a little more liberal, maybe more feminized – to emerge. Now a court challenge is equally likely. One may see all this as an expression of ever increasing arrogance by the lobby, something which is ultimately an unelected and publicly comparatively unaccountable repository of beliefs and passions. I prefer to regard it as an enriching of democracy and also believe that it has further to go. A reliance on the lobby has crept in. It will not go away.

In New Zealand, for example, the absence of a second Parliamentary chamber for the past 50 years was for some decades a contributor to governmental arrogance in the first-past-the-post electoral system. Eventually public frustration boiled over, one party leader promised a Royal Commission on the Electoral System, another leader promised to put the result to a referendum, and first-past-the-post was replaced by a mixed member proportional system, in which voters had both a party and candidate vote. The outcome has been permanent coalition government and a vastly enriched select committee system, which has become a de facto second chamber in which lobby organizations and ordinary members of the public have considerable input and influence. It is inconceivable to imagine that such a reform could be reversed and this may well be a sign of things to come as other nations struggle to sustain and improve the integrity of their democracies.

Other influences are also appearing worldwide. The traditionally clarified powers of the nation state are being slowly enhanced ('replaced' would probably be a more honest word) by supranational bodies. The African and the European Unions, the World Trade Organization, and the United Nations, in all its many forms, are all examples of this. With such developments comes the demand for ever more sophisticated lobbies and often a growing exasperation with the truncated democratic accountabilities of such bodies. They are truly bureaucracy driven and lobby frustrations can boil over in the absence of accessible politicians prepared to answer for the system.

Legal systems are not immune to all this. Access to legal remedies has been made easier, through both state interventions (such as legal aid systems) and specialist state support (e.g. for environmental test cases). As lobbies have attracted public donations, so they have been better able to access the legal system to challenge perceived injustice. As they have scored wins, so the donations have flowed more easily. All this comprises a distinct and, I believe, sustainable shift in power from traditional political centers of power towards civil society.

CONCLUSION

The purpose of this chapter was to trace the developing political and legal environment within which change movements are operating. My conclusion is that we live in a dynamic world where lobbies and broader civil society, within which most such lobbies reside, are now developing a real coherence and an essential purpose. In time, their ability to express viewpoints will become as essential to good governance as a good legal system, a representative Parliament, and a constitution. The clue in all that, for those now seeking to lobby, is to recognize that the system needs the lobby as much as the lobby needs the system, that the system is increasingly inviting to lobbies, and that work for change is an extraordinarily valid activity. The world awaits...

Modern cultural environments

Jacqueline Kerr and Constanze Rossmann

INTRODUCTION

Why is it so hard to promote health? Several countries set health targets for the year 2000, but few of these have been achieved at a national level. Instead of declining, obesity is on the increase, attempts to augment population activity levels have repeatedly failed, and smoking rates in some countries and in some groups are on the rise. Previous chapters have outlined the multiple social, psychological, and physical determinants of health behavior which partly explain why health promotion is so difficult. This chapter will show that a consumer-led society may not be entirely conducive to healthy living. Further, as national trade boundaries are breached by the Internet and globalization, traditional cultural influences on health, such as religion, race, ethnicity, and family structure, may diminish. This chapter will therefore focus on the implications of current popular Western culture, driven by consumerism and the media, on health promotion activities.

i see C1, B1

Primarily, health promoters have to compete with companies selling unhealthy products: cigarettes, junk food, and alcohol, for example. Companies spend billions of dollars to ensure we buy their products, which we do, even though we know that they may be bad for our health. Sometimes the health effects of such products are not made public and this will be considered. Health promoters must be aware, however, that advertising is only one promotional tool and advertising bans may be ineffective. Also, unhealthy behaviors are endorsed not only by society accepting and adopting them but by the media which both reflect and drive behavioral norms.

In addition to being avid consumers of the latest product, we want to be kept up to date and entertained. Thus, amongst other things, the media have the role of entertaining and informing; dramatically reporting on the newest, biggest, or fastest developments and dispelling reality with fantasy and fiction (Nelkin 1996). This conflicts with health promotion in several ways. First, disease may be a gradual process that poses no immediate risk. Second, the benefits of healthy behavior are often delayed or not even visible. Further, health promotion, often taking the form of health education, tends to focus on informing rather than entertaining. A tendency to focus on the negative also threatens health promotion and the reporting of health issues. Further, since governments are partly responsible for the health of the nation and in different ways for health services, health is also a political animal. It is therefore subject to the vagaries of those in temporary power and to the scrutiny of the press. In the same way that the general public is influenced by the media and behavioral norms, so too are policy makers. The role of the media in public perceptions will therefore be discussed in this chapter.

As a consequence of the powerful commercial influences on society, health promoters have to realize that they are in the business of promoting good health and, like any business, need to make easily available an effectively promoted product that appeals to consumers, at the right price. Further, like any commercial enterprise, health promoters need to identify threats to their business, turn these into opportunities, and compete in a cut-throat market. Later chapters will indicate various strategies to achieve this end, such as persuasion, education, social marketing, and interpersonal and mediated communication.

SALES OF UNHEALTHY PRODUCTS

A recent report commissioned by the World Health Organization and the Food and Agricultural Organization criticized the food and drinks industry for heavy marketing of energy-dense, micronutrient-poor products (WHO 2002a). Such products are sold using traditional marketing techniques of product, packaging, price, promotion, and place, i.e. product availability. Health 'promotion' seems to focus mainly on only one of these elements. This chapter will demonstrate how each element can contribute to the popularity of unhealthy goods.

Promotion

Most people automatically think of advertising when considering promotion. Advertising is a key marketing tool. In 1989 the Surgeon General identified seven reasons why tobacco advertising increased cigarette consumption (CDC 1989).

1 By encouraging children or young adults to experiment with tobacco and thereby slip into regular use.
2 By encouraging smokers to increase consumption.
3 By reducing smokers' motivation to quit.
4 By encouraging former smokers to resume.
5 By discouraging full and open discussion of the hazards of smoking as a result of media dependence on advertising revenues.

6 By muting opposition to controls on tobacco as a result of the dependence of organizations receiving sponsorship from tobacco companies.

7 By creating through the ubiquity of advertising, sponsorship, etc. an environment in which tobacco use is seen as familiar and acceptable and the warnings about its health risks are undermined.

As a result, tobacco advertising has been banned in many countries. The Australian government has also recently threatened restrictions on junk food advertising, following a report that 99% of television food commercials during children's viewing periods were for sweets and drinks of little nutritional value (Zinn 2003). Such advertising may not directly cause obesity, but it may affect children's perceptions of food choice (Nestle & Jacobson 2000). A recent report concludes that advertising to children does have an effect on their preferences, purchase behavior, and consumption (Hastings et al 2003). There may be no proof of this, but there seems sufficient evidence to indicate an effect. Advertising of alcoholic drinks may also affect children's behavior. In the UK there are only voluntary restrictions on the advertisement of alcoholic drinks. In Austria, Finland, Sweden, and Denmark, for example, television and radio advertising of some alcoholic drinks is prohibited. Drinks manufacturers claim that they are not targeting under-18 year olds in particular. Research has shown, however, that drinks adverts do appeal to teenagers (IAS 2003).

Advertising spend is also important. The 10 biggest spenders on food advertising have increased their advertising budgets by £100 million in the last 10 years (Uhlig 2003). In contrast, the annual spend for the National Cancer Institute '5-fruit n veg' a day campaign is about $1 million (Nestle & Jacobson 2000). The UK government has also recently launched a £2.1 million campaign against low-tar cigarettes. It is estimated, however, that tobacco companies spend about £113.5 million on advertising in Britain each year. Clearly, these differences are enormous and have implications for the success of public health campaigns. It is therefore important for health promoters to be aware of advertising terms, such as 'share of voice': how many people you have reached for the money you have spent and how this compares with other advertisers in your sector.

STEALTH MARKETING

Advertising, however, is only one communication medium. Bans on cigarette advertising have led to a new form of marketing called 'stealth marketing' which transcends traditional media. Due to litigation against the tobacco industry and government enquiries, data have become available which reveal the range of the tobacco industry's promotion strategies. Tobacco company relationships with the film industry were made public in this way (Mekemson & Glantz 2002). Hastings & MacFayden (2000) also analyzed internal documents in a report entitled *Keep smiling: no one's going to die.* Another source of 'negative' tobacco industry information is Action on Smoking and Health (ASH 1998; www.ash.org.uk), including a brainstorming by an advertising agency to identify loopholes in the tobacco legislation (Vickers 1997) and a briefing on 'brand stretching' (ASH 1998). The WHO (2002b) also produced a booklet entitled *Tobacco Sponsorship of World Sport.* These are the main sources for the following examples.

Although cigarette advertising is banned in many countries, manufacturers continue to receive media coverage through sponsoring sports and cultural events, by announcing successful sponsorship contracts, and by advertising other products which carry the cigarette name. Table C5.1 shows some of the main promotional activities which increase cigarette consumption and build brand imagery. Sports sponsorship particularly helps to build brand image and receives mammoth media coverage. Because of this, Formula 1 motor racing sponsorship is being restricted. Point-of-sale promotion may also become more important. In future, there may be special cigarette departments in stores or tobacco outlets decorated in brand colors. The colors, like football team colors, are very binding – gold for Benson & Hedges, purple for Silk Cut, red for Marlboro, for example. Retailers and shop assistants may also receive bonuses for increased sales. Dedicated tobacco-related shops may also appear. Marlboro Classics clothing, for example, is the second largest mail order brand in the USA, with over 1000 stores in Europe and Asia. Smoking is also strongly related to coffee drinking and newspaper reading. Newspaper stands could be branded and coffee is already sold under cigarette branding. A new 'Expresso' cigarette has been suggested which ties in with the new café culture. It would provide an unobtrusive quick fix in a world where places to smoke in public are becoming scarce. Alternative 'ambient' media, such as golf holes, petrol pump handles, umbrellas, beer mats, urinals, egg shells, etc., may in future carry cigarette branding. New media such as the Internet may also be open to exploitation through dedicated websites or sponsored sites. Some already exist.

Perhaps more concerning is not what may take place but what may already be common practice, such as political contributions and product placement in films, television programs, music videos, and computer games. There is some evidence that tobacco companies hired special companies to find opportunities for product placement (Mekemson & Glantz 2002). These activities may have included paying for products to be used in a film and working the product into the film script. Particularly successful placements were Lucky Strike in *Beverly Hills Cop,* Camel in *Who Framed Roger Rabbit,* and Marlboros in *Me, Myself, and Irene.* Billboards, merchandise, trucks, lighters, caps, T-shirts, and logos may also be provided as props and background scenery. To encourage personal and public use and placement in films,

Table C5.1 Additional promotional activities by the tobacco industry (ASH 1998, WHO 2002b)

Sports sponsorship (excluding Formula 1)	Cultural sponsorship	Brand stretching
Rugby League Challenge Cup, UK	Renaissance Silk Cut Grand Tour (nightclub-style parties)	
Whitbread Round the World Yacht Race	Cambridge Footlights, UK	
Sportsman Kakungulu Soccer Cup, Uganda	Sportsman of the Year award, Uganda	
John Player Gold Leaf sailing boat, India	Cambridge University Chair in International Relations, UK	
Badminton, boxing, basketball, Indonesia	Nottingham University International Centre for Corporate Social Responsibility, UK	
Motorbike racing, Indonesia	Gold photography competition, UK	
International Golf Open, UK	Hogzone Nightclub tour (electronic kiosks and lightshows)	
Master Snooker Tournament, UK	Gay Pride day, UK	
Cricket Cup, UK	Lighten Up comedy tour, UK	
NASCAR motor racing, USA	Ulster Orchestra, Ireland	
World Championship Snooker, UK	National Union of Students show guide, UK	
Welsh Open Snooker	Rolling roadshow at music festivals and nightclubs, UK	
Soccer M-League & national team, Malaysia		

the tobacco industry may give free cigarettes and merchandise to celebrities, actors, script writers, producers, and studio events. Further, special photographers may have been hired to snap celebrities smoking.

These examples illustrate the wide influence of the tobacco industry in society and serve as a warning to health promoters that their anti-smoking campaigns have to compete with multi-billion dollar spending on multiple fronts.

The product

The product itself is also important; low-tar cigarettes, for example, were introduced to appeal to women and those trying to quit smoking. Other health behaviors also depend on the particular product. The increase in teenage drinking is currently being attributed to a new range of products called alcopops. Despite being higher in alcohol content than most beers, they appeal to younger drinkers because of their sugary fruit flavours. The strong taste of alcohol would previously have been a barrier to some children, whereas alcopops are easy to drink (Alcohol Concern 2003a,b). Even before the introduction of alcopops, however, there was a significant increase in teenage drinking. At first, little was spent on marketing the drinks and their popularity was unprecedented. As the chairman of Zenith International market research commented on one alcoholic lemonade: 'Its early success defied all the basic marketing rules. It was achieved without research, advertising or even adequate supplies'. This suggests that the product itself appealed to drinkers and word of mouth played an important role.

Particular products can also help to promote healthy behaviors. The introduction of car safety belts, for example, has reduced traffic accident injuries. New forms of exercise, such as aerobics, yoga, snowboarding, scooters, and in-line skating, have all become popular activities in recent times. The question remains whether these new fads increase population physical activity levels or simply replace other forms of activity. Physical activity promoters must be aware of such new trends and include them in surveys of activity levels. Further, new forms of exercise may also carry new health risks, such as injury. Importantly, the health effects of some new consumer products are not always established before mass use. The health consequences of mobile phone use, for example, are still being investigated.

The diffusion of innovations theory (elaborated on later) suggests that some groups have a pro-innovation bias, irrespective of whether the innovation has positive or negative consequences, and that we tend to be more influenced by fads and fashion and the desire for conformity than rational arguments (Nutley et al 2002). Health promoters should also therefore consider branding their health behavior as a product and marketing it in a relevant way.

Price, place, and availability

It is now socially acceptable to eat anywhere, at any time. The price and availability of products are therefore important. Fruit and vegetables, for example, are more expensive than chocolate. Unhealthy foods are most easily available through the 170 000 fast-food restaurants and 3 million soft drink vending machines in the USA (Nestle & Jacobson 2000). Americans also spend half their food budget on meals outside the home where nutritional content may be less regulated. Further, there is a tendency for larger amounts of food to be better value for money. This is problematic because not only have portion sizes increased over the last few decades, but controlled trials indicate that people unconsciously consume increasingly larger portions and do not reduce their consumption elsewhere, resulting in higher total calorie intake (American Institute for Cancer Research 2003). Experts from the International Obesity Taskforce and the World Cancer Research Fund have recently called for a consumer revolt against oversized portions of food.

Importantly, some health-protecting behaviors involve buying additional products. In contrast to giving up smoking, taking up exercise, or choosing to eat alternative foods, sun skin protection involves buying an additional product: sunscreen. Health promoters must rely on the sunscreen industry for the products they make, the packaging and labeling, the promotion, availability, and price. The advantage to safe sun campaigners is that they are both aiming to increase sun cream use and some health campaigns are even supported by particular brands. However, a recent survey by a supermarket, announced as part of a press release promoting cheaper creams, indicated that sunscreen prices are very high and that consumers are not using adequate amounts due to the cost. Moreover, sunscreen is only one element of safe skin care. Avoiding the sun and covering up are more important. The sun cream industry, however, actively promotes sun bathing and makes tans seem attractive. In this way, they are also working against health promoters.

Responsibility

The question remains, therefore, who is responsible for the health effects of consumer products: the individual or the manufacturer? Legal cases against the tobacco industry, for example, have been successful when they could demonstrate that the smoker was unaware of the health effects. There is some suggestion that the health risks of smoking were not widely published because newspapers and magazines were reliant on the advertising income from cigarette manufacturers (Brown & Walsh-Childers 1994). Similar legal action against fast-food outlets has been unsuccessful because nutritional values are provided and consumers are generally aware of the potential health effects. Product labeling is clearly important but the legal requirements vary in different countries. The Plain English Campaign recently criticized food labeling, particularly for salt and sugar, suggesting that sugar content should be given in teaspoons (not sucrose, glucose, dextrose, and syrup) and salt (not sodium) as a percentage of the 6 g daily allowance (Maher 2003). The European Commission is also due to rule on the use of such terms as 'high fibre', 'low fat', and 'sugar free'. If consumers have to contend with misleading and poorly labeled products, it is much harder to ensure they are buying healthy items.

Some companies, however, are becoming more health conscious and consumer friendly. A large food manufacturer recently announced that it would overhaul its range of products to make them less unhealthy, reduce the size of single portions, provide more nutritional information, and stop all in-school marketing. Health promoters should encourage companies to review their products and marketing, to protect consumer health, and avoid legal action.

Diffusion of innovations

Clearly, product development is essential to hold consumers' interests and compete for sales. In addition to the marketing mix, the diffusions of innovations theory may explain 'the process by which an innovation is communicated through certain channels over time among the members of a social system' (Rogers 1995, p. 5). Central to the theory is what makes a product, organization, person, or process innovative (its structure or attributes), how initial knowledge (explicit and tacit) of innovations is communicated, and through which channels (interpersonal and mediated). The role of opinion leaders, change agents, and diffusion networks, the process of implementing innovations, the rate of adoption and utilization, the characteristics of adopters, and the consequences of adoption are also important.

Five key attributes of an innovation are relative advantage, compatibility, complexity, trialability, and observability. The process of adoption is said to pass through the following stages: knowledge, persuasion, decision, implementation, and confirmation. The theory also identifies two channels of communication: interpersonal (or local) and mass media (or cosmopolitan). Mass media channels are relatively more important at the knowledge stage, particularly for early rather than late adopters, whereas interpersonal channels may be more important at the persuasion stage (Nutley et al 2002). Although this indicates that the mass media are not the only communication medium, the media may also influence the content of interpersonal communication; we often talk about what we have seen on television, for example. The media are also a particularly vital source of information for health matters because few people have direct experience of illness until it is too late.

THE ROLE OF THE MEDIA IN HEALTH

Media interests

The media must be understood as a business which has to sell its products and stand out from its competitors. It may therefore be motivated by market demands more than public duty. In contrast, the British Broadcasting Corporation, for example, is a public service broadcaster and perhaps should be more responsible for informing and educating the public in health matters (Harrabin et al 2003). Most other countries in the European Union also have public service channels (other than Luxemburg), for example ARD in Germany and Canal 1 in Portugal. This chapter will focus on two of the media's roles: entertaining and informing. Straight entertainment, i.e. television entertainment programs, involves fiction which naturally results in a distorted view of reality. This is important if it affects our perception of what is normal and acceptable. News coverage involves both information and entertainment and is driven by newsworthiness. Table C5.2 shows the factors defined by news factor theorists as important (Schulz 1976). We must remember that the media is not solely responsible for what it publishes. It publishes news that will sell. It is the general public, however, who are responsible for what is bought.

One of the main news factors leading to higher publication rates is negativity, which also plays a role in the context of health information. A recent selective study of health news coverage indicated that health scares (e.g. SARS and BSE) and NHS crises occupy the British press more than public health issues (Harrabin et al 2003). This has implications particularly for the concept of health promotion. First, scares and crises are immediate and out of the ordinary, attracting greater interest. In contrast, public health is a long-term proposition. Scares and crises are also negative representations of health. Ill health is easier to feel, see, describe, and relate to than good health. It can also lead to specific actions; thus curing disease is newsworthy but preventing it is not. Further, health problems are a stick with which to beat the government of the day. If the media focuses on patient waiting times, for example, an immediate problem, the government is pressurized to respond. Or for example, press coverage of train crashes in the UK may have led to increased investment in the rail system, even though more deaths on the road could be avoided for less cost. In this way, the media sometimes helps to set the health agenda and long-term health issues of greater magnitude are sidelined. Further, news coverage of health issues, such as the mumps, measles, and rubella (MMR) combined vaccine and BSE crisis, because they involve the government, may be more widespread.

There are similar conflicts between newsworthiness and scientific accuracy. A journalist's priority is newness and originality. Scientific health findings, however, are concerned with replication and continuity.

Table C5.2 Factors contributing to newsworthiness

Dimension	Factor	Example
Time	Duration	Short occurrence of flu vs enduring wave of flu
	Continuity	Information about an unidentified disease vs continuous coverage of cancer
Proximity	Regional	A wave of flu in London is more likely to be published by a British editorial office than a wave of flu in Germany
	Political	A new law about the prohibition of smoking in public areas in Germany is more likely to be published by a British editorial office than a new law in Third World countries
	Cultural	New findings of an American research team are more likely to be published by British media than findings of a research team from Turkey
	Relevance	A lethal virus affecting many people is more likely to be published than a harmless virus affecting only a few
Status	Regional centrality	Political decisions in London vs decisions in small towns
	National centrality	New research findings of an American research team vs those of an Austrian research team
	Personal influence	Political decisions of the president vs those of a rural mayor
	Prominence	Report on rhinoplasty with Michael Jackson as an example
Dynamics	Unexpectedness	Report on a new virus (e.g. SARS) vs coverage of cancer, coverage of the separation of Siamese twins
	Structure	Covering simple relationships between people's lifestyle and a heart attack rather than complex medical research findings
Valence	Conflict	Report on a demonstration against abortion
	Criminality	Reports on the rising distribution of illegal drugs
	Damage	Report on medical malpractice causing a patient's death, report on lethal diseases
	Success	Ground-breaking research on a new medication to treat HIV patients
Identification	Personalization	A story about a certain woman coping with breast cancer vs enumeration of possible causes of breast cancer in women's lives
	Ethnocentricity	Coverage of medical treatment of people in industrial countries vs medical treatment of Aborigines

Hence scientific findings are seldom reported (Bartlett et al 2002) and when they are, an isolated negative result may be given coverage, as happened with the MMR vaccination and autism (Bellaby 2003). Scientists must emphasize the uncertainty of their results, whereas journalists want their stories to reflect the newest, biggest, and fastest advancement (Nelkin 1996). Their reports have to be short, simple, and readable which may, of course, result in oversimplification. The diffusions of innovations theory, for example, suggests that innovators (such as academics) are usually dissimilar to the broad mass of potential innovation adopters and therefore have communication and credibility problems (Nutley et al 2002). An intermediary, such as a health communicator, can bridge the gap between technical experts and their public. Further, words such as 'epidemic', 'evidence', 'predisposition', and 'risk' have different meanings in science and popular understanding (Nelkin 1996). Importantly, absolute and relative risks must be presented in the media. For example, one 'pill scare' in the UK arose because some pills were said to double the risk of blood clots. The absolute risk, however, was minimal (Brody 1999). Further, the risk of getting a blot clot, through pregnancy from not taking the pill, was much higher (Bellaby 2003).

With this focus on the unusual and the extreme, the number of stories on particular health problems seldom reflects the population risk of a disease (Harrabin et al 2003). The risk of autism caused by MMR is insignificant; the risk of variant CJD from BSE is real but probably small; the risk of a child being injured in a road crash is real and large; the British media, however, focus on the former (Bellaby 2003). Breast cancer is also an interesting example. Breast cancer is frequently covered in the media as it involves emotion, conflict, drama, and politics, and because survival rates are now relatively high, there are many breast cancer advocates seeking media coverage. Other diseases which strike later in life and with worse prognoses have fewer campaigners. This media coverage, however, may result in a disproportionate fear of breast cancer. For example, a recent British Heart Foundation report found that women were more worried about breast cancer than heart disease although they were four times more likely to suffer the latter (British Heart Foundation 2003). Further, young breast cancer patients are frequently shown in the media, whereas older patients are at greater risk (Gill 2003).

Media may affect perception and behavior

Media presentations may not only affect our perception of reality and what is acceptable and normal but also our behavior. Advertising forms a large part of media representations and has been shown to influence behavior. Despite much criticism, cultivation theory, focusing on television violence, indicates that television entertainment presents a distorted world-view with small but constant effects on the public's perception (Gerbner & Gross 1976).

Research in the health field has shown that portrayals of doctors and nurses do not reflect reality and that this distorted picture of medical staff influenced patients' perceptions. Heavy viewers reported more positive impressions of hospital staff (Rossmann 2002). The presentation of body ideals and their relationship with eating disorders has also been studied (Berel & Irving 1998). Content analyses have confirmed the emergence of a slim body ideal in the media (Silverstein et al 1986) and studies have shown that this ideal impacts public perceptions and aspirations (Botta 1999). This contrasts starkly with present reality – an obesity epidemic. Cosmetic surgery depictions in the media may also be unrepresentative and encourage greater use (Minkewitz 2003). The media coverage of MMR immunization questioned the UK government recommendation. Fewer children are now being immunized (Harrabin et al 2003). There is likely to be some relationship here, if not causal. The media may have misrepresented the risk, but they did not force parents to boycott the program. Trust in the government was already low and parents' concerns may have rubbed off on health professionals (Bellaby 2003). Even in countries not affected by BSE, beef consumption dropped, such is the power of the media and the irrationality of risk perception (Bellaby 2003, Weitkunat et al 2003).

Endorsement of behaviors by role models is a key part of health behavior change models. Celebrities, for example, are influential role models and their activities are frequently covered by the media. George Bush's colorectal cancer screening appointment was widely publicized and may encourage others to attend screening. Even Tony Blair's recent heart scare resulted in advice in the newspapers on how to prevent heart disease. Unfortunately, the focus is more often on celebrities' drinking, smoking, drug use, or extreme dieting. The presence of smoking in films and television has already been highlighted. In Germany, for example, a study found that the average television viewer may see nine scenes per hour involving alcohol (Lampert & Hasebrink 2002).

As well as presenting unhealthy behaviors, the media present a certain view of health care. Recently, medical dramas have become very popular viewing. Such entertainment programs, however, present an unrealistic view of illnesses, their causes, and the health system, leading to a belief in the 'magic of medicine' which may have consequences for health behavior and patient relationships with medical staff (Gerbner et al 1981). In the same way that the public are affected by media images, policy makers may also believe that what is in the press reflects public opinion and behavioral norms. Public health, which is seldom addressed, is therefore unlikely to be high on policy makers' agendas (Harrabin et al 2003).

Although the entertainment media tend to portray unhealthy behaviors, television narratives, such as soap operas, sitcoms, or dramas, can

Table C5.3 Modern cultural threats to and opportunities for health promotion, e.g. increasing population levels of physical activity (PA)

		Threat	Opportunity
Interpersonal	Peers	Laugh when you say you're going for a run.	Encourage you to go even if it's raining.
	Parents	Say it is not safe to go to the park.	Take you to the park and buy you the appropriate footwear.
	Partner	Moans when you get up early to go to the gym.	Suggests an evening walk together instead.
Organizational	School	No PA in school curriculum. No PA facilities.	Opens school facilities to community out of school hours.
	Workplace	No time allowed to use facilities, if available.	Provides showers for active commuters.
	GP	Does not prescribe physiotherapy for exercise injuries.	GP referrals to fitness programs.
	Health care	Insufficient focus on preventive medicine.	Subsidized exercise facilities.
	Government	Encourage mostly competitive sports.	More PA in national curriculum.
	Politicians	Accept pressure to build more roads.	Run/cycle in public.
Commercial industries	Car	Makes cars a prestige item and encourages road building.	Sponsors bike paths.
	Pharmaceutical	Promotes drugs for heart disease instead of PA.	Sponsors fun runs.
	Equipment	Encourages sales of superfluous PA gadgets.	Donates equipment to local schools.
	Fashion	Makes trainers expensive fashion item.	Makes 'blading' fashionable.
	Film	Glamorizes dangerous sports.	Shows the positive side of minority sports, e.g. women's football.
	Computer	Promotes energy-saving devices.	Develops running machines with virtual reality environments.
Media	Internet	Encourages armchair shopping.	Provides exercise tips. Networks exercise buddies.
	News coverage	Testicular cancer during Bike Awareness Week.	Supports exercise promotion campaigns.
	Advertising	Suggests eating healthy cereals is easier than jogging.	Promotes exercise as fun.
	Magazines	Features unachievable exercise goals.	Gives reduced-cost ad space to health campaigns.
	Soap operas	Shows sedentary pub life as the norm.	Shows girls from 'Friends' program jogging every day.

also be used to promote healthier lifestyles. This method, often called entertainment education, in many cases has proven more effective than conventional persuasive efforts (Slater 2002). The Harvard Alcohol Project, for example, convinced studio executives, writers, and producers to include story lines that promoted safe drink driving practices and resulted in an increase in the reported use of designated drivers (Montgomery 1993).

CONCLUSION

Modern culture is seldom supportive of health promotion attempts. Consumerism, media scandal, and immediate gratification currently dominate Western thinking and behavior. These are threats which health promoters must recognize. Renee Lyons coined the term 'enemy mapping' as the practice of identifying threats to health promotion campaigns (personal communication).

This chapter has discussed the many occasions when unhealthy behaviors are actively promoted by very influential groups. Table C5.3 summarizes some of these threats using the example of physical activity promotion. Later chapters will indicate strategies to address such barriers. The table also indicates how the same groups which threaten physical activity behavior could provide positive support. Perhaps some of the tactics that cigarette, drinks, car, and fast-food manufacturers use may also be harnessed by health promoters. Health promoters should not be afraid to be creative, for example. If not, they will help to perpetuate the image of health as boring and do more harm than good. To gain media coverage, novelty, drama, and strong visual content are required. Although health is a long-term proposition, short-term benefits may be sold more successfully. If being healthy were fashionable, even temporarily, some people may also be converted for the long term. People need regular reminders and a fresh angle to hold their interest. Additionally, companies and the media could be encouraged to take more responsibility for public health. Health promoters should at least be aware of new cultural trends, in order to measure their impact on health and to better understand the population with whom they are trying to communicate.

References

Action on Smoking and Health (ASH) 1998 Briefing on brand-stretching. Available online at: www.ash.org.uk

Alcohol Concern 2003a Factsheet 35. Alcopops. Alcohol Concern, London. Available online at: www.alcoholconcern.org.uk

Alcohol Concern 2003b Factsheet 36. Alcopops: the story so far. Alcohol
    Concern, London. Available online at: www.alcoholconcern.org.uk
American Institute for Cancer Research 2003 Awareness and action: surveys
    on portion size, nutrition and cancer risk. American Institute for Cancer
    Research, Washington
Bartlett C, Sterne J, Egger M 2002 What is newsworthy? Longitudinal study of
    the reporting of medical research in two British newspapers. British
    Medical Journal 325:81-84
Bellaby P 2003 Communication and miscommunication of risk: understanding
    UK parents' attitudes to combined MMR vaccination. British Medical
    Journal 327:725-728
Berel S, Irving L M 1998 Media and disturbed eating: an analysis of media
    influence and implications for prevention. Journal of Primary Prevention
    18:415-430
Botta R A 1999 Television images and adolescent girls' body image
    disturbance. Journal of Communication 49:22-41
British Heart Foundation 2003 Take note of your heart: a review of women
    and heart disease. British Heart Foundation, London. Available online at:
    www.bhf.org.uk
Brody J E 1999 Communicating cancer risk in print journalism. Journal of the
    National Cancer Institute Monographs 25:170-172
Brown J D, Walsh-Childers K 1994 Effects of media on personal and public
    health. In: Bryant J, Zillmann D (eds) Media effects: advances in theory and
    research. Lawrence Erlbaum Associates, Mahwah, pp 389-415
Centers for Disease Control (CDC) 1989 Reducing the health consequences of
    smoking. A report of the Surgeon General. US Department of Health and
    Human Services, Public Health Service, Centers for Disease Control, Center
    for Health Promotion and Education, Office on Smoking and Health,
    Washington
Gerbner G, Gross L 1976 Living with television: the violence profile. Journal of
    Communication 26:173-199
Gerbner G, Gross L, Morgan M et al 1981 Special report: health and medicine
    on television. New England Journal of Medicine 305:901-904
Gill L 2003 Cancer treatment: knickers to ageist attitudes. The Times,
    September 23
Hastings G, MacFayden L 2000 Keep smiling: no one's going to die. An
    analysis of internal documents from the tobacco industry's main UK
    advertising agencies. Centre for Tobacco Control Research, Strathclyde
Hastings G, Stead M, McDermott L et al 2003 Review of research on the
    effects of food promotion to children. Food Standards Agency, London
Harrabin R, Coote A, Allen J 2003 Health in the news: risk, reporting and
    media influence. King's Fund, London
Institute of Alcohol Studies (IAS) 2003 Fact sheet: alcohol and
    advertising. Institute of Alcohol Studies, St Ives. Available online at:
    www.ias.org.uk
Lampert C, Hasebrink U 2002 Alkohol im Fernsehen – Ergebnisse einer
    Programmanalyse. In: Aufenanger S, Große-Loheide M, Hasebrink U et al
    (eds) Alkohol, Fernsehen, Jugendliche. Programmanalyse und
    medienpädagogische Praxisprojekte. Vistas, Berlin, pp 33-188
Maher C 2003 The real world. Plain English Campaign Newsletter 56:7

Mekemson C, Glantz S A 2002 How the tobacco industry built its relationship with Hollywood. Tobacco Control 11:81-91

Minkewitz N 2003 'Medien-Krankheiten'. Eine Studie zur Kultivierung durch medizinische Inhalte im Fernsehen. Unpublished Masters thesis, University of Munich

Montgomery K C 1993 The Harvard Alcohol Project: promoting the designated driver on television. In: Backer T E, Rogers E M (eds) Organizational aspects of health communication campaigns: what works? Sage, Newbury Park, pp 178-202

Nelkin D 1996 Medicine and the media. An uneasy relationship: the tensions between medicine and the media. Lancet 347:1600-1603

Nestle M, Jacobson M F 2000 Halting the obesity epidemic: a public health policy approach. Public Health Reports 115:12-24

Nutley S, Davies H, Walter I 2002 Learning from the diffusion of innovations. Research Unit for Research Utilisation, University of St Andrews, St Andrews

Rogers E M 1995 Diffusion of innovations. Free Press, New York

Rossmann C 2002 Die heile Welt des Fernsehens. Eine Studie zur Kultivierung durch Krankenhausserien. Fischer, München

Schulz W 1976 Die Konstruktion von Realität in den Nachrichtenmedien. Analyse der aktuellen Berichterstattung. Alber, Freiburg im Breisgau

Silverstein B, Perdue L, Peterson B et al 1986 The role of mass media in promoting a thin standard of bodily attractiveness for women. Sex Roles 14:519-532

Slater M 2002 Entertainment education and the persuasive impact of narratives. In: Green M C, Strange J J, Brock T C (eds) Narrative impact. Social and cognitive foundations. Lawrence Erlbaum Associates, Mahwah, pp 157-181

Uhlig R 2003 Adverts blamed for poor diet of children. The Telegraph, September 26

Vickers A 1997 How the tobacco industry will exploit loopholes in an advertising ban. ASH Paper 1. Available online at: www.ash.org.uk

Weitkunat R, Pottgiesser C, Meyer N et al 2003 Perceived risk of bovine spongiform encephalopathy and dietary behavior. Journal of Health Psychology 8:365-373

WHO 2002a Report of the Joint WHO/FAO Expert Consultation on Diet, Nutrition and the Prevention of Chronic Diseases. WHO, Geneva

WHO 2002b Tobacco sponsorship of world sport. WHO, Geneva

Zinn C 2003 Australian ministers threaten restrictions on junk food advertising. British Medical Journal 327:380

SECTION D

Creating Behavior Change

Intervention strategies

Ralph DiClemente, Laura Salazar, Richard Crosby, and Gina Wingood

INTRODUCTION

This chapter focuses on illuminating the issues related to creating behavior change within the context of health promotion and disease prevention. The first part describes the underlying determinants and mediators of health behavior, examines the role of theory in creating change, discusses strategies for creating change, and delineates potential levels in which to position intervention programs (individual, familial, community, and societal). Because many health issues have causal roots that reach across multiple levels with some degree of intersection, intervening successfully and effectively depends upon a reconceptualization of intervention strategies. This implies an expansion from targeting behavior change at a single change level to using a socio-ecological framework that links several change levels. Finally, the chapter touches upon several pertinent issues for health promotion practitioners to consider when devising an overall intervention strategy. Specific issues considered will be identifying behavior type (e.g. one-off, such as getting vaccinated, or daily, such as healthy eating), matching intervention strategy to behavior type (e.g. awareness campaign, skills development), and choosing a sufficient dosage. Consequently, program designers will better understand the process involved in devising custom-tailored approaches that will promote health and prevent disease.

HEALTH BEHAVIOR IS A COMPLEX PHENOMENON

Understanding individuals' behavior is unquestionably a formidable challenge. To a large extent, a single virus, gene, or physiological process does not determine individual behavior. Rather, an individual's health behavior is reciprocally determined by myriad internal and external influences that result from the individual's interaction with their environment (Bandura 1986). Overall, an individual's health behavior is the end result of a complex process. This process weighs physiological processes, cognitions, and emotional responses, behavior, the environment, and interpersonal, social, economic, and psychological influences within a cultural context that is superimposed over traditions, values, and patterns of social organization. Such a complex process, which must be addressed to optimize and sustain behavior change, is not likely to be understood in simplistic, one-dimensional, or linear terms.

THE GRADIENT OF HEALTH BEHAVIOR CHANGE

Health behavior is inherently a broad concept that encompasses a broad spectrum of behaviors. Notwithstanding the fact that all behavior change requires some degree of effort, specific health behaviors may be differentially challenging or resistant to change. For instance, health behaviors that are highly relevant to people (i.e. their level of perceived threat is high) and require relatively little effort to modify (e.g. being vaccinated against the flu at the worksite) may be lower on the gradient of change. Conversely, other health behaviors may be more complex and, therefore, are higher on the gradient of change (pose a tremendous number of challenges to change). Health behaviors that have become an ingrained part of a person's lifestyle (e.g. dietary and exercise habits), for instance, are especially resistant to modification. Moreover, health behaviors that have a physiological substrate (i.e. are physiologically addictive, such as heroin use), serve a 'functional purpose' (e.g. are psychologically addictive) or both (e.g. smoking) can be resistant to change and may pose particular challenges in evoking change. Also, if change occurs at all, it may be short-lived.

Thus, achieving significant and sustainable changes in health behaviors represents a formidable undertaking. To better understand how best to create health-promoting behavior change, we need to understand the fundamental relationship between determinants, mediators, health behaviors, and health outcomes.

DETERMINANTS, MEDIATORS, HEALTH BEHAVIORS, AND HEALTH OUTCOMES

Diseases and health conditions are influenced by determinants which can be described as factors that are external to a person and are associated with their health behaviors. Examples of determinants may include, but are not limited to, demographics, social structures, peer pressure, and media influences (see Table D1.1). Modifying these external factors can influence the health of populations and is a central element in health promotion strategies. Because these external factors may be distal to the health behavior, they may be more challenging to modify compared with mediators.

Table D1.1 The core of a behavior change strategy

Determinants/mediators	Change levels	Change goals	Change activities
Internal	Individual	Awareness	**Self-monitoring**
Personality	Family	Motivation	Goal setting
Beliefs	School	Attitudes	Cost–benefit analyses
Attitudes	Workplace	Intention	Stimulus control
Expectations	Community	Skills	Conditioning
Readiness	Society	Behavior change	Implementation intentions
Past behavior		Political change	
Perceived risk		Commercial change	**Interpersonal communication**
Self-efficacy		Environmental change	Counseling
Control			Modeling
			Persuasion
			Education
			Skills training
External			
Demographics			**Mediated communication**
Socio-economic status			Written, audio, visual
Culture			Press, radio, television, Internet
Social support			Leaflets, posters, newsletters
Social networks, cohesion			Advertising, PR, edutainment, sponsorship
Built structures			Ambient media, e.g. golf holes, stair cases
Community design			Social marketing
Accessibility and availability			Lobbying and advocacy
Peer pressure			Passage of policy (organization, institution)
Media influences			Passage of law (societal)

Mediators are often defined as factors that are internal to a person and are associated with their health behavior. Examples of mediators may include a person's beliefs, attitudes, expectations, perceived risk, and self-efficacy. There are often many mediators associated with a particular health behavior. Because mediators are typically internal factors that are proximal to the actual health behavior, they may be easier to modify relative to external influences. Many health promotion programs are based on modifying mediators to enhance the likelihood of a person adopting healthy behaviors or decreasing unhealthy behaviors.

Health behavior refers to the actions of individuals, organizations, and groups that are designed to improve physical and mental health. As noted earlier in this chapter, a health behavior may be a single preventive action, such as seeking a vaccination, or it may be a lifestyle behavior, an action that should be maintained over the life course to stay healthy (e.g. regular exercising). Because health behaviors are contextually defined, it is imperative to consider the target audience for behavior change (adolescents, adults, ethnic minorities) and the social environment in which the desired behavior change will occur (at home, school, community, church, worksite, etc.). It is important to specify the behaviors targeted for change to maximize the potential impact on the health outcome(s) of interest. The health outcome is the consequence of performing or engaging in specific health behaviors.

Many different behaviors can lead to the same health outcome. For example, a health outcome such as reducing body weight may be achieved by behaviors such as exercising or changing one's dietary practices. Health outcomes may include diseases, such as HIV/AIDS, cancer, diabetes, or hypertension. Health outcomes may include conditions, such as pregnancy and obesity. More recently, public health researchers have also conceptualized quality of life as an important health outcome. The relationship between determinants, mediators, health behaviors, and health outcomes is schematically illustrated in Figure D1.1.

For illustrative purposes, if we were to apply the model in Figure D1.1 to understand factors associated with the health outcome of teen pregnancy, determinants may include lack of access to contraception, limited parental monitoring, and having an older male partner. Mediators may include having limited knowledge about pregnancy prevention,

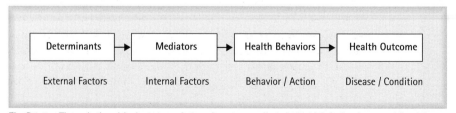

Fig D1.1 The relationship between determinants, mediators, health behaviors, and health outcomes

being less efficacious in using birth control, and having a low perceived risk for becoming pregnant. The associated health behaviors may include use of birth control pills, use of injectable contraception, condom use during sexual intercourse, or sexual abstinence. Thus, identifying determinants and mediators of health behaviors is important because they correspond to different change levels that specify various types of intervention strategies that can be designed to enhance the health of a person or the public.

The relationship specified in Figure D1.1 provides a useful heuristic for understanding the association among determinants, mediators, health behaviors, and health outcomes. Often, however, challenges arise that make accurate measurement of the associations among determinants, mediators, and a specific health behavior problematic. Health promotion researchers and practitioners have not identified, enumerated, or operationalized the full complement of determinants and mediators associated with a specific health behavior. Thus, undefined and unmeasured determinants and mediators may potentially exert influence on the health behavior, distorting the observed relationship between any one determinant or mediator and the specific health behavior. However, in the absence of a complete mapping of theoretically important determinants and mediators of specific health behaviors, it is still possible to change health behavior through a targeted health promotion intervention. Ideally, program designers should prioritize intervention activities and strategies toward those factors that have empirically demonstrable evidence of an association with the specific health behavior.

CHANGE LEVELS, GOALS, AND ACTIVITIES

Change levels can be conceptualized as representing different domains of influences that affect the health behavior of an individual, group, community, or organization. In this chapter we have delineated five change levels, in ascending order of hierarchy: individual level, family level, organizational level, community level, and societal level (see Fig D1.2). It is important to note, however, that there is no consensus in the field of health promotion regarding the nomenclature used to describe these change levels.

The most basic change level is that of the individual. The goal of *individual-level* interventions is to modify an individual's knowledge, awareness, motivation, intentions, and skills related to a health behavior. Examples of interventions at this level include: group or individual counseling and educational programs. Individual-level interventions often employ behavior change strategies, such as modeling, skills training, and goal setting.

Beyond individual-level interventions are *family-level* interventions. Although there are many definitions of family, family can be more

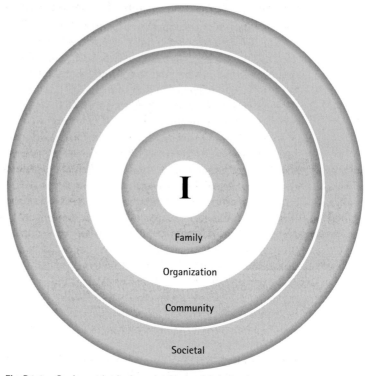

Fig D1.2   Socio-ecological model for health behavior

broadly conceptualized as any network of mutually supportive affilia-
tions and commitments. Thus, within this broader conceptualization,
family-level interventions would include consanguine relationships,
such as nuclear or extended families, and intergenerational families
that may include grandmothers parenting their grandchildren.
However, in addition to the family of origin it is also important to
include other family configurations, such as families of choice. Families
of choice may be more similar because they select each other based on
shared values and interests. Families of choice may include dyadic relationships, such as romantic relationships or social networks in which an
individual is embedded in a web of socially supportive relationships. The
goal of family-level interventions is to help families, however config-
ured, to provide support for one another, foster familial norms, and
create a healthy family environment. Examples of interventions at this
level include parent–child interventions, couple and family counseling,
and social network interventions.

Organizations may include schools, faith-based institutions, and
worksites. The goal of *organizational-level* interventions is to improve
organizational performance and quality of life to facilitate behavior
change. These goals are generally achieved through interventions

directed at modifying the norms of entire organizations, transform-ing organizational processes and structures, and enhancing the performance of workers. Examples of organizational-level interventions may include school-based nutrition programs, promoting breast can-cer detection in churches, or worksite policies requiring the use of protective work gear.

Community-level interventions are designed to foster community norms, supportive of healthy behaviors, or to improve commu-nity resources to achieve a healthier environment. Examples of community-level interventions may include neighborhood safety pro-grams, distribution of print media, or construction of billboards in a community to increase residents' awareness of local health services. Community-level interventions are most effective when engaging the community as a participant and partner. Community participation is the process of involving community residents in the decisions that affect their lives. Partnership with the community implies that the community has a voice in problem definition, designing the health intervention and applying the results to address community needs.

Societal-level interventions attempt to modify policies and influence laws. Examples of interventions at this level include taxing alcohol to reduce consumption, outlawing smoking in public venues, lobbying, and advocacy. For example, Mothers Against Drunk Driving is an effec-tive lobbying effort that was instrumental in the passage of drink-driv-ing legislation in the United States. Effective health promotion depends on researchers and practitioners marshaling the most appropriate theory and practice strategies that target particular change levels to optimize intervention efficacy.

i see C4

ROLE OF THEORY IN CREATING BEHAVIOR CHANGE

Theories are a set of interrelated concepts, definitions, and propositions that present a systematic view of events or situations by specifying relationships among variables in order to explain and predict the events or situations (Kerlinger & Lee 2000). A fully developed theory is a completely closed deductive system of propositions that identifies the interrelationships among the concepts in a systematic view of the phenomenon.

Theories that attempt to explain why people do or do not engage in specific behaviors that lead to health outcomes vary according to psy-chological, psychosocial, and political terms. The range of theoretical approaches discussed in this book is a reflection of the many disciplines aligned within the field itself, such as psychology, sociology, anthropol-ogy, and public health. A variety of theoretical approaches has been utilized in conducting basic research, as well as in the implementation of behavior change programs. Some theories of human behavior are not

i see B2-B5, D3

necessarily antithetical, but rather interact and provide more complex perspectives for directing individual and social change.

A theory that has been applied to a particular context can be described as a 'model' and forms the foundation for affecting behavioral change. Many theories have been amply tested and found to be useful models in the context of explaining and changing health behaviors. From a pragmatic perspective, it is important to consider different theories because the consequences of adopting one theory over another may affect how a problem behavior is conceptualized and, subsequently, the type of intervention approach that may be most efficacious in modifying that behavior (Seidman 1983).

Theory should play a significant role in the planning, implementation, and evaluation of health promotion interventions. From a behavior change perspective specifically, theories are composed of modifiable constructs or factors that are associated with the health behavior. Thus, a theory serves as a 'blueprint' or 'roadmap' for altering health behaviors. Health promotion interventions grounded in a particular theory are designed to impact those determinants and mediators that are hypothesized, within that particular theoretical framework, to impact specific health behaviors and, subsequently, culminate in changing the targeted health behavior. In general, the current armamentarium of theories has been demonstrably effective in providing intervention frameworks for promoting health behavior change. Acknowledging the manifold change levels that influence an individual's behavior, a socio-ecological model may be effective in optimizing behavior change and reinforcing, amplifying, and sustaining behavior change over protracted time periods.

THE IMPORTANCE OF A SOCIO-ECOLOGICAL MODEL IN MODIFYING HEALTH BEHAVIOR

More recently, researchers and practitioners in health promotion have ushered in a new era and begun to embrace the value of a multilevel approach (DiClemente & Wingood 2000, 2003, DiClemente et al 2003). Acknowledging a pluralism of determinants and mediators across change levels has resulted in a search for more holistic theoretical models of health behavior that transcend a single change level. One such paradigm is a modification of the seminal work of Bronfenbrenner (1979) (see Fig D1.2).

Examining the figure, we can understand that the innermost sphere represents the individual and includes individual characteristics and behaviors. The family, organizational, and community spheres suggest that interactions between individuals and family members, intimate partners, organizational factors, and peers also influence behavior. The outermost sphere (society) indicates that societal characteristics (e.g. socio-economic status, health-care policies, media, gender, and racial/ethnic discrimination) provide a broader context in which individuals, organizations, and communities are embedded and, thus, may have a powerful effect on individual behavior.

A socio-ecological approach may provide insight into the competing and reciprocal relationships between these influences and, furthermore, enhance our understanding of how these dynamics may affect individual risk behaviors and disease acquisition. It is hoped that this more complex theoretical model may have a synergistic impact on health behavior outcomes.

Examining the array of hypothesized determinants and mediators within this model, it becomes clear that they vary in their degree of impact on the health behavior, individual volition, and control over behavior and their environment, and whether the determinants and mediators directly or indirectly affect the specific behavior. Furthermore, health behaviors also vary in the degree to which they are associated with health/disease outcomes.

It is important to note that multifocal targeting of intervention strategies and activities, simultaneously across a range of change levels, may enhance the likelihood of achieving significant and long-lasting health behavior change. To address adequately the range of determinants and mediators that exist across the different change levels, multicomponent health promotion programs that include activities and strategies designed specifically to address the different sources of influence on health behavior are of critical importance.

SELECTING AN APPROPRIATE THEORETICAL FRAMEWORK TO GUIDE INTERVENTION PROGRAM DESIGN AND IMPLEMENTATION

Theory selection is a process. The process of selecting a theory, even within a specific change level, can be a daunting challenge. Clearly, there are numerous theories that may be applicable to a particular change level, so theory selection involves several critical steps. The first step is the specification of the health behavior targeted for modification. Second, clearly specifying the target audience and the setting in which the intervention will be administered. Third, identifying, through a thorough review of the empirical literature, the determinants and mediators of the specific health behavior in the target population. The culmination of this process is the selection of a theoretical framework that:

- incorporates empirically appropriate determinants and mediators of the target health behavior
- provides a framework for understanding the mechanism through which these empirically appropriate determinants and mediators produce the targeted health behavior
- provides guidance in the selection of applicable health behavior change strategies

- is appropriate for the target population
- has demonstrated effectiveness in modifying health behavior at the targeted change level.

INTERPRETING THE RESULTS OF HEALTH PROMOTION INTERVENTIONS AT THE DIFFERENT CHANGE LEVELS

Caution should be exercised when interpreting the effectiveness of different levels of interventions. For instance, interpretation of the effectiveness of community-level interventions should be based on different criteria from those used for individual-level interventions. Community-level interventions are likely to observe smaller changes in individual health behaviors than are individual-level interventions, with motivated volunteers. For example, Rose (1992) suggests that when risks are widely distributed in the population, small changes in the behavior of many individuals in the population are likely to have a greater impact on risk reduction than large changes among smaller groups of high-risk individuals. Smaller change at the population level, therefore, may lead to larger effects on health outcomes.

CHOOSING THE CORRECT DOSAGE TO ACHIEVE BEHAVIOR CHANGE

When resources available for health promotion programs are scarce, it is a challenge to design a program that will generate the most 'bang for the buck'. The number of program sessions, the session length, spacing of sessions, and the duration of the program constitute a program's 'dosage'. Unlike medical procedures and medications, however, calculating the optimal dosage is often not precise, mainly due to an individual's propensity to change their behavior and the different trajectories of change inherent in diverse health behaviors.

Several other external factors also dictate the dosage, such as risk level of population, budget constraints, scheduling constraints, and political barriers. Cultural factors will perhaps have the most profound effect on the dosage requirement. Although dosage is therefore very difficult to measure (and, by extension, to 'prescribe'), it may nonetheless be prudent to determine a *minimum dosage* that is necessary for reaching the change goals. This 'threshold' should then be thought of as the starting point for increased efforts as demanded by the numerous factors listed here.

Making decisions regarding dosage is not easy. Previous research, if available, may be helpful in determining a sufficient dosage. Metaanalyses and literature reviews are a first step in making this decision; however, not all evaluations include dosage as a term. Moreover, depending upon the particular health issue, there may be conflicting results: sometimes 'less is more' may be more effective, whereas at other times evidence suggests a 'dose–response' relation (i.e. increased dosage results in better outcomes) is more effective. For example, Kerr et al (2001) found that 42 × 30 cm sized point-of-choice posters (tested in two different styles and locations) did not encourage stair use whereas a larger poster (42 × 60 cm) did. Advertising research has also shown that effectiveness may be tied to the number of times an advert is aired (Howell & Dipboye 1982). However, Campbell & Keller (2003) found that advert repetition was associated with effectiveness, but only for adverts whose brands were familiar to participants. Adverts in which unfamiliar brands were promoted resulted in decreased effectiveness. Also, Nordhielm (2002) revealed that how the adverts are processed (i.e. shallow or deep) influences the relation between repetition and effectiveness. In a similar vein, Edleson & Syers (1990) found no significant difference in reassault rates between a 12-week, 12-session batterers' treatment program and a 16-week, 32-session program. Cunningham et al (1995) found that two formats of an educational program for cancer patients (six weekly 2-hour sessions versus a weekend intensive course) produced similar outcomes as well. Yet, Fallowfield et al (2002) revealed evidence of a dose–response relation in their communication skills training course for oncologists. They found that 'upping' the dosage of communication training resulted in better outcomes. For example, their pilot studies showed that a 3-day and a 2.5-day training for doctors was significantly better than shortened 1.5-day or half-day training modules.

Given the divergence of evidence, there appears to be no definite recommendation regarding proper dosage other than to examine the empirical evidence available as a starting point and gauge the parameters to the particular constraints. In addition, and further complicating this issue of dosage, is the possibility that although the program may be effective in reaching its targeted goals in the short-term, the effects may dissipate over time (a phenomenon referred to as 'intervention decay'). To sustain positive outcomes, supplemental or adjuvant interventions designed to sustain, reinforce, and amplify primary intervention effects are necessary and warranted.

CONCLUSION

This chapter has described mechanisms that create health behavior change. In doing so, we emphasized the need for a broader contextual perspective in examining the diverse array of factors that may influence health behavior. Further, we stressed the need for contextual interventions that can create preventive synergy within a community. We also discussed the core components of a behavior change strategy and highlighted the decisions that must be determined for devising effective health promotion programs.

The field of health promotion is dynamic and complex and so too are the theories and intervention strategies. The field continues to evolve, albeit slowly. Moreover, a continuum of research needs exists. Finally, for health promotion to advance as a science, a comprehensive and coordinated infrastructure is needed to conceptualize, stimulate, and support the continuum of research necessary to understand health behavior, design innovative health behavior change interventions, and develop strategies to sustain and amplify intervention efficacy.

References

Bandura A 1986 Social foundations of thought and action: a social cognitive theory. Prentice-Hall, Englewood Cliffs

Bronfenbrenner U 1979 The ecology of human development. Harvard University Press, Cambridge

Campbell M C, Keller K L 2003 Brand familiarity and advertising repetition effects. Journal of Consumer Research 30(2):292-304

Cunningham A, Jenkins J, Edmonds C et al 1995 A randomized comparison of two forms of a brief, group, psychoeducational program for cancer patients: weekly sessions versus a 'weekend intensive'. International Journal of Psychiatry in Medicine 25(2):173-189

DiClemente R J, Wingood G M 2000 Expanding the scope of HIV prevention for adolescents: beyond individual-level interventions. Journal of Adolescent Health 26(6):377-378

DiClemente R J, Wingood G M 2003 HIV prevention for adolescents: windows of opportunity for optimizing intervention effectiveness. Archives of Pediatrics and Adolescent Medicine 157:319-320

DiClemente R J, Wingood G M, Crosby R 2003 A contextual perspective for understanding and preventing STD/HIV among adolescents. In: Romer D (ed) Reducing adolescent risk: toward an integrated approach. Sage, Thousand Oaks, pp 366-373

Edleson J, Syers M 1990 The relative effectiveness of group treatments for men who batter. Social Work Research and Abstracts 26:10-17

Fallowfield L, Jenkins V, Farewell V et al 2002 Efficacy of a cancer research UK communication skills training model for oncologists: a randomized controlled trial. Lancet 359:650-656

Howell W C, Dipboye R L 1982 Essentials of industrial and organizational psychology. Dorsey, Homewood

Kerlinger F N, Lee H B 2000 Foundations of behavioral research. Harcourt, Fort Worth

Kerr J, Eves F, Carroll D 2001 The influence of poster prompts on stair use: the effects of setting, poster size and content. British Journal of Health Psychology 6:397-405

Nordhielm C L 2002 The influence of level of processing on advertising repetition effects. Journal of Consumer Research 29(3):371-382

Rose G 1992 The strategy of preventive medicine. Oxford University Press, Oxford

Seidman E 1983 Unexamined premises of social problem solving. In: Seidman E (ed) Handbook of social intervention. Sage, Beverly Hills, pp 48-67

Target audiences and target behaviors

D2

Robert Donovan

LOCATING TARGET AUDIENCES AND TARGET BEHAVIORS

Commercial organizations spend a great deal of money identifying and understanding subsegments of the population that will be most profitable for them to target. Not surprisingly, then, market segmentation and target marketing are emphasized in the literature describing the application of marketing techniques to public health campaigns (e.g. Donovan & Owen 1994, Egger et al 1993, Hastings & Haywood 1991).

The communication process

Following McGuire's (1985) hierarchical model, Rossiter & Percy (1997) developed a simplified six-step model relating advertising exposure to company objectives and profits (see Fig D2.1). Although developed in a commercial advertising context (Rossiter et al 1991), the model applies to all communication methods and in any context or setting.

Communication begins with a person's *exposure* to a message. Messages may be delivered in a variety of ways (advertising, publicity, edutainment, etc.), through a variety of media and media vehicles (face to face, teleconferencing, websites, newspapers and magazines, television, billboards, radio, soap operas, hit songs, etc.) and in a variety of settings (homes, worksites, schools, hospitals, sporting events, etc.).

Messages that attract attention will be *processed* in short-term memory. This involves comprehension of the message, often some emotional arousal, and perhaps acceptance or rejection of the message content. Message execution (i.e. the use of music, color, and graphics), who delivers the message (a celebrity, scientific expert, or peer group member), and where the message is encountered (e.g. in *The Times* broadsheet newspaper or *The Sun* tabloid) all influence how the message is processed.

Processing of the message (and subsequent related messages) results in *communication effects* in long-term memory. These are beliefs

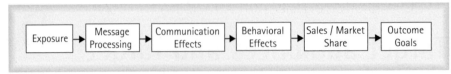

Fig D2.1   A six-step communication process

about, attitudes towards, and intentions with respect to the message topic or promoted behavior (e.g. a belief that marijuana use may trigger depression and a tentative disposition to reduce use). When recalled during decision making, the desired communication effects facilitate *behavioral effects*, such as rejecting the offer of a 'joint', purchase of a product (pedometer), trial of the recommended behavior (e.g. trying a low-alcohol beer), or intermediate behavioral effects, such as seeking further information about where to get help (i.e. calling a men's domestic violence helpline).

These behavioral effects amongst the target group result in the achievement of *objectives and goals*, which in commercial terms are usually sales and market share objectives that contribute to profit goals. In the health area, these objectives may be stated in terms of participation rates or prevalence rates (e.g. a smoking prevalence goal of 20% by 2005), while overall goals might include health cost reductions and improved quality of life-years for the target population.

The sequence is reversed when developing a communication strategy. That is, the campaign planner asks – and then sets out to answer – the following questions.

1 *What is our overall goal that the campaign must help achieve?* (e.g. a reduction in male-to-female intimate partner violence; improved physical and mental well-being amongst women who experience such violence.)

2 *What specific objectives do we want this campaign to achieve?* (e.g. enroll 200 violent or potentially violent men in counseling programs.)

3 *Who do we need to impact to achieve our goal?* (e.g. violent and potentially violent men who accept that they need help.) *What do we want them to do?* (e.g. call a men's domestic violence helpline and accept a referral to counseling.)

4 *What beliefs and attitudes do we need to create, change, or reinforce to have them behave this way?*

5 *What sorts of messages do we need to create to have them adopt these beliefs and attitudes?*

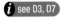

6 *Where, how often and in what form do we need to expose these messages to reach these people?*

This chapter focuses on step 3: *Who do we need to impact to achieve our goals and what do we want them to do?*

TARGET AUDIENCE DELINEATION AND SEGMENTATION

Given that a comprehensive approach involves targeting individual, community, and structural change, there will be a number of target groups. For example, a comprehensive approach to reduction in tobacco use will need to target smokers (the primary target group) to quit; legislators for advertising bans and restrictions on smoking in public places; general practitioners (GPs) to intervene with smoking patients; teachers to include antismoking messages in health curricula; and so on. These secondary target groups are usually targeted to facilitate the primary target group's adoption of the desired behavior. In this chapter we focus mainly on the primary target group, although the principles are the same for targeting all groups.

Primary and secondary target groups are rarely homogeneous and different segments exist within these groups (e.g. social versus addicted smokers; legislators already in favor of smoking restrictions in public places; GPs who feel confident about tackling lifestyle behaviors versus those who don't; precontemplators versus later stages of change, etc.). However, we rarely have the resources to develop approaches for all these groups. Hence we develop messages that appeal to a number of subsegments or select and concentrate only on one or two subgroups.

Segmenting target audiences

Segmentation refers to the division of the population into relatively homogeneous but distinct segments. Target marketing refers to the selection and concentration of resources on one or more of these segments. Market segmentation is one of the most important principles of marketing (Lunn 1986). This principle acknowledges that different strategies and approaches may be necessary to reach (locate), communicate with, or motivate different subgroups:

- different target audiences may be reached by different channels, inhabit different geographical areas, or attend different types of entertainment
- different target audiences may have different values, attitudes, and lifestyles, and hence different communication styles may be necessary to attract their attention and establish rapport
- different target groups may be motivated to achieve the desired behavioral reaction by different factors.

For example, lower socio-economic status (SES) groups may be more avid TV watchers and consumers of print media than upper SES groups, but a message about child immunization can be communicated in the same style and tone of language to both groups and both may be motivated by the same factor (protection of their children). In this case, we need only select different media vehicles to locate the different groups.

Box D2.1	Bases for market segmentation
Demographic	e.g. age, sex, income, education, religion, ethnicity, occupation
Geographic	e.g. state, region, urban, suburban, rural, remote, climate, local government area
Psychographic	e.g. values, lifestyle, personality
Sociodemographic	e.g. social class
Epidemiological	e.g. risk factor prevalence
Behavioral	e.g. perform–not perform, frequency, intensity
Attitudinal	e.g. positive, neutral, negative
Benefits sought	e.g. avoidance of illness, positive health benefits
Readiness stage	e.g. stage of change

In other cases, communications styles may have to be very different or the motivations to comply may be quite different.

Box D2.1 lists the ways in which segments can be described or profiled. Health promoters often begin with a basic *risk factor status* (e.g. smokers, inactives, heavy drinkers, drug users, etc.), often in combination with a demographic grouping that epidemiological data show are at high risk (e.g. blue collar groups for smoking; sedentary occupations for physical activity; Aborigines for diabetes, etc.) (Donovan & Henley 2003).

However, these segmentations are purely 'diagnostic' – they provide little direction for developing campaign interventions. On the other hand, attitude–behavior segmentation (e.g. Sheth & Frazier 1982) and stage of change segmentation (Prochaska & DiClemente 1984) are 'prognostic' segmentations, as both methods emphasize an understanding of the beliefs and attitudes of the target groups.

 see B2, B5

Attitude–behavior segmentation

Sheth & Frazier's (1982) model of strategy choice is based on the concept of attitude–behavior consistency/discrepancy. When attitudes and behavior are consistent and in the desired direction, Sheth & Frazier state that a reinforcement strategy is appropriate, to ensure the desired behavior continues. The strategy can involve reinforcing the attitude, rewarding the behavior, or both. For example, teenagers who do not binge drink should be reminded of all the benefits for not doing so; adult non-smokers can be reinforced by insurance premium discounts;

**SKIN CANCER
HAVE YOU BEEN CHECKED?**

The ....LIONS CLUB has organized a FREE skin cancer screening. Specialists from the LIONS CANCER INSTITUTE will be available to examine people who feel they are at risk of having skin cancer.

If you are 16 years of age or older and have one or more of the following:
- A family member who has had a malignant melanoma
- Five or more moles (not freckles) on your arms
- Previously had moles or skin cancers removed
- A mole or freckle that is changing in size or color
- Fair skin that burns rather than tans
- Had blistering sunburn as a child
- Any inflamed skin sores that do not heal

**then please phone .... to make an appointment.
Venue: ....
Date: ....**

If you are concerned but cannot attend the screening on that date please express your interest with the **LIONS CANCER INSTITUTE** and see your family doctor.

Fig D2.2 Targeting by risk factor profile: an example (Katris et al 1996)

non-smokers should congratulate their smoker friends for attempting to quit; road safety campaigns should feed back that the campaigns have successfully reduced crashes; and people can in fact reward themselves for reaching various milestones.

Where people hold positive attitudes towards a behavior (e.g. most sedentary people believe that increased physical activity would be a 'good thing to do') but do not carry out the desired behavior, an incentive strategy is required. These strategies are aimed at facilitating the desired behavior by minimizing or removing organizational, socio-economic, time, or place constraints to make it easier for the positive attitude to be translated into action. For example, providing changing rooms at the worksite to facilitate lunchtime or before/after-work exercise; providing well-lit walkways and parks to encourage walking; providing 24-hour helpline counseling for violent men in remote geographic areas; making condoms available in nightclub washrooms.

Where the behavior is being performed but the attitude is negative (e.g. mandatory attendance at counseling; use of public transport only

Table D2.1	Attitude–behavior segmentation model		
	Behavior		
Attitude	Strongly perform desired behavior	Moderately perform	Do not perform desired behavior
Positive	Cell 1	Cell 4	Cell 7
Neutral	Cell 2	Cell 5	Cell 8
Negative	Cell 3	Cell 6	Cell 9

when the car is out of action; using a litter bin only when others are watching), Sheth & Frazier propose that rationalization needs to occur to shift the individual into a positive frame of mind.

The most difficult-to-impact group consists of those negative to, and not performing, the desired behavior. In this case, behavioral confrontation (e.g. punitive legal sanctions) or psychological confrontation (e.g. face-to-face interrogative counseling) may be necessary to achieve change.

The Sheth–Frazier Model as described above is based on a 2 × 2 contingency table of positive versus negative attitude by perform versus not-perform the desired behavior. However, many behaviors are more usefully classified as at least trichotomous (e.g. physically active at a level sufficient for cardiovascular benefits; physically active sufficient for health benefits; insufficiently active for any health benefits; alcohol consumption beyond recommended levels; alcohol consumption at or below recommended levels; no alcohol consumption) and there are many issues for which some people do not have a view one way or the other, either because they simply don't care or they know little about the issue. In Table D2.1, the Sheth–Frazier framework is extended to a more comprehensive and realistic nine cells.

Survey methods with appropriately designed questionnaires are used to determine the proportions falling into each of the segments and to profile each segment in terms of their demographics, media habits, lifestyle variables, risk factor profiles, and other relevant health beliefs and attitudes (Donovan & Owen 1994).

 see B, C

A stage approach to segmentation

The author has suggested elsewhere (Donovan & Owen 1994, Egger et al 1993) the potential utility of Prochaska & DiClemente's (1984) stages of change concept as a segmentation base in health promotion and social marketing. This approach divides the total target segment (for example, all smokers, all non-exercisers) into subsegments depending on their stage in progression toward adoption of the desired behavior (i.e. quitting smoking, taking up exercise). As for the attitude–behavior segmentation, the model is prognostic in that different strategies are deemed appropriate for people in the different stages of change. Although the various processes applicable to each of the stages are perhaps not always properly understood (Whitelaw et al 1999), the model is nevertheless very useful as a segmentation method for formative research and targeting. For example, the Western Australian Freedom From Fear campaign targets men who are violent toward their female intimate partner. The primary target group is defined as men in the contemplator and ready for action stages (Donovan et al 2000). These are described as men who are aware of their problem, accept responsibility for their actions, and accept that it is up to them to seek help. The Freedom From Fear campaign facilitates this help-seeking behavior by providing a confidential helpline staffed by non-judgmental counselors (Donovan et al 1999a).

The stages of change concept is dealt with elsewhere in this book and hence is not elaborated further here (see Donovan & Henley 2003).

Choosing target audiences when resources are limited: TARPARE

Given an attitude–behavior segmentation, such as that in Table D2.1, or a stage of change segmentation (e.g. precontemplators, contemplators, and preparers for action), the next step is to select one or more segments to target. Donovan et al's (1999b) TARPARE analysis is a useful and flexible method for assessing the potential viability of interventions directed at each segment. The analysis is particularly useful when, as is usually the case, there is a need to prioritize segments in terms of available budgets.

The TARPARE model appraises the segments on the following criteria.

- **T:** *the Total number of persons in the segment.* This criterion is very important where small percentage shifts on risk factors in large proportions of the population yield substantial benefits (Rose 1985, 1992) (e.g. reductions in driving speed to 50 km per hour in built-up areas; population cholesterol shifts and heart disease).
- **AR:** *the proportion of 'At Risk' persons in the segment.* This involves an assessment of risk factors associated with the primary issue and the total expected benefits of risk reduction in the segment. For example, different subsegments of heavy smokers might have higher obesity levels, lower levels of physical activity, and a higher incidence of diabetes.
- **P:** *the Persuasibility of the target audience.* Segments with a higher proportion of persons neutral or positive to the desired behavior would yield better intervention outcomes than segments with a high proportion very negative to the desired behavior change.

- **A:** *the Accessibility of the target audience.* Where target segments are more easily reached at a reasonable cost (whether via mass communication or other channels, such as worksites, community centers, entertainment venues, schools, or other institutional settings), the more likely an intervention is to be successful and cost effective.
- **R:** *Resources required to meet the needs of the target audience.* Some segments can be directed towards current services and facilities, whereas others might only be attracted to adopt the desired behavior via additional resources. For example, various segments might be motivated to engage in increased physical activity only if an indoor running track or heated swimming pool were available within 5 km of their home; violent men may only enter a counseling program if the cost is heavily subsidized by the health authority.
- **E:** *Equity.* Social justice issues must always be considered. Groups like travelers and homeless teenagers might constitute a very small proportion of the population, but for equity reasons warrant special programs.

TARPARE can be usefully applied qualitatively and can also be represented as a weighted multi-attribute model, where each segment's overall score is the weighted sum of its scores on each of the attributes, where the weightings reflect the relative importance of each attribute:

Segment priority = $f (T.w_t + AR.w_{ar} + P.w_p + A.w_a + R.w_r + E.w_e)$

where w_i represents the weight attached to each factor, and:

T = Total number in segment
AR = % at (high) risk
P = Persuasibility
A = Accessibility
R = Additional resources required
E = Equity factor.

Cross-cultural targeting

Targeting subcultural groups has always been a dilemma for health promoters. Developing campaigns for a large number of small-sized ethnic groups would be prohibitively expensive and, in fact, is not always necessary. Pasick et al (1996), using a five-phase intervention model of problem identification, objective setting, theory, evaluation design, and implementation, proposed that the extent of cultural tailoring required depended on the relative importance of cultural versus other variables in each of these phases. For example, in applying the model to underage drinking amongst Aboriginal and non-Aboriginal youth in Australia, Donovan et al (1997) found a number of differences between non-Aboriginal youth and Aboriginal youth. However, they concluded that the problem identification, objective setting, and theoretical models for underage drinking were largely independent of cultural differences, but that cultural differences were important in expressing the content of the intervention materials and were crucial for implementation.

Individual tailoring

Prior to mass communications and supermarkets, personal selling predominated in all product and service areas, especially in non-urban areas. Good salespersons, while selling the same product to every customer, tailored their pitch to the idiosyncrasies of individual customers. After a few questions about the potential customer's lifestyle and hobbies, a car salesperson could emphasize the roominess of a station wagon for golf bag and buggy, or a child's bassinette and toys, or trade tools and equipment, depending on the potential customer's previously established needs and lifestyle. While each customer might receive a common sales pitch about certain aspects of the vehicle, each also received a customized or, in today's language, tailored sales pitch about how the vehicle met their individual needs.

The advent of computers and interactive technology has stimulated the development of tailored messages, as individual information can be entered and analyzed, and a customized message constructed and delivered in the one session.

The individual usually completes a questionnaire covering their beliefs, attitudes, and behavior with respect to the issue, usually based on some model of attitude–behavior change, and particularly the stage of change model. The program then matches the individual's responses with a number of predeveloped messages that incorporate the individual's information. Kreuter et al (2000) report that, in general, tailored messages outperform non-tailored messages, but not always, and not always substantially enough to warrant tailoring. More recent studies are investigating the type of tailoring that would be most effective.

TARGET BEHAVIORS

Each target group member is required to perform some action, the sum total of which leads to achieving the desired goal. Smokers are required to try to quit; legislators are required to vote for restrictions on smoking; GPs are required to ask their smoking patients to try to quit and offer a brief intervention; and so on. However, target behaviors can be looked at in a number of ways and formative research is necessary to establish what behaviors should be targeted.

 see D9

Intermediate behaviors versus end behaviors

Different target groups will have different behavioral objectives. For example, for condom use for sexually transmitted disease (STD) and unwanted pregnancy prevention, there are several target behaviors: condom purchase for those reluctant to publicly buy the product; carrying a condom or having a condom readily available for those who have purchased but feel uncomfortable carrying the condom; suggesting the use of a condom by those who have a condom available in spite of feeling they might then be accused of suggesting the intended partner might have an STD; actual use of the condom by those who are asked to use one; and so on.

Similarly, there are many situations where interventions are designed to attract people to seek assistance or further information about an issue. For example, people may be asked to attend a Tupperware-type gathering to learn how to prepare foods with a minimum of saturated fat; smokers may be asked to call a helpline for tips on quitting; inactive people might be asked to come along to a physical activity exposition and try some of the activities available.

With respect to this last point, it is useful to remember that in many cases the behavioral objective is 'trial' rather than 'adoption'. That is, we want smokers to *try* to quit, we want inactives to *try* to do more exercise, we want food preparers to *try* to change their cooking methods, and so on. In the same way, we want those already carrying out the desired behavior to *continue* to do so.

The 'Healthy Blokes' ad (see Fig D2.3), placed in the sporting news section of the daily newspaper, was designed to motivate blue collar men over 40 to have a regular health check (the project also aimed to increase awareness of the main risk factors for heart disease, cancer, and diabetes: poor diet and physical inactivity). Qualitative research indicated that men would respond to a car maintenance analogy and that health assessment 'scores' were likely to trigger action (Donovan & Egger 2000).

Ancillary or skilled behaviors

In many cases, the end behavior (e.g. quitting, condom use, cessation of violence) requires the acquisition of skills and knowledge without which the individual could not achieve the desired change. While most smokers quit without assistance beyond mass media advertising (and encouragement from other persons), other smokers benefit from helpline counseling, booklets with quit tips, or attending a quit program. Similarly, many young people would benefit from having negotiation skills when suggesting condom use and cessation of violence rarely occurs without formal counseling interventions that both teach skills and reframe attitudes.

i see D4, D6

Take five minutes to give your body a road test.

COMPLETE THIS QUIZ TO SEE IF YOU'RE DUE FOR A SERVICE!

Circle the number that answers each question best for you. Then add up your score at the end of each column.

NUTRITION

How many days a week do you eat at least 2 pieces of fruit?

Seven	4	
Five to six	3	One to two	1
Three to four	2	None	0

How many days a week do you eat a meal which includes vegetables?

Seven	4	
Five to six	3	One to two	1
Three to four	2	None	0

How do you spread butter or margarine on your bread?

Don't have	2	Thickly	0
Thinly	1		

How often do you eat fatty foods eg pies, pasties, sausage rolls ?

Seldom or never	3
Once or twice a week	2
Three or four times a week	1
Daily or almost daily	0

PHYSICAL ACTIVITY

How many days a week do you participate in physical activity that makes you puff?

Seven	4	One to two	1
Five to six	3	None	0
Three to four	2		

How long do you do physical activity each time?

Thirty minutes or more	3
Fifteen up to thirty minutes	2
Up to fifteen minutes	1
I do not exercise at all	0

How many hours do you sit each day (include home and work)?

Zero to eight hours	2
Eight to twelve hours	1
Twelve or more hours	0

How often do you drive the car when you could walk?

Daily or almost daily	0
Three or four times a week	1
Once or twice a week	2
Seldom or never	3

How often do you walk the dog or the family?

Daily or almost daily	3
Three or four times a week	2
Once or twice a week	1
Seldom or never	0

THE CHECK UP

When was the last time you had a check up with your doctor?

Within the last year	4
One or two years ago	3
Three or four years ago	2
More than four years ago	1
Never	0

Do you know the result of your last cholesterol check?

Yes	1
No/Haven't had one done	0

Do you know the result of your last blood pressure check?

Yes	1
No/Haven't had one done	0

Do you know the result of your last blood glucose check?

Yes	1
No/Haven't had one done	0

Do you know if you are in the healthy weight range?

Yes	1
No	0

7-8:   You are the full bottle about you — excellent!
3-6:   A check up in the near future is a good idea.
0-2:   Definitely make an appointment to see your Doctor.

11-13: You are doing well keep up the healthy diet.
5-10:   Umm...you could probably eat a bit better.
0-4:   You need help. Definitely call for information.

11-15: Well done — you must be a fit guy.
5-10:   There is always room for improvement.
0-4:   Leave the remote and go for a walk — NOW!

HEALTHY BLOKES

Disclaimer: The purpose of this quiz is to raise awareness only of your risk factors for cardiovascular disease and type 2 diabetes and certain types of cancer. Evidence proves that early intervention can make a difference.

Your body is like a car and the older it gets, the more important it is to get it serviced regularly. Start by using this quiz to see if you're in need of an overhaul. If your score is low, see your doctor for some practical advice or call 13 11 20.

Fig D2.3   Take five minutes to give your body a road test (reprinted with permission from the Cancer Foundation of Australia)

217

Strategies for increasing desirable behaviors versus decreasing undesirable behaviors

Many health promotion campaigns are aimed at *decreasing* the frequency of, or ceasing altogether, undesired behaviors: reduce excess alcohol consumption; don't drink and drive; don't speed; eat less fat; quit smoking; and so on. Other campaigns are aimed at *increasing* the frequency of or adopting desired behaviors: eat more fruit and vegetables; drink more reduced-alcohol products; walk to the bus stop/up the stairs/to the shop, and so on. In some cases the behaviors are directly inversely related; but not always so, and the question arises as to whether the emphasis should be on increasing the desired behavior or on decreasing the undesired behavior. For example, for targeting obesity in children, should we focus on reducing the time spent watching TV and playing video games (i.e. reduce inactivity) or increasing the children's level of physical activity? The answer will be supplied in most cases by research. However, regardless of the answer, behavior modification/applied behavioral analysis suggests that different strategies are appropriate for increasing behaviors versus decreasing behaviors.

Behavior modification is defined as 'the systematic application of principles derived from learning theory to altering environment-behavior relationships in order to strengthen adaptive and weaken maladaptive behaviors' (Elder et al 1994, p. 128). Table D2.2 delineates two methods for increasing a behavior (*reinforcement* strategies) and two ways of decreasing a behavior (*punishment* strategies) (Donovan & Henley 2003).

Two strategies *increase* the likelihood of a behavior being repeated.

- A pleasant consequence is experienced following the behavior (e.g. socializing with friends after exercising).
- Relief from an unpleasant experience follows the behavior (e.g. guilt and shame reduced after calling a men's domestic violence helpline).

Two strategies *decrease* the likelihood of a behavior being repeated.

- The behavior is followed by an unpleasant consequence (e.g. drug use followed by nausea; speeding attracts an on-the-spot fine).

Table D2.2 Behavior modification strategies		
Consequence	**Deliver consequence**	**Remove consequence**
Good experience	Positive reinforcement increases response	Negative punishment decreases response
Bad experience	Positive punishment decreases response	Negative reinforcement increases response

- The behavior is followed by removal of a positive benefit (e.g. exceeding the allowable blood alcohol level while driving leads to a loss of license and consequent limitations on mobility and socializing).

Other behavior modification implications are that a desired behavior will decrease if previously received rewards are no longer given (e.g. walking may decrease if aesthetic features of the environment are removed) and an undesired behavior may strengthen or reemerge if a punishment is discontinued (e.g. speeding behavior returns after enforcement by speed camera usage declines).

While these strategies apply primarily to direct behavioral interventions, all can be depicted and modeled in communication materials – most commonly as threat appeals.

CONCLUSION

Health promoters generally do not have the resources to develop campaigns and specific interventions for all subgroups of a target population. Where target groups do not differ in basic motivations, targeting can occur via different media channels and via different executional styles. However, where the target groups differ in basic motivations or require different products and services, then different campaigns or programs must be developed for optimal effectiveness. The most effective way to segment a population is via attitudes and behaviors with respect to the issue, because this more clearly defines the necessary communication and behavioral objectives for each target group.

Once the target groups are identified, it is essential to be clear about just what behavior is being targeted by the campaign. Communication campaigns, in most cases, can impact only on intermediate behaviors. Face-to-face interventions are generally necessary for end-behavior outcomes, many of which might involve skills learning.

References

Donovan R J, Egger G 2000 Men's health beliefs: a qualitative research report to the 'Healthy Blokes' project. Center for Behavioural Research in Cancer Control, Bentley, West Australia

Donovan R J, Henley N 2003 Social marketing: principles and practice. IP Publishing, Melbourne

Donovan R J, Owen N 1994 Social marketing and population interventions. In: Dishman R K (ed) Advances in exercise adherence. Human Kinetic Books, Champaign, pp 249-290

Donovan R J, Mick L, Holden S J S et al 1997 Underage drinking amongst Aboriginal and islander youth in the Northern Territory. Report to Northern Territory Department of Health, Donovan Research, Perth

Donovan R J, Paterson D, Francas M 1999a Targeting male perpetrators of intimate partner violence: Western Australian 'Freedom From Fear' campaign. Social Marketing Quarterly 5(3):127-144

Donovan R J, Egger G J, Francas M 1999b TARPARE: a method for selecting target audiences for public health interventions. Australian and New Zealand Journal of Public Health 23(3):280-284

Donovan R J, Francas M, Paterson D et al 2000 Western Australian 'Freedom From Fear' campaign targeting male perpetrators of intimate partner violence. Health Promotion Journal of Australia 10(2):78-83

Egger G, Donovan R J, Spark R 1993 Health and the media: principles and practices for health promotion. McGraw-Hill, Sydney

Elder J P, Geller E S, Hovell M F et al 1994 Motivating health behavior. Delmar, New York

Hastings G, Haywood A 1991 Social marketing and communication in health promotion. Health Promotion International 6:135-145

Katris P, Donovan R J, Gray B N 1996 The use of targeted and non-targeted advertising to enrich skin cancer screening samples. British Journal of Dermatology 135:268-274

Kreuter M, Farrell D, Olevitch L et al 2000 Tailoring health messages: customising communication with computer technology. Lawrence Erlbaum Associates, Mahwah

Lunn T 1986 Segmenting and constructing markets. In: Worcester R M, Downham J (eds) Consumer market research handbook. New Holland, Amsterdam, pp 287-424

McGuire W J 1985 Attitudes and attitude change. In: Lindsey G, Aronsen E (eds) The handbook of social psychology, vol II, 3rd edn. Random House, New York, pp 233-346

Pasick R J, D'Onofrio C N, Otero-Sabogal R 1996 Similarities and differences across cultures: questions to inform a third generation for health promotion research. Health Education Quarterly 23(suppl):142-161

Prochaska J O, DiClemente C C 1984 The transtheoretical approach: crossing the traditional boundaries of therapy. Dow-Jones/Irwin, Illinois

Rose G 1985 Sick individuals and sick populations. International Journal of Epidemiology 14(1):32-38

Rose G 1992 The strategy of preventive medicine. Oxford University Press, Oxford

Rossiter J R, Percy L 1997 Advertising communications and promotion management. McGraw-Hill, New York

Rossiter J R, Percy L, Donovan R J 1991 A better advertising grid. Journal of Advertising Research 31:11-22

Sheth J N, Frazier G L 1982 A model of strategy mix choice for planned social change. Journal of Marketing 46:15-26

Whitelaw S, MacHardy L, Reid W et al 1999 The stages of change model and its use in health promotion: a critical review. Health Education Board of Scotland Research Centre, Edinburgh

Motivating personal change　**D3**

Brian McMillan and Mark Conner

INTRODUCTION

The majority of theories applied to health-relevant behaviors examine the factors motivating individuals' behavior. If we can understand the factors motivating individuals to behave in certain ways, then we can theoretically influence these factors in ways that will either empower individuals who wish to behave more healthily (*control motivation*) or motivate those who do not, but would benefit from doing so (*choice motivation*). This chapter examines the differences between choice motivation and control motivation. We also outline the main models of behavior that have been applied to the area of health promotion and discuss how these models incorporate three kinds of expectancies: situation–outcome expectancies, action–outcome expectancies, and self-efficacy expectancies. We also examine the nature of control motivation and the implications for behaviors that require regular repetition or sustained effort. Potential shortcomings of these approaches are discussed along with suggestions for future research.

MOTIVATION AND VOLITION

A number of researchers have suggested that there are two processes involved in motivation (Heckhausen & Gollwitzer 1987, Kuhl 1984). Kuhl (1984) defines 'choice motivation' as the motivation to select a particular behavioral alternative and 'control motivation' as the motivation to expend effort to perform this behavior. In a similar vein, the Rubicon Model (Heckhausen & Gollwitzer 1987) suggests that action is best considered in terms of predecisional and postdecisional phases, both of which have associated mindsets. Taylor & Gollwitzer (1995) presented evidence to suggest that in the predecisional stage individuals are less biased in their evaluations of goals than they are in the postdecisional stage. In addition, after individuals have decided upon a goal, more attention is paid to information regarding the implementation of that goal than to other types of information, such as goal desirability.

Such findings suggest that attempts to motivate personal change should take a two-pronged approach: one that motivates individuals to choose healthier behaviors and another that enables them to enact these choices. The following sections consider the extent to which current theoretical approaches address these separate yet intertwined issues.

MODELS OF BEHAVIOR

Recent years have seen a proliferation of models that can be applied to understanding, predicting (Conner & Norman 1995, Norman et al 2000), and changing health behavior (Norman et al 2000, Rutter & Quine 2002). An in-depth description of each of these models is beyond the scope of this chapter and readers are instead referred to Conner & Norman (1995), Norman et al (2000), and Rutter & Quine (2002). Many of these theories propose similar accounts of the precursors of

motivation.

Table D3.1 shows the psychosocial theories most widely applied in the area of health behavior and illustrates the overlapping constructs within these theories. With the exception of the Transtheoretical Model (TTM) and the Health Action Process Approach (HAPA), these models are primarily concerned with the factors underlying choice motivation.

i see B5, B2

One major group of factors used to explain choice motivation in these theories fits under the umbrella of expectancies, and it is these that we consider next.

EXPECTANCIES

It is useful to consider expectancies in terms of situation–outcome expectancies, action–outcome expectancies, and self-efficacy expectancies (Bandura 1986). Situation-outcome expectancies are based on the perception that some consequences are determined by the environment. Action–outcome expectancies refer to beliefs about the consequences of performing a particular behavior, and self-efficacy expectancies refer to beliefs about one's ability to perform a behavior. Thus, in order to be motivated to change, an individual must believe:

- that not changing will pose a threat to their health (i.e. situation–outcome expectancy)
- that changing will reduce this threat (i.e. action–outcome expectancy), and
- that they are capable of changing (i.e. self-efficacy expectancy).

Many popular health interventions target the potential outcomes of not changing particular behaviors (i.e. situation–outcome expectancies); for example, the 2001 UK government TV campaign depicted a rear seat passenger killing his mother during a crash because he was not

Table D3.1 Summary of the overlapping constructs within theories widely applied to health behavior

Theory	Reference	Overlapping constructs			
		Outcome expectations	Control/Self-efficacy	Commitment to goal pursuit	
Health Belief Model (HBM)	Janz & Becker 1984	Perceived severity of illness, perceived benefits of action	Self-efficacy	General health motivation	
Theory of Reasoned Action (TRA)	Ajzen & Fishbein 1980	Outcome beliefs, normative beliefs		Intention	
Theory of Planned Behavior (TPB)	Ajzen 1991	Outcome beliefs, normative beliefs	Perceived behavioral control	Intention	
Protection Motivation Theory (PMT)	Rogers 1983	Advantages and costs of behavior	Self-efficacy, response efficacy	Protection motivation	
Social Cognitive Theory (SCT)	Bandura 1986	Outcome expectations	Self-efficacy	Proximal goals	
Transtheoretical Model (TTM)	Prochaska & DiClemente 1984	Contemplation stage	Preparation stage	Preparation stage, action stage	
Precaution Adoption Process Model (PAPM)	Weinstein & Sandman 1992	Deciding about acting	Decided to act	Acting stage, maintenance stage	
Health Action Process Approach (HAPA)	Schwarzer & Fuchs 1995	Outcome expectancies	Self-efficacy	Action plans	

wearing a seatbelt. Situation–outcome expectancies can be generated or modified through campaigns such as these, which focus on vicarious learning (see Bandura 1986) or through personal experience. The 'cues to action' component of the Health Belief Model (HBM) (Janz & Becker 1984) suggests that situation–outcome expectancies can also result from internal cues such as physical symptoms that may lead individuals to believe they might develop an illness if they do not change their behavior. The cues to action component also refers to situation–outcome expectancies that result from external sources, such as advice from a doctor. Interventions aimed at motivating personal change obviously need to stipulate sensible alternatives to inaction. One such example was a study by Jones et al (1991), which incorporated cues to action into their intervention aimed at motivating individuals to schedule and keep hospital appointments. They found that those receiving the intervention were three times more likely to schedule and keep appointments than a control group.

i see B3

Social cognitive theories of behavior typically focus on the expected outcomes of performing a behavior (action–outcome expectancies). The Theory of Planned Behavior (TPB) differentiates between normative outcome expectancies (i.e. the social approval or disapproval that a behavior would generate) and outcome beliefs (other potential consequences of performing a behavior). Several interventions have focused on the outcome beliefs component of the TPB in order to try to motivate personal change (see Hardeman et al 2002 for a review). Armitage & Conner (2002), for example, carried out an intervention that included a component aimed at strengthening positive beliefs and refuting negative beliefs about the outcomes of eating a low-fat diet (e.g. weight control and general health) and found that the proportion of fat consumed decreased by more than 1% in high-fat consumers. Even such a seemingly small reduction in dietary calories derived from fat could result in 10 000 lives saved in the USA alone (Armitage & Conner 2002). Parker (2002) included a normative belief video condition in her intervention aimed at reducing drivers' speeding and found that participants perceived others would be more disapproving of speeding after watching the video. Future interventions could usefully target significant others in attempts to change actual levels of disapproval, as well as targeting perceived levels of disapproval.

i see B2

Rewards also tap into the power of action–outcome expectancies to motivate change and have been used effectively to motivate a number of health behaviors, including increased consumption of fruit and vegetables (e.g. the 'Food Dudes' study: Tapper et al 2003). The authors of this study point out, however, that rewards should be used with caution, since rewards for a particular behavior can undermine the intrinsic motivation for that behavior. In their theory of self-determination, Deci & Ryan (1987) note that those who characteristically adopt an autonomous motivation towards a goal will remain task focused and task involved in the face of setbacks. Bearing this in mind, programs using rewards need to be designed in such a way as to suggest that the target behavior is both high status and enjoyable (Tapper et al 2003).

Action–outcome expectancies have also been targeted in interventions employing stages of change theories, such as the Precaution Adoption Process Model (PAPM: see Weinstein & Sandman 1992). For example, Weinstein & Sandman (1992) reasoned that a focus on possible outcomes would be effective in shifting individuals forward from the 'deciding to act' stage. They found that a video which aimed to convince individuals they had a moderate to high risk of finding unhealthy radon levels in their homes was more effective in shifting individuals forward from the 'deciding to act' stage than it was in shifting those who were already in the 'decided to act' stage. This suggests that, in terms of motivating people to change, information about the potential outcomes of a behavior may be less effective at strengthening control motivation than it is in stimulating choice motivation.

Self-efficacy expectancies are determined by factors such as mastery experience, vicarious learning, verbal persuasion, and physiological feedback (Bandura 1986). In this respect, self-efficacy differs from unrealistic hopes about possible success in that it is based more firmly on feedback from actual events and personal competencies. Self-efficacy has been incorporated into several theories of human behavior, including Protection Motivation Theory (PMT) and the TPB. In line with the suggestions of these theories, many interventions aimed at motivating personal change target self-efficacy or perceptions of control. For example, Lev et al (2001) found that a nurse-administered self-efficacy intervention, given to women receiving chemotherapy for breast cancer, improved self-reported quality of life and decreased symptom distress. Other successful interventions have included activities aimed at increasing perceptions of control over behaviors, such as condom use (Jemmott et al 1998) and testicular self-examination (Murphy & Brubaker 1990). Weinstein & Sandman (1992) found that providing individuals with a video showing how to test their homes for radon and an order form for a testing kit was successful in moving individuals forward from the 'decided to act' stage to the 'acting' stage.

i see B2

When attempting to motivate personal change, we should therefore aim to devise strategies that will enable individuals to change more easily, and do so in such a way that their perceptions of control will be heightened. However, individuals may feel a high degree of control over performing a behavior before they start, but find as they continue and reassess the situation that their perceptions of control diminish. The importance of self-efficacy beyond initiation of a behavior remains an issue of some debate (Weinstein et al 1998). The mechanisms by which individuals can maintain levels of motivation throughout a task are the concern of a later part of this chapter, but it is important to emphasize that individuals will not be motivated to change simply because they believe they can. The next part of this chapter is concerned with how individuals combine situation and action–outcome expectancies in deciding whether to act.

COST–BENEFIT ANALYSIS

It makes little sense to consider the potential and actual outcomes of a particular behavior without examining how individuals engage in a cost–benefit analysis of these outcomes. This part of the chapter examines how inaccurate cost–benefit analyses may motivate unhealthy behavior, how some of the major theories have explained the cost–benefit analysis process, and how encouraging individuals to engage in such analyses may be a useful tool for motivating personal change.

Unrealistic optimism is concerned with inaccurate situation and action–outcome expectations and refers to the finding that individuals generally believe negative events are more likely to happen to others than to themselves (Weinstein 1980). Several interventions have aimed at 'debiasing' this unrealistic optimism in order to motivate change. For example, Myers & Frost (2002) attempted to 'debias' smokers' unrealistic optimism by asking them to imagine a situation where they developed a severe health problem and to describe the consequences of this on their personal, social, and work life. They found that those who were originally comparatively optimistic did not display comparative optimism about developing heart disease and bronchitis post intervention.

The hedonic axiom that individuals strive to maximize desirable outcomes and minimize aversive outcomes underpins most theories of human motivation. The TRA/TPB, HBM, PMT, HAPA, and Social Cognitive Theory (SCT) all incorporate cost–benefit analysis components. While some theories, such as the HBM, have been criticized for not being specific enough about how this cost–benefit analysis takes place (Sheeran & Abraham 1995), the mechanisms proposed by others have also been called into question. The TPB, for example, employs the expectancy value framework to describe the cost–benefit analysis of positive and negative outcome beliefs, although many interventions based on the TPB have not examined multiplicative composites when deciding which beliefs to target (see Hardemann et al 2002). This is unfortunate, as the manner in which individuals weigh up the pros and cons of following a particular course of action may hold the key to understanding what motivates individuals to change. Bandura (1986) argues that the effects of outcome expectancies on intentions and behavior are partly governed by self-efficacy expectancies: even if outcome expectancy is high, performance of a behavior is unlikely if self-efficacy is low. This suggestion is echoed in Gollwitzer & Oettingen's (2000) account of the emergence of goals, which we consider next.

The assumption underlying theories such as the TPB is that humans are rational beings who will make use of the information available to them and that this in turn will influence intention, which is a reflection of motivation to act in a particular way. Gollwitzer & Oettingen (2000) argue that this conceptualization of motivation is unsatisfactory, partly because individuals do not always make use of all the information available to them and partly because an intention to act in a particular way may bear more similarity to a wish than a commitment. Their account of the emergence of goals offers an interesting alternative as it is concerned with how individuals may think about *states* rather than specific *behaviors*. Figure D3.1 is a simplification of Gollwitzer & Oettingen's (2000) conceptualization of the emergence of goals and has been included here as it offers useful insights into how we may be able to motivate personal change.

To help with the illustration, we will consider a state that an individual may wish to change (being overweight). Figure D3.1 depicts four possible paths that the overweight individual may follow. The first path, represented by the bottom box in the figure, is where the individual does not consider their current negative state nor do they engage in

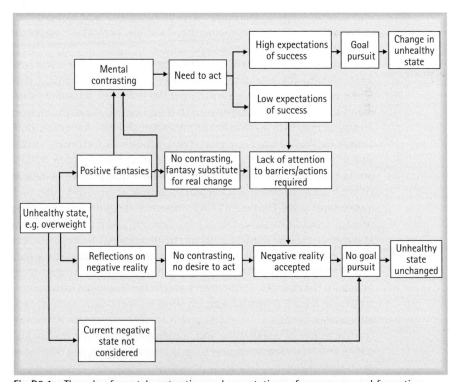

Fig D3.1   The role of mental contrasting and expectations of success on goal formation (based on Gollwitzer & Oettingen 2000)

positive fantasies about an alternative future. In this condition, no goal formation occurs and the individual's unhealthy state remains unchanged. The second path, represented in the figure as the line of boxes directly above this, is where the individual reflects upon the negative state that they are in, but does not consider the options. In this condition, individuals are not spurred to action by considering the options and thus accept their current negative state, do not form goals, and their unhealthy state remains unchanged. The third path is where an individual engages in positive fantasies about the future (e.g. being a healthy weight, being more attractive) but does not contrast these with the current negative reality. Gollwitzer & Oettingen (2000) note that although engaging in positive fantasies is encouraged by much of the 'self-help' literature, it can in fact be counterproductive. In this condition, an individual may enjoy their positive fantasy (such as being thin and attractive), an activity which Gollwitzer & Oettingen (2000) term 'anticipatory consumption', but because this fantasy is not contrasted with the current negative reality, a need to act is not generated. The final path, represented by the top row in the figure, is where an individual engages in both positive fantasies and reflections on the negative reality. In this condition the individual mentally contrasts these two options and this produces a need to act. However, Gollwitzer & Oettingen (2000) argue that this need to act will only be transformed into goal pursuit if an individual has high expectations of success. If an individual has low expectations, they face the unpleasant option of once again accepting their negative reality.

A number of studies have provided support for the suggestions outlined already. For example, Oettingen & Wadden (1991) found that obese women who engaged in positive fantasies lost around 11 kilograms less than those who engaged in reflections on the negative reality and women with positive expectations lost about 12 kilograms more than those with negative expectations. Studies by Oettingen (1996) found that children with gastrointestinal disease who engaged in more positive fantasies had higher disease levels and that positive fantasy in children with leukemia and lymphoma hampered recovery rate. In a longitudinal study, Oettingen (1996) measured the professional success of university students in terms of job offers and salaries. This study also found that positive fantasies hampered professional success whereas high expectations facilitated it. Other studies have suggested that encouraging individuals to engage in mental contrasting can spur them to action. For example, Oettingen et al (2001) encouraged mental contrasting in female students by asking them to think about an important interpersonal problem. They were asked to alternate between listing a positive aspect of a resolution and negative aspects of the current situation and their expectations of success were also measured. Other students were asked only to engage in positive fantasizing or ruminate on the negative reality. Those in the mental contrasting condition, who had the highest expectations of success, were subsequently found to initiate actions towards resolving the problem earlier than in the other conditions.

These findings suggest that if we wish to encourage individuals to form goals that will subsequently be turned into actions, there are a number of factors we should consider. It is not enough to simply encourage individuals to imagine what life could be like (if, for example, they were a non-smoker), and this on its own may in fact be counterproductive. Individuals who merely ruminate on the present undesirable situation may be equally unmotivated to act. Encouraging individuals to contrast the way things could be with the way things are, combined with strategies that heighten their expectations of success, on the other hand, would appear to be a useful way forward. Here we can see similarities between the work of Gollwitzer & Oettingen (2000) and Ajzen's (1991) TPB, where perceptions of control are thought to be directly predictive of behavior when they accurately reflect actual levels of control. The next part of the chapter considers how we might increase individuals' motivation throughout the process of changing.

CONTROL MOTIVATION

Many health behaviors (such as exercise) require regular repetition in order to be effective. Despite this, many theories provide unsatisfactory accounts of how motivation is maintained to ensure the consistent regular performance of a behavior over a prolonged period of time. The TRA/TPB, for example, suggests that intentions need to remain stable over time for a behavior to be maintained. Research supports the idea that stable intentions predict health behaviors over considerable periods of time (e.g. Conner et al 2002) but provides comparatively little insight into the determinants of intention stability. Similarly, the HBM seems better suited to predicting and explaining simple one-off behaviors. Although stage models seemingly deepen our understanding of the processes underlying personal change, many contain important flaws, such as definitions of stages based on arbitrary time periods (Weinstein et al 1998). Models are emerging, however, that acknowledge the need to consider the mechanisms underlying control motivation in more depth (e.g. the HAPA emphasizes the role of self-efficacy in maintenance: Schwarzer & Fuchs 1995).

Rothman (2000) has argued that there are different motivational processes underpinning the initiation and maintenance of health behaviors. As noted earlier, being motivated to initiate a behavior may be based on holding optimistic *action–outcome expectations* regarding future outcomes of performing that behavior. On the other hand, Rothman (2000) argues that the decision to maintain a behavior is more concerned with the desirability of the received outcomes associated with one's new pattern of behavior. Thus, remaining motivated to maintain a behavior is based upon the *perceived satisfaction* with the received outcomes. An important implication is that interventions that aim to heighten optimistic expectations of adopting a health behavior may increase the likelihood of initiation, but may also lead to reduced satisfaction when the optimistic expectations are not met and so undermine maintenance. In contrast, interventions to promote maintenance would need to increase perceived satisfaction with the received outcomes of a behavior change. Further work testing these different predictions is clearly needed.

Kuhl (1985) describes six self-regulatory strategies relevant to control motivation:

1 active attentional selectivity
2 encoding control
3 emotion control
4 motivation control
5 environment control, and
6 parsimony of information processing.

Attentional selectivity ensures that information relevant to the current intention is processed and that information regarding competing options is ignored. Those wishing to eat a healthier diet could, for example, ensure that they do not stop to examine the cakes and sweets aisle when doing their weekly shop. Encoding control refers to the selective encoding of aspects of a behavior that support the intention. For example, someone who is highly motivated to maintain his or her daily morning jog may retain the positive aspects of this experience (such as feeling refreshed afterwards) in memory, rather than the negative aspects (such as being out of breath). Emotion control refers to the need to promote emotional states consistent with the behavior and inhibit emotions that are inconsistent. Motivation control is similar to attentional selectivity except that it focuses specifically on strengthening the motivation to maintain the intention. Kuhl (1985) suggests that individuals may think about the consequences of not carrying out an intention as a strategy to maintain motivation (e.g. 'If I do not go jogging this morning I will feel guilty for the rest of the day').

Environment control refers to strategies that manipulate the environment to maintain motivation, such as entering into 'buddy' agreements or removing all smoking-related materials when trying to quit smoking. Finally, parsimony of information processing refers to the idea that individuals must know when to stop weighing up the pros and cons of a particular behavior in order to avoid being trapped in endless deliberation.

A number of Kuhl's ideas have been incorporated into Gollwitzer's (1993) work on implementation intentions. Implementation intentions are concerned with plans about when, how, and where an intention will be translated into behavior (e.g. I intend to exercise every morning between 8 a.m. and 8.30 a.m. by cycling from my house to work), and represent a greater degree of involvement than intentions alone. There is mounting evidence that encouraging individuals to form implementation intentions significantly increases the likelihood that they will perform a given behavior (e.g. Orbell et al 1997). What remains to be seen is if the idea of implementation intentions can also be used to motivate individuals to change unhealthy behaviors, such as smoking, and their effectiveness in maintaining behavior change.

CONCLUSION

Individuals are motivated to change by a wide variety of factors. Being aware of the potential negative consequences of a behavior is not enough to prevent that behavior being performed and being aware of the potential beneficial consequences of a behavior is not enough to ensure action. Simple behavior change approaches, which provide information about the risks and hazards or benefits of particular behaviors, are therefore likely to fail. Self-empowerment techniques, which include participatory learning such as the drama-based intervention described by Evans & Norman (2002), are more likely to succeed as they encourage individuals to become personally involved and develop self-regulatory strategies to increase their likelihood of success. Individuals' behavior, however, does not occur in a social vacuum. To motivate personal change, we need not only to empower individuals, but also to create a social and political climate that fosters personal change. Interventions need to focus on both choice motivation and control motivation if they are to bring about lasting change.

References

Ajzen I 1991 The theory of planned behavior. Special Issue: Theories of Cognitive Self-Regulation. Organizational Behavior and Human Decision Processes 50:179-211

Ajzen I, Fishbein M 1980 Understanding attitudes and predicting social behavior. Prentice-Hall, Englewood Cliffs

Armitage C J, Conner M 2002 Reducing fat intake: interventions based on the Theory of Planned Behavior. In: Rutter D, Quine L (eds) Changing health behavior. Open University Press, Buckingham, pp 87-104

Bandura A 1986 Social foundations of thought and action: a social cognitive theory. Prentice-Hall, Englewood Cliffs

Conner M, Norman P 1995 Predicting health behavior: research and practice with social cognition models. Open University Press, Buckingham

Conner M, Norman P, Bell R 2002 The theory of planned behavior and healthy eating. Health Psychology 21(2):194-201

Deci E, Ryan R M 1987 The support of autonomy and the control of behavior. Journal of Personality and Social Psychology 53:1024-1037

Evans D, Norman P 2002 Improving pedestrian road safety among adolescents: an application of the Theory of Planned Behavior. In: Rutter D, Quine L (eds) Changing health behavior. Open University Press, Buckingham, pp 172-192

Gollwitzer P M 1993 Goal achievement: the role of intentions. In: Stroebe W, Hewstone M (eds) European review of social psychology, vol 4. John Wiley, Chichester, pp 141-185

Gollwitzer P M, Oettingen G 2000 The emergence and implementation of health goals. In: Norman P, Abraham C, Conner M (eds) Understanding and changing health behavior: from health beliefs to self-regulation. Harwood, Amsterdam, pp 229-260

Hardeman W, Johnston M, Johnston D W et al 2002 Application of the Theory of Planned Behavior in behavior change interventions: a systematic review. Psychology and Health 17(2):123-158

Heckhausen H, Gollwitzer P M 1987 Thought contents and cognitive functioning in motivational versus volitional states of mind. Motivation and Emotion 11:101-120

Janz N K, Becker M H 1984 The Health Belief Model: a decade later. Health Education Quarterly 11:1-47

Jemmott J B, Jemmott L S, Fong G T 1998 Abstinence and safer sex HIV risk-reduction interventions for African American adolescents. Journal of the American Medical Association 279(19):1529-1536

Jones S L, Jones P K, Katz J 1991 Compliance in acute and chronic patients receiving a health belief model intervention in the emergency department. Social Science and Medicine 32(10):1183-1189

Kuhl J 1984 Volitional aspects of achievement motivation and learned helplessness: toward a comprehensive theory of action control. In: Maher B A (ed) Progress in experimental personality research, vol 13. Academic Press, New York, pp 99-171

Kuhl J 1985 Volitional mediators of cognition-behavior consistency: self-regulatory processes and action versus state orientation. In: Kuhl J, Beckman J (eds) Action control: from cognition to behavior. Springer Verlag, New York, pp 101-128

Lev E L, Daley K M, Conner N E et al 2001 An intervention to increase quality of life and self-care self-efficacy and decrease symptoms in breast cancer patients. Scholarly Inquiry for Nursing Practice 15(3):277-294

Murphy W G, Brubaker R G 1990 Effects of a brief theory-based intervention on the practise of testicular self-examination by high school males. Journal of Social Health 60:459-462

Myers L B, Frost S 2002 Smoking and smoking cessation: modifying perceptions of risk. In: Rutter D, Quine L (eds) Changing health behavior. Open University Press, Buckingham, pp 172-192

Norman P, Abraham C, Conner M 2000 Understanding and changing health behavior: from health beliefs to self-regulation. Harwood, Amsterdam

Oettingen G 1996 Positive fantasy and motivation. In: Gollwitzer M, Bargh J A (eds) The psychology of action: linking cognition and motivation to behavior. Guilford, New York, pp 236-259

Oettingen G, Wadden T A 1991 Expectation, fantasy, and weight loss: is the impact of positive thinking always positive? Cognition Therapy and Research 15:167-175

Oettingen G, Pak H, Schnetter K 2001 Self-regulation of goal-setting: turning free fantasies about the future into binding goals. Journal of Personality and Social Psychology 80(5):736-753

Orbell S, Hodgkins S, Sheeran P 1997 Implementation intentions and the theory of planned behavior. Personality and Social Psychology Bulletin 23(9):945-954

Parker D 2002 Changing drivers' attitudes to speeding: using the Theory of Planned Behavior. In: Rutter D, Quine L (eds) Changing health behavior. Open University Press, Buckingham, pp 138-152

Prochaska J O, DiClemente C C 1984 The Transtheoretical Approach: crossing traditional boundaries of therapy. Dow Jones Irwin, Homewood

Rogers R W 1983 Cognitive and physiological processes in fear appeals and attitude change: a revised theory of protection motivation. In: Cacioppo J T, Petty R E (eds) Social psychophysiology: a source book. Guilford Press, New York, pp 153-176

Rothman A J 2000 Toward a theory-based analysis of behavioral maintenance. Health Psychology 19(1)(suppl):64-69

Rutter D, Quine L 2002 Changing health behavior. Open University Press, Buckingham

Schwarzer R, Fuchs R 1995 Changing risk behaviors and adopting health behaviors: the role of self-efficacy beliefs. In: Bandura A (ed) Self-efficacy in changing societies. Cambridge University Press, Cambridge, pp 259-288

Sheeran P, Abraham C 1995 The Health Belief Model. In: Conner M, Norman P (Eds) Predicting health behavior: research and practice with social cognition models. Open University Press, Buckingham, pp 23-61

Tapper K, Horne P J, Lowe C F 2003 The Food Dudes to the rescue! The Psychologist 16(1):18-21

Taylor S E, Gollwitzer P M 1995 Effects of mindset on positive illusions. Journal of Personality and Social Psychology 69(2):213-226

Weinstein N D 1980 Unrealistic optimism about future life events. Journal of Personality and Social Psychology 39(5):806-820

Weinstein N D, Sandman P M 1992 A model of the Precaution Adoption Process: evidence from home radon testing. Health Psychology 11(3):170-180

Weinstein N D, Rothman A J, Sutton S R 1998 Stage theories of health behavior: conceptual and methodological issues. Health Psychology 17(3):290-299

Learning habits and skills

D4

Vivian Stevens

INTRODUCTION

This chapter will discuss the many considerations and methods for helping individuals make health-related behavioral changes over the short- and long-term. While there are various theories of health behavior – often with similar concepts and some with greater empirical support than others – a unifying theory of behavior change does not exist. Thus an integrated approach utilizing concepts from various theories will be discussed. Despite the range of theories, several areas of importance to health behavior change do emerge: the provider–patient relationship, patient motivation and perceived importance of change, self-efficacy, social support, and knowledge of specific skills, all factors which can be potentially affected by the intervention process.

Behavior change interventions rest on two basic assumptions:

- that behavior is affected by affective, cognitive, and environmental factors, and
- that maladaptive behavior can be unlearned and adaptive behavior learned.

Behavior change may involve acquiring a new set of behaviors, increasing or decreasing the frequency of existing behaviors, and maintaining changes over time. While the acquisition of new behaviors generally requires repetition, the rewarding aspects of some health risk behaviors (e.g. tobacco use) present particular challenges to health behavior change. Research on smoking has shown that successful long-term change is usually preceded by multiple change attempts (Fiore et al 2000) and, as noted by Schacter (1982), while a single attempt at health behavior change may be unsuccessful, over the course of a lifetime successful outcomes are possible. Even with an appreciation that behavior change typically takes time, clinicians may not get to observe such change among their patients, as it may come weeks, months, or years later. With successful outcomes often out of sight, it may feel futile to help, but even minimal intervention, such as brief physician advice to quit smoking, can lead to substantial change (Russell et al 1979). Among those who are not interested in change, intervention aimed at producing a shift across the 'stages of change' (Prochaska et al 1992) is a step in the right direction. This contemporary approach offers liberation from definitions of success based solely on behavioral end-points and creates an atmosphere in which the process of change itself is valued. Discouragement about the usual slow course of change can be replaced with realistic expectations and thoughtfully crafted interventions that meet individuals along their own trajectory of change.

It is also crucial to remember that it is the individual who must do the 'work' of change, with all that it entails (e.g. effort, personal discomfort, family disruption). A person's decision to initiate or maintain change is typically affected by many factors in addition to a health-care provider's specific recommendation (e.g. what effect will this change have on the quality of my life? Do I have the ability to change?). An appreciation of the multitude of factors influencing change, such as attitudes, cognitions, motivation, confidence, and the environment, can go a long way in developing an understanding of an individual's situation, in building a positive rapport, and in determining an appropriate course of action.

While influences on change are complex and multiple, this chapter will focus on the change process primarily within the context of the provider–patient relationship. Certain theories are emphasized in light of their prominence in the health behavior literature (Glanz et al 2002) and as a means to illustrate the application of theoretical principles to behavior change interventions. Many of the strategies used to promote and sustain behavioral change are rooted in learning theory and, more recently, cognitive theory. The next part of the chapter will review basic theories of learning and their application to the modification of behavior.

CLASSICAL CONDITIONING

A 33-year-old woman, who quit smoking 4 days ago, attends lunch with friends at a favorite restaurant, an activity she has not pursued since quitting. Upon being seated at the table, she experiences her most intense urge to smoke since cessation. She wrestles with the urge, trying to employ coping strategies that have worked in the past, but finds herself unprepared for the strength of her craving. She decides to give in to the urge to smoke on 'this one occasion', obtains a cigarette from her companions and lights up.

This scenario describes an example of classical conditioning: the urge to smoke has been classically conditioned to the cues in the restaurant environment and neutral stimuli that otherwise would not elicit an urge to smoke, through their repeated pairing with smoking, now have the capacity to do so.

Ivan Pavlov first described the phenomenon of classical conditioning while studying the digestive system. Pavlov observed that dogs would salivate when stimuli (i.e. a bell) that had been repeatedly presented just prior to meat powder were later introduced on their own. A reflex (i.e. salivation) was elicited by a stimulus (the bell) that otherwise would not naturally elicit this reflex. In this case, the meat powder is the unconditioned stimulus (UCS), salivation the unconditioned response (UCR), the bell a conditioned stimulus (CS), and salivation the conditioned response (CR).

Responses that are classically conditioned are sensitive to extinction: after a period in which the conditioned stimulus (i.e. the bell) is no longer paired with the unconditioned stimulus (i.e. meat powder), the CS will no longer elicit the conditioned response (i.e. salivation), and the CR will disappear. Assuming the woman above remains a non-smoker, a decrement in urges to smoke in response to restaurant cues would follow as this environment becomes disassociated with smoking. Stimulus generalization describes the phenomenon by which stimuli similar to the conditioned stimulus (e.g. bells with different sounding tones) elicit the conditioned response, even though there has been no pairing of these stimuli originally with the unconditioned stimulus (e.g. the smoker above experiences an urge to smoke when visiting a restaurant for the first time).

Counter-conditioning is a process in which a new response to a stimulus, through repeated pairings, replaces a previous response (e.g. rather than smoke in response to a craving, a man practices relaxation; a patient with a dental phobia learns to relax in response to a fear-evoking image of dentist's drill, thus replacing an anxiety response). Aversive conditioning is a process in which an unpleasant stimulus is repeatedly paired with an undesired behavior, resulting in a decrement in the behavior (e.g. an alcoholic takes medication that will cause nausea if alcohol is consumed).

 see B1

OPERANT CONDITIONING

Within several days of her initial smoking lapse, the woman resumes smoking at the rate of a pack per day. A month later she decides to make another quit attempt but experiences irritability and strong cravings upon cessation. Feeling unequipped to manage these symptoms, she abandons her goal of abstinence and lights up. Within moments, she experiences the pleasures of the ritual of smoking.

Operant conditioning, formulated by B F Skinner, is based on the concept that behavior is functionally related to its consequences. Behavior followed by positive consequences (reinforcement) will likely increase in frequency, while that followed by negative consequences (punishment) will likely decrease in frequency. In the above vignette, the woman's behavior of smoking is strengthened through its effect on removing an aversive stimulus, the unpleasant symptoms associated with nicotine cessation; this effect is known as negative reinforcement. Similarly, the pleasure she derives from smoking strengthens this behavior; this effect is known as positive reinforcement.

Not only do the consequences that follow behavior affect its course, but so does the pattern or schedule of reinforcement received. Acquisition of new behavior is most quickly achieved when reinforcement is immediate and continuous – that is, given immediately upon and with each performance of the desired behavior. Once behavior is established, intermittent reinforcement can be employed to maintain behavior; intermittent reinforcement is most effective at preventing the decay of behavior (Gambrill 1977). In the health-care setting, attention and praise by the clinician represent potent social reinforcers. However, opportunities to reinforce behavior are primarily limited to occasions when the patient is seen rather than with each occurrence of the behavior so reinforcement is at best intermittent. Similarly, the delivery of reinforcement is not likely to be given immediately after the desired response. To aid in developing new behavior and to sustain individual motivation, building in short- and longer term rewards can be useful (e.g. a man rewards himself by listening to his favorite music each day he exercises and then by purchasing a new CD at the end of the week). Discriminative stimuli are antecedents to behavior and cue whether reinforcement will likely follow a response.

When a behavior is no longer followed by positive consequences, it decreases and eventually extinguishes; this is known as extinction. Prior to reaching extinction, an extinction burst occurs, observed as an increase in the behavior that occurs when reinforcement is initially withdrawn. Two additional procedures are shaping and stimulus control. Shaping is a procedure in which successive approximations of a desired behavior are rewarded and stimulus control refers to engineering the environment in such a way as to govern behavior.

SOCIAL COGNITIVE THEORY

Determined to reach her goal of cessation, the woman seeks help from her physician. After discussing additional coping strategies and reflecting on her brief earlier successes with quitting (performance attainments), the woman feels confident (self-efficacy) that she can quit again and renews her commitment to do so. Although she again gets off to a rough start, she focuses on the benefits of cessation and remains smoke free a month later.

Social cognitive theory (SCT) (Bandura 1986) posits that behavior is reciprocally influenced by personal factors, the environment, and behavior. It also delineates methods useful in the modification of behavior, such as goal setting, reinforcement, and self-monitoring. A central premise of SCT is that learning can occur by observing others and in the absence of emitting a response or direct reinforcement. Observational learning (modeling) can efficiently transfer knowledge about behavior and its consequences, without the trial-and-error learning inherent in operant conditioning. Also central to SCT is self-efficacy, the belief that an individual can successfully engage in a behavior. Self-efficacy is a powerful determinant of behavior; greater self-efficacy leads to greater persistence in the face of obstacles. Enactive attainments (engaging in a behavior) are most influential in shaping self-efficacy judgments. Mastery experiences enhance self-efficacy, while failure can lower self-efficacy.

i see D6

i see B2, D3, D7

BEHAVIORAL ANALYSIS

As previously discussed, behavior is influenced not only by stimuli that precede it but also by its consequences. Behavioral analysis is a systematic attempt to uncover the functional relationships among antecedents (stimuli that act as triggers or cues for the occurrence of a behavior), behavior, and its consequences (responses following behavior). This assessment is an important step in planning behavioral interventions and provides an acute examination of the internal and external factors which influence behavioral chains. A behavioral analysis of the case vignette is shown in Figure D4.1.

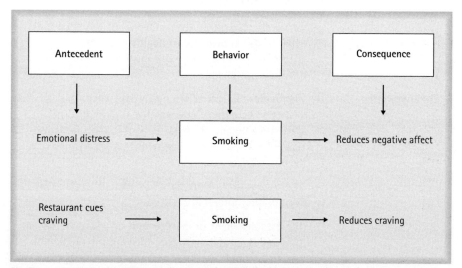

Fig D4.1   Behavioral analysis of cigarette smoking

STRATEGIES FOR BEHAVIOR CHANGE

The next part of the chapter describes behavioral and cognitive strategies that can be employed to promote health behavior change (See Meichenbaum & Turk 1987 for further discussion). Their use is likely to be maximized in the presence of other co-factors for change, several of which are shown in Box D4.1. 'Teachable moments' also create useful contexts in which to promote health behavior change and offer opportunities when individuals may be more receptive to the idea of change (Currie & Beasley 1982).

Individuals progress through specific stages during the course of change and it is important to recognize a person's stage of change when designing an intervention (Prochaska et al 1992). This part of the chapter presents a general overview of strategies to assist individuals who are considering change (contemplation stage) who have committed to change and are preparing for it (preparation stage) and who have undertaken change and are actively working to maintain change (action and maintenance stages). For those not ready to change (precontemplation stage), it is tempting to argue with them or otherwise try to convince them of the need for change, but this approach often results in greater defensiveness rather than openness to discuss a problem. Another approach, motivational interviewing (Miller & Rollnick 2002), is a client-centered approach that creates opportunities for individuals to articulate their own reasons for change, rather than confronting 'resistance' head-on. Motivational interviewing was originally developed for use with addictive disorders but is gaining popularity in addressing various health-related behaviors (Emmons & Rollnick 2001, Resnicow et al 2002).

i see B5

Box D4.1   Several factors which promote behavior change

Patient knowledge:	An awareness within the individual of the need for change and knowledge of health-relevant information (a necessary but insufficient condition for behavior change).
Collaboration:	A provider–patient relationship that values and respects the patient's perspective and invites the patient to be an active participant in care. Enhances patient satisfaction and adherence to health recommendations.
Readiness for change:	The recognition of the patient's stage of change in formulating intervention goals.
Social support:	The establishment or involvement of a support system that will buoy the individual through the predictable tides of change.

Specific skills

> The woman's friends comment on her success and ask how she was able to quit. She admits that talking with her physician improved her understanding of the risks to her health with continued smoking, which heightened her feelings of vulnerability to illness and strengthened her motivation to quit. She states that this encounter, combined with the use of specific cessation strategies, such as learning about her smoking triggers (self-monitoring), setting specific tasks (goal setting), and modifying her environment (stimulus control), proved beneficial to her. She adds that the positive attention (reinforcement) from family was also a 'nice bonus'. (See Box D4.2.)

SET GOALS

Goals should be realistic, specific, and measurable and of a short- and long-term nature. Proximal goals offer signposts from which self-evaluations of progress can be made and motivation strengthened for distal aspirations (Bandura 1986). Challenging attainable goals is more effective than simpler goals when individuals have the requisite skills (Meichenbaum & Turk 1987).

Box D4.2 Behavior change checklist

Be selective in determining target behaviors:	Making several changes at once can undermine change.
Elicit commitment:	Secure a public commitment, if possible.
Review past successes and problems:	Determine what helped, what did not.
Set specific goals:	Create goals that are specific, realistic, and measurable.
Plan a course of action:	Discuss specific skills and plans for change; offer choices where possible.
Anticipate problems before they arise:	Discuss expected obstacles and any previous relapse conditions.
Enlist support:	Identify individuals who can provide support.
Reinforce progress:	Reward steps towards change.
Be flexible where possible:	Individualize interventions, modify as necessary.
Maintain follow-up:	Assess progress; create accountability.

EMPLOY SELF-MONITORING

Self-monitoring can promote greater awareness of a behavior, reveal its antecedents and consequences, and also provide an interventional effect (Johnson & White 1971). For example, an individual's use of a smoking diary (in which the time, situation, mood, and intensity of smoking urges are recorded) might reveal consumption of a cigarette 5 minutes earlier. Based on this information, the individual might decide to postpone smoking and thus the act of self-monitoring has created a 'pause' in the usual behavioral chain and, in this instance, has brought a habitual event under greater self-control.

CREATE A HELPFUL ENVIRONMENT

Stimulus control refers to arranging the environment in such a way that it controls behavior. This can be achieved by incorporating cues in the environment that promote change and reducing cues that hamper change. Examples include removing smoking paraphernalia from sight, posting a sign on the refrigerator to be reminded of a personal weight loss goal, and eating meals only at the table rather than other areas of the house.

ENLIST SUPPORT

Social support can benefit the process of behavior change, as shown in the smoking cessation literature (Fiore et al 2000, Mermelstein et al 1986). Support may be derived from within the treatment setting (e.g. health-care professionals) or beyond it (e.g. family, friends, a change 'buddy').

MAXIMIZE OPPORTUNITIES FOR SUCCESS; ENHANCE SELF-EFFICACY

Drawing from SCT, it is not hard to appreciate how creating opportunities for success can enhance self-efficacy and thus facilitate change. Thus, creating goals that are likely to be met with success and breaking tasks into manageable steps when needed deserve consideration.

SUPPORT INCREMENTAL CHANGE

Based on the concept of shaping, incremental steps can be developed and rewards given for behaviors that approximate the eventual goal.

USE REINFORCEMENT

Reinforcement can help sustain motivation during the change process. Develop both short-term and long-term rewards. Rewards can be derived externally (e.g. family) and internally (e.g. improved self-esteem).

ENGAGE IN BEHAVIORAL REHEARSAL

Rehearsal of a desired behavior can provide 'practice runs', identify problems, and instill confidence.

EMPLOY CONTINGENCY CONTRACTING

A contingency contract creates a formal plan which outlines the reinforcement contingencies for behavior. It specifies the targeted behavior, identifies rewards and consequences, and articulates other aspects of the change plan, such as support persons to be involved.

ENCOURAGE INDIVIDUALS TO REFLECT ON THEIR PERSONAL REASONS FOR CHANGE AND THE BARRIERS TO CHANGE

Helping individuals to reflect on the pros and cons of change may tip the decisional balance in favor of change and uncover change barriers which can then be addressed.

PREVENTING RELAPSE

After 3 months of abstinence, the woman buys a pack of cigarettes after receiving some upsetting news (high-risk situation). She smokes throughout the day, feels guilty about doing so, and begins to have doubts about her ability to remain smoke free (abstinence violation effect). Craving a cigarette when drinking her morning coffee the next day and anticipating the pleasurable effect of smoking, she reaches for her cigarette pack. Within days, her cigarette use climbs to her pre-quit rate of consumption (relapse).

Successful health behavior change is frequently followed by a return to the undesired behavior. The commonality of relapse among health risk behaviors, specifically substance use, was reported by Hunt et al (1971), who noted similar relapse curves among persons treated for heroin addiction, alcohol abuse, and smoking: nearly two-thirds of the relapses occurred within 3 months of treatment. These observations underscore the need for clinicians to prepare themselves for the likelihood of patient relapse, as well as to aid patients in the development of skills for maintaining change.

Relapse prevention is a self-control program, developed by Marlatt & Gordon (1985), which focuses on the maintenance phase of behavior change. This program prepares individuals for potential lapses by identifying high-risk situations and developing coping strategies for managing these experiences. It aims to prevent a lapse from slipping into a full-blown relapse.

Research reveals that lapses are more likely to occur under certain situations: in the presence of negative affective states (e.g. anxiety, depression, boredom), interpersonal conflict, and social pressure (Marlatt & Gordon 1985). The 'abstinence violation effect' refers to the process that occurs with transgression to an undesired behavior. Whether a lapse progresses into a complete relapse is affected by the individual's response to this event. Responses that involve feelings of guilt and self-blame increase the likelihood of a relapse. Anticipating high-risk situations ahead of time, arming individuals with strategies for coping with these situations, and helping individuals to view a lapse, should it occur, as a learning opportunity rather than as a sign of personal inadequacy are useful methods for addressing lapse experiences.

ADHERENCE TO BEHAVIOR CHANGE RECOMMENDATIONS

The last part of this chapter will address the problem of non-adherence to health-care recommendations. Generally, rates of non-adherence increase for long-term and preventive regimens and those involving lifestyle changes (DiMatteo 1997, Meichenbaum & Turk 1987).

While many factors influence adherence, the importance of the provider–patient relationship in enhancing adherence is well documented in the adherence literature (Meichenbaum & Turk 1987). Adherence improves when patients are satisfied with the health-care provider and satisfaction increases when patients feel they have been listened to, treated respectfully, and are involved in their care. Other factors affecting adherence include (see Meichenbaum & Turk 1987 for a review):

- attitudinal factors (e.g. the perceived cost of adherence is too high)
- regimen-related factors (e.g. the regimen is too complex)
- illness-related factors (e.g. no apparent symptoms)
- knowledge-related factors (e.g. inadequate or incorrect knowledge)
- environmental factors (e.g. unavailability of clinic, no transportation)
- psychiatric factors (e.g. depression).

When behavior change stalls, examining adherence-related factors may get things back on track. The approach used to inquire about adherence is also important. Adherence problems are more likely to be detected through sensitive questioning (Nockowitz 1998) and statements that normalize adherence problems may be useful (Modest 2001); for example, 'Many people have problems keeping up with regular exercise routines when the weather gets cold. How has this been going for you?'.

CONCLUSION

Helping individuals make behavioral changes can be likened to a dance: if one person moves too far ahead of the other, the dance runs the risk of disintegrating. But if both partners move with an appreciation of the steps to be practiced, the distance to be covered, and the speed at which to proceed, then the dance is more likely to flourish and survive some missteps along the way.

This chapter has presented methods for use in promoting and maintaining health behavior change. While these methods are widely applicable to health behavior change efforts, the focus of their use in this chapter has been primarily within the context of the patient–provider dyad. The change process is affected not only by the individual but also by what the provider brings to this exchange. Showing respect, developing interventions consistent with agreed goals (where possible), expressing willingness to help when individuals are ready, and conveying hope in the capacity for change are basic aspects of this process.

References

Bandura A 1986 Social foundations of thought and action: a social cognitive theory. Prentice-Hall, Englewood Cliffs

Currie B F, Beasley J W 1982 Health promotion in the medical encounter. In: Taylor R B, Ureda J R, Denham J W (eds) Health promotion: principles and clinical applications. Appleton-Century-Crofts, Norwalk, pp 152-153

DiMatteo M R 1997 Adherence. In: Feldman M D, Christensen J F (eds) Behavioral medicine in primary care: a practical guide. Appleton and Lange, Stamford, pp 136-140

Emmons K M, Rollnick S 2001 Motivational interviewing in health care settings: opportunities and limitations. American Journal of Preventive Medicine 20(1):68-74

Fiore M C, Bailey W C, Cohen S J et al 2000 Treating tobacco use and dependence, clinical practice guideline. US Department of Health and Human Services, Public Health Service, Rockville

Gambrill E 1977 Behavior modification: handbook of assessment, intervention, and evaluation. Jossey-Bass, San Francisco

Glanz K, Rimer B K, Lewis F M 2002 Theory, research, and practice in health behavior and health education. In: Glanz K, Rimer B K, Lewis F M (eds) Health behavior and health education, 3rd edn. Jossey-Bass, San Francisco, p 31

Hunt W A, Barnett L W, Branch L G 1971 Relapse rates in addiction programs. Journal of Clinical Psychology 27(4):455-456

Johnson S M, White G 1971 Self-observation as an agent of behavioral change. Behavior Therapy 2:488-497

Marlatt G A, Gordon J R 1985 Relapse prevention: maintenance strategies in the treatment of addictive behaviors. Guilford Press, New York

Meichenbaum D, Turk D C 1987 Facilitating treatment adherence: a practitioner's guidebook. Plenum Press, New York

Mermelstein R, Cohen S, Lichenstein E et al 1986 Social support and smoking cessation and maintenance. Journal of Consulting and Clinical Psychology 54(4):447-453

Miller W R, Rollnick S 2002 Motivational interviewing: preparing people for change, 2nd edn. Guilford Press, New York

Modest G A 2001 Medical adherence: the physician–patient relationship. In: Noble J (ed) Textbook of primary care medicine. Mosby, St Louis, pp 16-20

Nockowitz R 1998 Enhancing patient compliance with treatment recommendations. In: Stern T A, Herman J B, Slavin P L (eds) MGH guide to psychiatry in primary care. McGraw-Hill, New York, pp 565-574

Prochaska J O, DiClemente C C, Norcross J C 1992 In search of how people change: applications to addictive behaviors. American Psychologist 47(9):1102-1114

Resnicow K, Dilorio C, Soet J E et al 2002 Motivational interviewing in health promotion: it sounds like something is changing. Health Psychology 21(5):444-451

Russell M A H, Wilson C, Taylor C et al 1979 Effect of general practitioners' advice against smoking. British Medical Journal 2:231-235

Schacter S 1982 Recidivism and self-cure of smoking and obesity. American Psychologist 37(4):436-444

Persuasion

Robert Cialdini, Jon Maner, and Mary Gerend

INTRODUCTION

Why do some interventions aimed at increasing particular health-protective behaviors succeed while others fail? Why do some physicians enjoy high patient compliance rates while others watch as their patients continue a disturbing trend of non-compliance?

Health professionals, practitioners, and communicators consistently deliver large amounts of information to patients and their families, as well as others in the health industry. Information about the costs and benefits of using hormone therapy, a physical therapist's recommendations to his clients about how best to care for their injuries, and a doctor's instructions to her patients regarding how to get the maximum benefit from a new medication may all be extremely useful pieces of information for people making decisions about their health. It would be marvelous if people were like computers, able to absorb all of the relevant health information, process it rationally, and arrive at informed decisions about how to behave in the best interests of their health. However, as many people in the health industry can attest, people are anything but computers. They often disregard very important health communications. They fail to comply with their doctors' recommendations. And they even behave in obviously health-damaging ways.

Might there be ways to improve the communication of health information so that people would be more likely to behave in ways that protect their health? Social scientific research strongly suggests that the answer to this question is a resounding 'yes'. This research has identified many of the key factors that can help health professionals enhance their attempts at affecting positive behavior change.

When people have both the ability and the motivation, they often think deeply about health-related communications and subsequently weigh all the information to come to an informed decision about how best to behave. However, most people are bombarded daily by information about issues like whether or not a new diet really works, how much exercise people need to stay fit, and the differences between good cholesterol and bad cholesterol. There is simply too much information for people to register it all. As a result, people use cognitive shortcuts or rules of thumb to help them decide what to make of a communication and, in turn, whether to comply with the recommended action (e.g. Chaiken et al 1989, Petty & Cacioppo 1986). Understanding these cognitive shortcuts can provide tools to enhance the persuasiveness of messages ultimately aimed at increasing health-protective behavior.

These cognitive shortcuts fall naturally into six categories, shown in Table D5.1, that describe commonly used principles of social influence (Cialdini 2001). And each of these shortcuts relates to at least one of three basic human motives:

1 wanting to behave effectively; that is, wanting to make the 'right' choices
2 wanting to build and maintain positive social relationships
3 trying to manage the way we feel about ourselves (i.e. self-concept and self-esteem) (Cialdini & Trost 1998).

These motives will serve to organize our discussion of the six useful principles for persuading people to engage in (or avoid) certain health-related (or risky) behaviors.

BEHAVING EFFECTIVELY

Effective decision making is essential for achieving one's goals. Indeed, making the right choices is a prerequisite for living an effective, healthy, successful life. Making the right choices about our health is particularly important for our survival. Because people are required to make dozens of important choices each day, they are often forced to rely on cognitive shortcuts that on average will lead them to make good choices.

Authority

A nurse at the local hospital is frustrated with the lack of compliance she has been receiving from her patients. After an early morning appointment with a man being treated for heart problems, she finds that patients seem particularly attentive to her suggestions and more willing than usual to follow her orders. It is not until her afternoon break that she realizes that she forgot to take off her stethoscope from her first appointment.

What might be the connection between the nurse's stethoscope and the increased compliance observed in her patients? Social psychological research indicates that *people are more easily persuaded by individuals perceived to be legitimate authorities*. Physicians, for example,

Table D5.1 The six principles of effective persuasion

Principle	Definition	Implication
Authority	People are more easily persuaded by individuals perceived to be legitimate authorities	Make visible the credentials of those who deliver health-care recommendations
Social proof	People often look to the behavior of similar others for direction about what choices to make	Make salient to patients the health-promotive actions of similar patients
Scarcity	People typically overvalue things that are rare, dwindling in availability or difficult to acquire	Highlight scarce or limited opportunities for engaging in heath-protective behavior
Liking	People prefer to say 'yes' to those they like	Point out areas of similarity and give genuine compliments
Reciprocity	People feel obligated to repay, in kind, what has been given to them	Give patients new information regarding their disorder
Consistency	People feel strong pressure to be consistent within their own words and actions	Have people make active, public commitments to their health, preferably in writing

are afforded substantial authoritative power in our society. Because we tend to view authorities as credible sources of information, they are particularly effective as agents of behavior change. Indeed, research suggests that nurses who wear stethoscopes, an emblem symbolizing a physician's expertise, are viewed as more authoritative than those who do not (Castledine 1996).

To maximize patient compliance, it is crucial that health professionals, particularly physicians, make the most of their authority. For example, whenever possible physicians should directly communicate instructions to their patients, rather than passing them indirectly through people who may be viewed as less credible in the eyes of the patient (e.g. a nurse, physician assistant, medical technician, etc.). Because this may not always be possible, physicians can emphasize to their patients the credentials and expertise of their co-workers so that they are also viewed as credible sources of information. In turn, these health professionals can increase their credibility by prominently displaying their diplomas, awards, and certifications (Redelmeier & Cialdini 2002).

Because people look to health professionals for credible information, such professionals also act as direct examples for how to behave in healthy ways. Indeed, healthy professionals and practitioners serve as better role models for others than less healthy professionals and practitioners do (Redelmeier & Cialdini 2002). For example, if a physician were to tell her patients to quit smoking and then was caught sneaking out for a smoke break, this would likely undermine her credibility. And chances are that an exercise therapist will be taken far less seriously if he recommends to a client a vigorous exercise program that his own appearance indicates he is not doing.

Social proof

Suppose that this year you decide that you are going to lose 10 pounds by getting more exercise. But how do you choose the route to your goal? Should you join an aerobics class or a yoga class or should you just take a run every morning? If you decide to join a health club, should you undertake the stationary bike or the treadmill? Most likely, you'll look outside yourself for at least part of the answer.

When uncertain and trying to make correct decisions about our health, *we often look to the behavior of similar others for direction about what choices to make.* Social psychologists refer to what people commonly do in a given situation as a *descriptive norm.* Descriptive norms typically provide people with useful information about which courses of action to take – if you find that the weekly yoga classes are generally popular, chances are that yoga would not be a bad choice. Looking

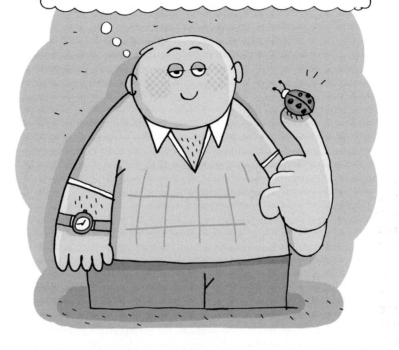

PERHAPS SPiDERS WOULD HANG AROUND PEOPLE MORE, iF THEY HAD PRETTY SPOTS...

to see what other people are doing is a quick and easy tool for making decisions in uncertain circumstances (Festinger 1954). Indeed, social proof has the greatest persuasive power when the 'right' choice in a given situation is somewhat ambiguous (Clark & Word 1972). For example, anxious people awaiting an anxiety-provoking medical procedure prefer to share a room with someone who has already undergone the procedure (Kulik & Mahler 1989), because such a person can provide useful information about what to expect (Kulik et al 1994). This finding should generalize to situations in which people have not yet decided whether or not to endure a difficult medical procedure. For example, physicians might recommend that a good candidate for a severe procedure speak with others (e.g. a support group) who have already been through the process – such people are in a special position to argue successfully that the procedure would be worthwhile.

Health communicators can also set their own descriptive norms by informing people that a particular behavior is normative. For example, a physician's declaration that most of his patients tend to choose the recommended activity over another option (e.g. 'Most of my patients opt for surgery over radiation therapy': see Crawford et al 1997) is likely to prove particularly persuasive. Evidence also suggests that people tend to seek information especially from those who are similar to them (Miller & Zimbardo 1997). Health professionals and behavior change specialists can use this knowledge to their advantage. For example, they might communicate that a particular behavior is increasing among a certain group of people ('More and more people *your age* are starting to take walks on their lunch breaks to squeeze in some exercise during the day').

When highlighting descriptive norms, however, it is important not to normalize potentially health-damaging behaviors by emphasizing their prevalence in the population. For example, there is evidence that, by having students repeatedly practice how to resist their peers' attempts to persuade them to use alcohol, some school-based alcohol prevention programs may have inadvertently increased students' perceived prevalence of drinking among peers. As a result, this prevention program appeared to have increased rather than decreased student acceptance of alcohol use (Donaldson 1995).

Scarcity

Imagine that you are sitting in your doctor's office and have just learned that you are at increased risk for developing diabetes. Sensing your distress, your doctor tells you about a new diabetes prevention trial beginning next month. After telling you this information she adds: 'I've recently learned that there are only a few spaces left, so I would call for information as soon as possible'. How might knowing that there are only a limited number of openings in the trial motivate you to make that call?

People typically associate greater value with things that are rare, dwindling in availability, or difficult to acquire. One reason for this is that people tend to reason that if something is scarce or hard to come by, many others must want it. Prompting the use of the mental shortcut of scarcity can motivate positive health behavior change (Redelmeier & Cialdini 2002). Whether it is the only remaining seat in a community nutrition class, exclusive information about a limited clinical trial, or the last lecture on the benefits of getting regular mammograms to detect breast cancer, knowing that something is scarce often makes it more desirable.

BUILDING AND MAINTAINING SOCIAL RELATIONSHIPS

Of all the motivations guiding people's behavior, fostering positive social relationships with others is perhaps the most far reaching. Wanting to be accepted and liked by others shapes a vast array of decision-making processes, from what to wear and what to eat to how we should exercise and take care of our health.

Liking

Imagine that while watching TV you see an advertisement touting the advantages of a new drug designed to alleviate allergy symptoms like those that afflict you. Depicted is a popular television actor who, despite sitting in a field of grass and pollen-laden flowers, seems quite content and clear headed. If you are like millions of people exposed to such advertising in the past few years, you might head for the nearest pharmacy to purchase the product.

It is, in fact, no coincidence that advertisers typically portray popular, attractive, well-liked individuals alongside their products. Put simply, people prefer to say 'yes' to those they like. What characteristics influence people's liking for others? First, people tend to like others who are similar to them (e.g. Suls et al 2000). For example, an exercise promoter wishing to persuade audience members to enhance their exercise regimens might point out areas of similarity she shares with her audience (e.g. like them, she was once not in the best physical shape but, like them, she wanted a healthy, well-rounded lifestyle). Second, people tend to like others who are physically attractive. Physically attractive people are generally thought to possess a variety of other positive characteristics (Eagly et al 1991), including more intelligence, authority, and expertise. Consequently, well-groomed, professionally dressed individuals tend to be more persuasive. Third, and above all, we like people who seem to like us (Cialdini 2001). As this evidence would suggest, friendly, charismatic, well-liked physicians tend to be particularly persuasive among patients and colleagues (Buston & Wood 2000, Davis et al 1995).

Reciprocity

Consider the following scenario. While you are walking on the street, a Red Cross volunteer approaches and asks if you would be willing to participate in a long-term blood donor program by donating a unit of blood every 60 days for the next 3 years. Thinking of the time this would require (and of the pile of work waiting for you on your desk) you tell the volunteer that, no, you don't think you can make such a commitment. The volunteer responds, 'I understand. In that case, would you be willing to help us with a one-time donation sometime this week?'. With some hesitation, you say 'okay' and agree to this more reasonable request.

A study by Cialdini & Ascani (1976) presented participants with this very scenario. What the researchers found was quite interesting. Those people who declined to participate in the long-term donor program (as nearly all did) subsequently agreed to the one-time donation substantially more often than people who were simply asked straight away to offer a one-time donation (49.2% vs 31.7%). This study exemplifies the principle of reciprocity: people feel obligated to repay in kind what has been given to them. In this case, the volunteer granted the potential donor a concession – retreating from the larger request to the smaller request. In turn, donors felt obligated to repay the volunteer with a reciprocal concession – agreeing to the smaller one-time donation. The power of reciprocity is unequivocal; not only did those people who reciprocated agree to the smaller donation more often than those who were only presented with the smaller request, when those people arrived at the donation center they were also more likely to volunteer for future donations (Cialdini & Ascani 1976).

In another version of the reciprocal concessions technique, a health practitioner might advise patients to engage in the most beneficial (likely also to be the most difficult) regimen appropriate for their condition (Sensenig & Cialdini 1984). If the practitioner finds that his patients fail to comply with the recommended plan, he might then suggest, as a concession, a somewhat easier regimen. In using this approach, there is the chance for two kinds of success. Some patients will comply with the most beneficial regimen, which is to everyone's advantage, but those who don't should be more likely to comply with the more moderate (but still effective) plan than they would had the practitioner suggested only that one.

The principle of reciprocity does not only apply to concessions – it pertains to the exchange of other types of resources as well. For example, in persuading her clients to adhere to a special diet, a nutritionist might provide them with the newest relevant information or even provide them with free referrals to other valuable fitness programs. There is one caveat to the principle of reciprocity: for it to be effective, people must be able to view one's favor or gift as sincere; if they see it simply as an attempt to persuade, the strategy can backfire.

MANAGING OUR SELF-CONCEPT

A ubiquitous part of human nature is that people strive to feel good about themselves. People generally behave in ways that help them maintain or enhance their self-esteem. This includes behaving in accordance with one's important values and beliefs; when our behavior is consistent with who we are and what we value, it makes us feel good (Sheldon & Elliot 1999).

Consistency

Imagine that you are a medical receptionist. A patient has just seen her
physician and is waiting to schedule a follow-up appointment. Should you
fill out the patient's reminder card or might it be better to have the patient fill
out the card herself?

Decades of social science research suggest why the latter procedure
should be preferred: *people feel strong pressure to be consistent within
their own words and actions* (Baumeister et al 1994, Festinger 1957).
Making a commitment ties a person's sense of self to a particular course
of action. Asking the patient to fill out her own form establishes a basis
for consistency – failing to return for her scheduled appointment
would be inconsistent with her earlier commitment (see Sensenig &
Cialdini 1984).

There are several conditions in which consistency tends to have maximum impact. First, the person's commitment should be *active* and
effortful (Aronson & Mills 1959, Bem 1967). Indeed, in the aforemen-
tioned example, having the patient fill out the card herself, rather than
simply handing one to her, should enhance her sense of commitment.
And in general, the greater the effort, the greater the resulting sense
of commitment will be. Second, the commitment should be public
(Deutsch & Gerard 1955). Watching the patient fill out her reminder card
should increase the probability of her return, whereas simply handing
her the card and allowing her to fill it out by herself in the waiting room
would likely be much less effective. Indeed, one of the linchpins of the
consistency principle is that people don't like to *appear* inconsistent to
others. Third, the commitment should be (or at least appear to be) freely
chosen (Freedman 1965). Commanding the patient to fill out her own
card would not be nearly as effective (since the commitment would not
be internally motivated) as suggesting to the patient that she write her
own reminder, giving her the sense that her action was freely chosen.

As another example, a physical therapist might ask his clients to
write a contract listing their recovery goals. This contract would then
serve as a public expression of each client's commitment. Along the
same lines, smokers wishing to rid themselves of their habit would be
well advised to make public their commitment to quitting, for example
by voicing their resolution to close friends and family (see Cialdini
2001). This public declaration would likely increase the probability of
the quitter's success.

Finally, if a particular health improvement process proves difficult,
one might use a strategy involving several small steps. For example, asking a physical therapy patient to start off with small, relatively easy
steps (e.g. starting with simple, painless exercises) should foster a sense
of commitment. Consequently, that sense of commitment should

increase the likelihood that the patient will see the therapy through to its completion.

CONCLUSION

There are five final points we would like to make regarding the use of the principles we have described. First, although these principles are conceptually distinct, health communications are likely to be most effective at fostering positive behavior change when integrating several of these principles at once. For example, consider a health practitioner who kindly offers her client one of a limited number of quickly disappearing slots in a special health intervention trial. She might also point out that in her expert opinion, the trial is a valuable opportunity and very much in line with the client's own health goals. In doing so, the practitioner is using each of the principles we have described: liking, reciprocity, social proof, scarcity, authority, and consistency.

Second, it should be clear that although people use these mental shortcuts when making decisions, this is not to say that it happens *consciously*. For example, someone is unlikely to say to himself, 'Well, I've gotten this far in my physical therapy. My sense of commitment dictates that I continue!'

Third, it is important to realize that the reason people use these shortcuts is because, on average and in most circumstances, they tend to appropriately steer people in the right direction. That is, people are not being stupid or making mistakes when they use these mental heuristics to guide their choices.

Fourth, because much health information is highly relevant to their goals, people may consequently be motivated (although not always able) to deeply process the content of these messages. Indeed, the effectiveness of a message will depend upon a combination of the substance of the message and the way that message is delivered. Thus, the principles we have discussed are not an alternative to providing people with substantive health information.

Finally, knowing how to harness these powerful principles of persuasion never gives license to use them unscrupulously. Indeed, in trying to persuade others, health communicators should ethically appeal to genuine authority figures, bona fide social proof, real similarities and compliments, sincere favors, true scarcity, and existing commitments to health-enhancing and protective goals.

References

Aronson E, Mills J 1959 The effect of severity of initiation on liking for a group. Journal of Abnormal and Social Psychology 59:177-181

Baumeister R F, Stillwell A M, Heatherton T F 1994 Guilt: an interpersonal approach. Psychological Bulletin 115:243-267

Bem D J 1967 Self-perception: an alternative interpretation of cognitive dissonance phenomena. Psychological Review 74:182-200

Buston K M, Wood S F 2000 Non-compliance among adolescents with asthma: listening to what they tell us about self-management. Family Practice 17:134-138

Castledine G 1996 Nursing's image: it is how you use your stethoscope that counts. British Journal of Nursing 5:882

Chaiken S, Liberman A, Eagly A H 1989 Heuristic and systematic processing within and beyond the persuasion context. In: Uleman J S, Bargh J A (eds) Unintended thought. Guilford, New York, pp 212-252

Cialdini R B 2001 Influence: science and practice, 4th edn. Addison Wesley Longman, Boston

Cialdini R B, Ascani K 1976 Test of a concession procedure for inducing verbal, behavioral, and further compliance with a request to give blood. Journal of Applied Psychology 61:295-300

Cialdini R B, Trost M R 1998 Social influence: social norms, conformity, and compliance. In: Gilbert D, Fiske S, Lindzey G (eds) The handbook of social psychology, vol 2, 4th edn. McGraw-Hill, New York, pp 151-192

Clark R D III, Word L E 1972 Why don't bystanders help? Because of ambiguity? Journal of Personality and Social Psychology 24:392-400

Crawford E D, Bennett C L, Stone N N et al 1997 Comparison of perspectives on prostate cancer: analyses of survey data. Urology 50:366-372

Davis D A, Thomson M A, Oxman A D et al 1995 Changing physician performance: a systematic review of the effect of continuing medical education strategies. Journal of the American Medical Association 274:700-705

Deutsch M, Gerard H B 1955 A study of normative and informational social influences upon individual judgment. Journal of Abnormal Psychology 51:629-636

Donaldson S I 1995 Peer influence on adolescent drug use: a perspective from the trenches of experimental evaluation research. American Psychologist 50:801-802

Eagly A H, Ashmore R D, Makhijani M G et al 1991 What is beautiful is good, but ... A meta-analytic review of research on the physical attractiveness stereotype. Psychological Bulletin 110:109-128

Festinger L 1954 A theory of social comparison processes. Human Relations 7:117-140

Festinger L 1957 A theory of cognitive dissonance. Stanford University Press, Stanford

Freedman J L 1965 Long-term behavioral effects of cognitive dissonance. Journal of Experimental Social Psychology 1:145-155

Kulik J A, Mahler H I M 1989 Stress and affiliation in a hospital setting: preoperative roommate preferences. Personality and Social Psychology Bulletin 15:183-193

Kulik J A, Mahler H I M, Earnest A 1994 Social comparison and affiliation under threat: going beyond the affiliate-choice paradigm. Journal of Personality and Social Psychology 66:301-309

Miller N, Zimbardo P 1997 Motive for fear-induced affiliation: emotional comparison or interpersonal similarity? Journal of Personality 34:481-503

Petty R E, Cacioppo J T 1986 Communication and persuasion: central and peripheral routes to attitude change. Springer, New York

Redelmeier D A, Cialdini R B 2002 Problems for clinical judgment: principles of influence in medical practice. Canadian Medical Association Journal 166:1680-1684

Sensenig P E, Cialdini R B 1984 Social-psychological influences on the compliance process: implications for behavioral health. In: Matarazzo J D, Weiss S M, Herd J A et al (eds) Behavioral health: a handbook of health enhancement and disease prevention. Wiley, New York, pp 384-392

Sheldon K M, Elliot A J 1999 Goal-striving, need satisfaction and longitudinal well-being: the self-concordance model. Journal of Personality and Social Psychology 76:482-497

Suls J, Martin R, Wheeler L 2000 Three kinds of opinion comparison: the triadic model. Personality and Social Psychology Review 4:219-237

Interpersonal communication

Donald Cegala

INTRODUCTION

The scope of this chapter is severely limited by the breadth and diversity of communicative functions and contexts, as well as other complex aspects of the interpersonal communication process. Regarding the former, communication skills interventions may be directed to a wide assortment of functions and contexts, among them individuals' informative skills; competence in persuasion, argumentation, negotiation, conflict management, or group decision making; skills in providing social support, establishing and/or maintaining romantic or friendship relationships; and interacting with children, to name only a few (Green & Burleson 2003). As for the latter, interpersonal communication is a complex process involving cognitive, affective, and behavioral components that vary both individually and situationally in ways that are not completely understood (Spitzberg 1986, Spitzberg & Cupach 1984).

Thus, no single chapter, or even volume, could possibly address all or even the most relevant issues to consider in developing behavioral interventions for changing a variety of interpersonal communication skills. At best, this chapter identifies a few basic principles to consider in developing interpersonal communication skills interventions and illustrates application of these principles within the context of communication skills training for physicians and patients.

While the principles are illustrated with reference to communication skills training for physicians and patients, it should be noted that interpersonal communication skills training has a much broader application in the health-related arena. For example, increasing attention is being paid to the role of interpersonal communication and alcoholism, especially within the family context (Jacob & Seilhamer 1987). Many alcoholics experience interpersonal problems, which are thought in turn to stimulate problem drinking. Interestingly, this relationship extends to work on substance abuse prevention with children and adolescents. Social skills training is often used to address problems in social functioning among children and adolescents who are prone to substance abuse. Other work has shown the importance of interpersonal communication and health promotion with such widely varying topics as dietary behaviors (Rimal 2003), adolescent diabetes (Seiffe-Krenke 2002), and giving advice about smoking during pregnancy (Dunn et al 2003). Overall, this research shows that communication skills training for family members, friends, and co-workers is often critical to promoting and maintaining healthy choices and lifestyles among target individuals.

IDENTIFYING AND DEFINING COMMUNICATION GOALS

Although significant parts of communication are sometimes enacted in a scripted fashion, somewhat 'mindlessly' or at least habitually (Langer 1978), there are many instances in which communication is reasonably consciously goal directed (O'Keefe & Delia 1982, Tracy 1991). Most of the interest in intervention development is concerned with these instances of conscious, goal-directed communication (e.g. skills in persuasion, negotiation, social support, etc.). Accordingly, it is fundamentally important to identify and specify the communication goals that are to be targeted in an intervention.

McFall (1982) offers an approach to social skills training that provides useful guidelines regarding functions and contexts, among other things. McFall developed his model in response to perceived pitfalls associated with trait and molecular approaches to social skills training. Among the useful ideas in McFall's model is his recommendation to conduct a *task analysis*, which consists of several steps. A brief description of these steps follows.

First, one must clearly specify the purpose for which a performance (in this case, communicative performance) is designed. Second, the constraints affecting a particular task's performance should be specified. For example, in designing an intervention to help patients ask questions of physicians during a medical interview, it is potentially important to determine a patient's knowledge of, say, treatment options associated with their medical problem and/or how comfortable the patient feels about asking a physician questions. Third, the setting in which the behavior is to be performed must be taken into consideration in assessing how the task may be most appropriately done. With respect to communication skills training, a significant part of any setting includes (but is not limited to) individual differences that are important to appropriate message adaptation, such as sex, age, ethnicity, and cultural factors. In training physicians to provide diagnostic and treatment information, for example, it may be necessary to address how ethnic and cultural factors influence patients' health beliefs about the causes and cures of disease. A related and fourth step is understanding the social rules governing a particular task. For example, status and power differences between patients and physicians may suggest that the rules for challenging a physician's treatment recommendation are different from the rules for disagreeing with a friend or relative. A fifth step in conducting a task analysis is identifying the criteria for distinguishing between adequate and inadequate task performances. The complexity and limited control over the sequential structure of interpersonal communication (Sanders 2003) underscore that there is usually more than one way to accomplish a task effectively. Thus, the definition of competent communication cannot be held to a single, rigid behavior or sequence of behaviors. The ultimate criterion is the outcome or effect of the message, within the limitations of appropriateness suggested by step four. Finally, McFall recommends that a task analysis be conducted from a systems perspective, meaning that one should examine how performance on one task relates to other aspects of an individual's life-system.

We used parts of McFall's (1982) model to guide our initial work in developing a communication skills training intervention for patients. The following is a description of the steps used in identifying and defining the skills that ultimately were addressed in an intervention called the PACE System (Cegala et al 2000a,b, 2001).

Several reviews of the literature in physician–patient communication suggested that the medical interview context has two primary communicative functions: information exchange and relational development. Since we were interested in developing patient communication skills, we focused on information exchange because virtually all of the attention to relational development is physician directed. Our direct observations of patients during medical interviews provided several ideas about what information exchange goals were appropriate for the intervention. The literature on patient communication skills training was also helpful, but unfortunately it is not nearly as extensive as research on physician communication (Anderson & Sharpe 1991, Cegala & Broz-Lenzmeier 2003). Indeed, the relative lack of attention to patient communication skills training suggested that additional work was needed.

Two of our preliminary studies proved to be important steps in identifying and confirming essential skills for the intervention (Cegala et al 1996, 1998). In Cegala et al (1996), we asked a sample of patients and physicians to rate self and other communication on a single, 7-point, Likert scale, then to provide a description of the behavior(s) that led them to the judgment they just made. The results confirmed the importance of information exchange skills in physicians' and patients' perceptions of self and other communication competence during a medical interview. The results also suggested that the goals of information provision, information seeking, and information verifying were central to perceptions of competent communication. We then used these results to develop the Medical Communication Competence Scale and administered it to a sample of physicians and patients (Cegala et al 1998). Together, these studies confirmed the utility of focusing on information provision, seeking, and verifying as the main goals of our intervention.

We were especially pleased that these communicative functions were seen by *both* physicians and patients as important aspects of information exchange during the medical interview. More recently, we replicated the Cegala et al (1996) study with a larger sample of physicians and patients and found continued support for the perceived relevance of the three primary communication skills (Cegala et al 2004).

In summary, it is essential to identify and define the behavioral goals of an interpersonal communication intervention. Doing this in more than one way is highly recommended. While literature reviews are necessary and often helpful, we found that surveying patients (and physicians) first in an open-ended manner then with a close-ended scale was most helpful in identifying and confirming relevant intervention goals for the context in which we were working. Additionally, by examining both physicians' and patients' views we were able to identify communication skills that were valued by the key parties in the communication context of interest.

One of McFall's (1982) suggestions is to conduct a task analysis from a systems perspective, emphasizing intra-individual relationships between intervention behaviors and other aspects of the trainee's life-system. While this is important, our approach in focusing on both physicians and patients suggests how a systems approach can be applied, with respect to inter-individual aspects of the context to which the intervention is directed. This may not always be possible but when it is, such an approach can provide valuable insight into the essential communicative (i.e. interactive) goals that an intervention should address.

COMMUNICATION SKILLS TRAINING REQUIRES MODELING AND PRACTICE

So much of our interpersonal communication is done in a taken-for-granted manner that its true complexity is often underestimated. Interpersonal communication skills training requires an intervention strategy that relies heavily on modeling and practice with feedback.

Modeling

Modeling is widely used among social skills trainers because it is an effective way to teach a complex social behavior, such as interpersonal communication (Liberman et al 1989). The function of modeling is to demonstrate effective and sometimes ineffective applications of behaviors and/or behavior sequences. Seeing others perform a behavior is a more effective way of learning what to do (or not do) than is merely reading about the behavior or listening to a lecture. Some reading or discussion about the behavior prior to seeing it modeled is often useful, and in some instances necessary, but this should serve more as introductory or background information rather than the primary means of teaching the skill.

Bandura (1997), Trower (1995), and others have offered several guidelines for increasing the likelihood of successfully promoting the acquisition of a new behavior through modeling. One suggestion is to employ multiple models demonstrating the same behavior or to use a single model repeating the behavior, perhaps in different contexts. Either approach takes advantage of repetition and, thus, tends to enhance learning. The use of multiple models has an added advantage of allowing trainees to see several people performing the behavior, thus lessening the belief that only a few, super-capable people are able to enact the skill.

A second guideline is to employ models that are similar to the trainee in age, sex, ethnicity, and other relevant characteristics. Models who are similar to trainees implicitly send a message indicating that they too are capable of performing the modeled behavior. A third guideline reflects a cornerstone of learning theory: when models are rewarded for their behavior, observers are more likely to enact the observed behavior (Bandura 1986). Thus, if modeling includes a second actor who rewards the modeler, the process will be more effective.

Finally, the model(s) should *not* produce a masterful performance, but instead should demonstrate an effective, though somewhat naturally flawed performance. The idea is to demonstrate effective coping, but with some difficulty. This kind of modeling is typically viewed by trainees as more realistic, less discouraging, and illustrative of perseverance in the face of difficulty. Although modeling is an important component of interpersonal skills training, it is most effective when used in conjunction with practice, preferably practice with feedback. Viewing a behavior, and even imitating it, is very different from producing the behavior on one's own account.

Practice

Research from numerous skill domains suggests that the most important aspect of practice is that it is focused on improving the trainee's performance, as opposed to, for example, how much time is devoted to practice or how many repetitions there are (Ericsson et al 1993). Thus, practice should be a highly structured activity, allowing the trainee to focus on the details of the required behavior with the goal of modifying and adjusting the performance as needed. This kind of deliberate practice requires clear specification, and often illustration, of behavioral goals, performance feedback, and task simplification.

The identification and definition of goals have already been discussed. With respect to practice, these goals must now be specified in ways that ensure trainees have a clear understanding of what they are supposed to do. As already indicated, modeling is an excellent way to show trainees exactly what they are expected to accomplish. Because a key purpose of practice is to promote needed modification and adjustment of the performance, feedback is an essential component of practice. Trainees' skill acquisition is facilitated when they are informed of what they did (i.e. knowledge of performance) and whether their performance met the criterion (i.e. knowledge of results). Trainees have little basis for adjusting their performance without this sort of feedback. This is especially true in the initial stages of skill acquisition where trainees have not yet acquired the ability to self-critique performance. Feedback may be especially valuable to trainees when it is provided by someone who participates in the practice exercise. For example, practice components in physician communication skills training interventions often involve the use of simulated patients. These are individuals who actually play a key role in the practice exercise (i.e. patients with a particular medical problem), but who then provide feedback to the physician trainees on what they did, and did not do, and how effective they were.

The complexity of interpersonal communication often warrants steps to simplify the task for practice. For example, a communication task might be segmented so components that would normally be performed sequentially are practiced individually. Or simplification might be accomplished by restricting practice to a subset of behaviors, rather than requiring the trainee to perform the entire set of skills at once. For example, in training physicians to use patient-centered interviewing skills we have found that it is usually better to break the entire interview into component parts (e.g. opening few minutes, history taking, examination, post examination) and develop practice exercises that focus on separate parts of the interview. Once skills have been mastered, or at least well practiced, then physicians can be given the opportunity to practice conducting an entire interview. We have found that, for interpersonal skills as complex as patient-centered interviewing, it is best to structure the entire intervention following principles of simplification. Thus, physicians are instructed in communication skills relevant to the first 3 minutes of the interview. They are then engaged in practice with feedback that focuses on the skills to be used during the first 3 minutes. Once this is accomplished, we move to the next unit (e.g. history taking) and repeat the process.

Although practice with feedback is an essential element of interpersonal skills training, it should not be assumed that practice will necessarily lead to the transference of skills. For one thing, different kinds of practice tend to facilitate or retard retention and transfer. As a general rule, practice routines that facilitate short-term acquisition may retard long-term retention and transfer, and vice versa. For example, practice that involves varied stimuli or responses tends to retard acquisition, but facilitates retention and transfer. Additionally, most interpersonal communication skills training requires some form of follow-up to reinforce behavior and promote retention and transfer.

In our physician communication skills training program we also provide communication skills training to the physician's patients. The physician and patient interventions are designed with a common model so the skills that are taught are complementary. In this way, each time a physician sees a patient, key aspects of the skills intervention are reinforced, for both the physician and patient. Of course, this is the ideal and likely does not always occur in reality. However, even if only a small percentage of patients follow our training guidelines, physicians are likely to experience sufficient exposure to key aspects of our model and thus facilitate reinforcement and retention of communication skills.

In summary, modeling via videotape or live performance and practice have been used extensively in communication skills training for physicians and, to a lesser extent, for patients. Anderson & Sharpe's (1991) metaanalysis found the largest effect sizes in studies that employed modeling and practice in communication training interventions for heath-care providers and patients. We found a similar pattern in physician and patient communication skills training studies published after Anderson & Sharpe's review (Cegala & Broz-Lenzmeier 2003). Thus, it is clear that modeling and practice are important, indeed essential, components of physician and patient communication skills training. This principle is easily generalized to virtually all interpersonal communication skills interventions.

INTERVENTION ASSESSMENT MUST MATCH COMMUNICATION GOALS

Recently, we reviewed published research on physician communication skills interventions (Cegala & Broz-Lenzmeier 2002). Selected aspects of 26 studies were examined and one finding of this review is especially relevant to interpersonal communication skills interventions in general. We found that in a large percentage of studies there was an incongruity between the stated objectives of a communication skills intervention and the instrument or procedure used to assess the communicative performance of participants (e.g. Baile et al 1999, Bowman et al 1992, Brown et al 1999, Greco et al 1998). Clearly, such mismatching significantly undermines one's ability to assess the effectiveness of the intervention and to make any necessary modifications in the content and/or procedures.

Of the studies we reviewed, Smith et al (1998) arguably did the best job of matching skills with assessment procedures. For example, one of the communication skills addressed in their intervention was 'encouraging patient responses'. Their assessment instrument included the item 'encourages responses', which clearly matches the communication skill. However, in their discussion of the alignment of assessment items and skills, they provide even more specificity:

Rating scales were anchored at the upper and lower ends with examples of criterial [sic] behaviors. For example, the upper end of 'encouraging patient responses' had examples, such as 'uses exploratory questions,' 'uses echoing', or 'uses paraphrasing'. Criteria for the lower end of the scale included such examples as 'uses directive questions' and 'dismisses patient's responses'. (Smith et al 1998, pp. 120-121)

This degree of specificity and alignment of skills with assessment is rare in research on physician communication skills interventions, but it serves as a good example of what should be done generally in assessing the effects of interpersonal skills interventions.

A related matter regarding the alignment of skills and assessment procedures is the likely relevance of timing; that is, *when* a particular communication skill is performed. Research into discourse and conversation analysis clearly shows that the exchange of information and meaning is unfolded *sequentially* as participants produce, interpret, and respond to communicative acts (Glenn et al 2003, Levinson 1983). Thus, the assessment of interpersonal communication skills should include considerations about the timing of a trainee's behavior. For example, while a physician communication skills intervention, developed by Joos et al (1996), overall enhanced physicians' elicitation of patient concerns, only 22% of the trainees elicited concerns at the beginning of the interview, where such elicitations are most effective. Most of the rest of the elicitations occurred at the end of the interview, where they are least effective. If Joos et al had not considered the relevance of the timing of elicitations in their assessment, potential weaknesses in the intervention may have gone unnoticed.

CONSIDERATIONS ABOUT THE METHOD OF DELIVERY

The role of modeling and practice in interpersonal communication skills training was discussed earlier, indicating that both were essential to the development of effective interventions. Yet, the inclusion of modeling, and to a greater extent practice, can pose a dilemma with respect to options for delivering the intervention to participants.

Modeling may be done in several ways, the most popular being live and videotaped presentations. CD and web-based formats may also be used effectively to display models, though these formats have not been used as widely as they may be in the future. Except for live presentations, these formats can be used to deliver instruction cheaply to large numbers of people, even in disparate geographical areas. Unfortunately, this is not the case for delivering guided practice opportunities. Practice with feedback is arguably the most critical component of any interpersonal communication skills intervention, but it is also the most expensive and least efficiently delivered. The most effective means of delivering guided practice is in person and tailored to individual participants. Current technology offers some possibilities for delivering a practice component and

Box D6.1 Principles of skills training		
Task analysis	**Modeling**	**Practice**
• Purpose	• Multiple models	• Deliberate practice
• Constraints	• Single model	• Feedback
• Setting	• Model similarity	• Segmentation
• Social rules	• Reward	• Simplification
• Criteria	• Non-masterful performance	• Transference
• Systems perspective		• Reinforcement

future technological developments will probably offer even more, but for the moment, delivering guided practice to large numbers of participants remains a challenge for interpersonal communication skills interventions.

CONCLUSION

Box D6.1 summarizes the key concepts discussed in this chapter. Some of the concepts, such as modeling and practice, are not only essential to learning interpersonal communication skills, but are also key in learning other skills as well.

Similarly, interpersonal communication skills are often central to an intervention, even when the focus of the intervention is not communication per se. Persons exposed to behavioral interventions often face challenges in maintaining their newly acquired behavior and many of these challenges come in the form of interpersonal communications from family, friends, co-workers, and others. Thus, intervention planners should consider how the addition of an interpersonal component might better prepare targets to resist such challenges.

References

Anderson L A, Sharpe P A 1991 Improving patient and provider communication: a synthesis and review of communication interventions. Patient Education and Counseling 17:99-134

Baile W F, Kudelka A P, Beale E A et al 1999 Communication skills training in oncology. Description and preliminary outcomes of workshops on breaking bad news and managing patient reactions to illness. Cancer 865:887-897

Bandura A 1986 Social foundations of thought and action. Prentice-Hall, Englewood Cliffs

Bandura A 1997 Self-efficacy: the exercise of control. Freeman, New York

Bowman F M, Goldberg D P, Millar T et al 1992 Improving the skills of established general practitioners: the long-term benefits of group teaching. Medical Education 261:63-68

Brown J B, Boles M, Mullooly J P et al 1999 Effect of clinician communication skills training on patient satisfaction. A randomized, controlled trial. Annals of Internal Medicine 131:822-829

Cegala D J, Broz-Lenzmeier S 2002 Physician communication skills training: a review of theoretical backgrounds, objectives, and skills. Medical Education 36:1004-1016

Cegala D J, Broz-Lenzmeier S 2003 Provider and patient communication skills training. In: Thompson T L, Dorsey A M, Miller K I et al (eds) Handbook of health communication. Lawrence Erlbaum Associates, Mahwah, pp 95-119

Cegala D J, Socha D, McGee K S et al 1996 Components of patients' and doctors' perceptions of communication competence during a primary care medical interview. Health Communication 8:1-28

Cegala D J, Coleman M T, Warisse J 1998 The development and partial test of the Medical Communication Competence Scale (MCCS). Health Communication 10:261-288

Cegala D J, Marinelli T, Post D M 2000a The effect of patient communication skills training on treatment compliance in primary care. Archives of Family Medicine 9:57-64

Cegala D J, McClure L, Marinelli T M et al 2000b The effects of communication skills training on patients' participation during medical interviews. Patient Education and Counseling 41:209-222

Cegala D J, Post D, McClure L 2001 The effects of patient communication skills training on the discourse of elderly patients during a primary care interview. Journal of the American Geriatrics Society 49:1505-1511

Cegala D J, Gade C, Lenzmeier B S et al 2004 Physicians' and patients' perceptions of patients' communication competence in a primary care medical interview. Health Communication 16:289-304

Dunn C L, Pirie P L, Hellerstedt W L 2003 The advice-giving role of female friends and relatives during pregnancy. Health Education Research 183:352-362

Ericsson K A, Krampe R T, Tesch-Romer C 1993 The role of deliberate practice in the acquisition of expert performance. Psychological Review 100:363-406

Glenn P, LeBaron C D, Mandelbaum J 2003 Studies in language and social interaction: in honor of Robert Hopper. Lawrence Erlbaum Associates, Mahwah

Greco M, Francis W, Buckley J et al 1998 Real-patient evaluation of communication skills teaching for GP registrars. Family Practice 151:51-57

Green J O, Burleson B R 2003 Handbook of communication and social interaction skills. Lawrence Erlbaum Associates, Mahwah

Jacob T, Seilhamer R A 1987 Alcoholism and family interaction. In: Jacob T (ed) Family interaction and psychopathology: theories, methods, and findings. Plenum, New York, pp 535-580

Joos S K, Hickam D H, Gordon G H et al 1996 Effects of a physician communication intervention on patient care outcomes. Journal of General Internal Medicine 113:147-155

Langer E J 1978 Rethinking the role of thought in social interaction. In: Harvey J, Ickes W, Kiss R (eds) New directions in attribution research. Lawrence Erlbaum Associates, Hillsdale, pp 35-58

Levinson S C 1983 Pragmatics. Cambridge University Press, Cambridge

Liberman R P, DeRisi W J, Mueser K T 1989 Social skills training for psychiatric patients. Pergamon Press, New York

McFall R M 1982 A review and reformulation of the concept of social skills. Behavioral Assessment 4:1-33

O'Keefe B J, Delia J G 1982 Impression formation and message production. In: Roloff M E, Berger C R (eds) Social cognition and communication. Sage, Newbury Park, pp 33-72

Rimal R N 2003 Intergenerational transmission of health: the role of intrapersonal, interpersonal, and communicative factors. Health Education and Behavior 301:10-28

Sanders R E 2003 Applying the skills concept to discourse and conversation: the remediation of performance defects in talk-in-interaction. In: Greene J O, Burleson B R (eds) Handbook of communication and social interaction skills. Lawrence Erlbaum Associates, Mahwah, pp 221-256

Seiffe-Krenke I 2002 'Come on, say something, dad!' Communication and coping in fathers of diabetic adolescents. Journal of Pediatric Psychology 275:439-450

Smith R C, Lyles J S, Mettler J et al 1998 The effectiveness of intensive training for residents in interviewing. A randomized, controlled study. Annals of Internal Medicine 1282:118-126

Spitzberg B H 1986 Issues in the study of communicative competence. Ablex, Norwood

Spitzberg B H, Cupach W R 1984 Interpersonal communication competence. Sage, Beverly Hills

Tracy K 1991 Understanding face-to-face interaction: issues linking goals and discourse. Lawrence Erlbaum Associates, Hillsdale

Trower P 1995 Adult social skills: state of the art and future directions. In: O'Donohue W, Krasner L (eds) Handbook of psychological skills training: clinical techniques and applications. Allyn and Bacon, Boston, pp 54-80

Education

Claus Vögele

INTRODUCTION

'It's far more effective to take a big company like ... to court than to – literally – educate millions of Americans.' This statement was recently made by John F Banzhaf on television, in an interview on one of his latest lawsuits to claim compensation for obese children from a well-known fast food chain. Banzhaf is Professor of Public Interest Law at George Washington University Law School in Washington DC and one of the most ardent legal activists against international companies in the fast-food and tobacco industries. The statement by Banzhaf cannot be regarded as qualified in scientific terms, but it serves to highlight the area of conflict in which health promotion and education take place in industrialized countries. What difference can educational campaigns make if big companies put all their effort into advertising and selling unhealthy products and lifestyles? What use are programs to raise awareness if global market forces exploit the entire armory of marketing strategies to coax the general public into consuming products that we know contribute to the high prevalence of all modern ailments? Is this not David against Goliath, a lost cause already?

i see C5

While these questions are legitimate and important, it is beyond the scope of this chapter to provide an adequate discussion platform, not to mention an answer. It is the purpose of this chapter to provide an up-to-date account of the theoretical background and the application of health education and promotion. While describing the potential and the limitations of this approach, it is important to bear in mind that health education and promotion are one valuable and efficient approach in initiating behavior change to advocate better health and that it is only in concert with other approaches that it will be able to reach its full potential.

At the heart of health education lies the assumption that humans are rational decision makers and, if properly informed, individuals will choose beneficial health behaviors over risk behaviors and health hazards. Health education aims, therefore, to increase individuals' knowledge about the factors impinging on health and illness. Through this route it is hoped that education contributes to prolonged life, improved quality of life, and the prevention or reduction of the effects of impaired physical and/or mental health, both in the individuals affected and in those who care for them.

While the wider term 'health promotion' is used to describe any process which facilitates the health status of individuals, groups, or populations, 'health education' concentrates on bringing about changes in individual behavior through changes in the individual's cognitions. This chapter will concentrate on the psychological factors involved in changing specific health cognitions, how to raise awareness, give a developmental perspective, provide examples on how to successfully design interventions, and finally discuss the limitations of this approach. First, however, we will describe similarities and differences of frequently used terms, such as health education, health promotion, and illness prevention.

DEFINITIONS

Health education and health promotion

Although there is no universally accepted definition of health education, most practitioners and researchers would agree that health education involves interventions designed to influence the incidence and prevalence of health-related behaviors in specific populations. The World Health Organization (WHO 1981) defines health education as all those planned activities that contribute to people wanting to be healthy (health motivation), to knowing how to achieve health (health knowledge), and to helping people to translate this knowledge into action (health behavior), alone or with the assistance of other people or organizations.

Health education is mostly understood as one component of the broader concept of health promotion. Health promotion takes into account that human behavior is not only governed by personal factors (e.g. knowledge, expectancies, competencies, and well-being), but also by structural aspects of the environment. Whether adolescents progress to develop a smoking habit is not only determined by their level of knowledge about the adverse consequences of tobacco smoking and their social competencies in declining an offer for a cigarette. It is also strongly affected by environmental factors, such as the availability of cigarette machines, whether cigarette smoking is advertised and how health warnings on the cigarette packages are designed, whether there are smoking zones, how expensive cigarettes are, and whether smoking is restricted in public buildings and community places. While health education, therefore, concentrates on the individual, health promotion, on the other hand, exceeds this approach by addressing the organizational, ecological, and political levels when designing interventions to further a healthy lifestyle.

i see D8

Health promotion and illness prevention

Health promotion and illness prevention are not simply two sides of the same coin. Illness prevention interventions are designed to achieve a reduction in the incidence of specific disorders through prophylactic measures. For example, taking fluoride tablets helps to reduce the incidence in tooth decay (caries). Health promotion, on the other hand, not only intends to reduce the incidence of specific disorders but aims to strengthen health much more extensively, i.e. physical, mental, social, and personal health (Perry & Jessor 1985). Through health promotion the individual is supposed to be enabled to live an active life in society. It is not only, therefore, through classic behavioral techniques that health promotion interventions aim to help people to acquire a healthier lifestyle (e.g. increase physical activity, healthy diet, and moderate alcohol consumption). In addition to health-related behaviors, such as diet and physical activity, health promotion interventions are designed to be more comprehensive in that they may target areas such as the development of a positive self-concept, may help with the acquisition of social skills and stress reduction techniques, support the pursuit of long-term goals, and even enhance the ability to enjoy life.

An illustration of such a comprehensive health promotion intervention is the Californian Department of Mental Health countrywide campaign 'Friends Can Be Good Medicine' (Hersey et al 1984). The campaign had three goals:

1 education of the general public about the important role of positive personal relationships for psychological and physical well-being
2 encouragement to spend more time and energy on maintaining and caring for personal relations
3 to create opportunities for meeting new friends and establish personal relationships.

The information materials used in this campaign ranged from television spots and radio broadcasts to self-test brochures, stickers, and slide shows. This example demonstrates how health promotion campaigns differ in target and scope from illness prevention programs.

THEORIES AND MODELS OF HEALTH PROMOTION

 see A2

The majority of preventable risk factors for chronic diseases are behavioral in nature. It is consistent with this finding that prevention programs seek to reduce behavioral risk behaviors (e.g. smoking, diet high in saturated fats, alcohol abuse) and to establish protective behaviors (e.g. physical activity, seatbelt use, medical adherence, stress reduction techniques). In order to make such interventions effective, however, it is crucial to have a sound knowledge of the relevant social and cognitive factors that are important for the development and maintenance of health behaviors. It is only plausible to assume that behavioral interventions would succeed in changing the causal chains of many chronic disorders if the relevant factors can be identified beforehand and assessed in relation to their ability to be modified.

In the literature on prevention research, four different types of theories can be distinguished that are used as theoretical foundations.

1 More general psychological models to explain human behavior (Theory of Reasoned Action, Theory of Planned Behavior, Social Cognitive Theory, Behavioral Decision Theory).

2 Specific models to explain health behaviors (Health Belief Model, Protection Motivation Theory, Systems Model for Health Behavior Change, Precaution Adoption Process, Health Action Process Approach).
3 Eclectic models (PRECEDE Model, Health Promotion Model).
4 Outcome-oriented models (Communications-Persuasion Model).

Important as the general and specific models (types 1 and 2) are for the theoretical underpinning and explanation of health behaviors, intervention designers much prefer technological (or eclectic) models (type 3) which show clearly what psychological or social variables should be targeted in order to achieve the desired behavior change. In contrast to models of type 1–3 which aim to change health behavior-related variables, outcome-oriented models (type 4) target factors important for the efficacy and effectiveness of interventions in order to optimize outcome (e.g. information campaigns).

CHANGING SPECIFIC HEALTH COGNITIONS

The majority of health promotion models agree that health behaviors – as long as they are under volitional control – are affected primarily by five factors: outcome expectancies, perceived self-efficacy, perceived susceptibility, perceived severity of the problem, and perceived social desirability (normative beliefs). Most interventions focus on the first three of these factors and they will, therefore, be discussed in more detail in the following sections.

Outcome expectancies

Outcome expectancies reflect the balance of perceived benefits and costs of a specific health behavior. For example, 'If I exercise regularly I will be less likely to catch a cold'. Many studies support the notion that this type of expectancy is a strong predictor of health behaviors, such as smoking, exercise, alcohol consumption, and diet. Outcome expectancies can be shaped by personal experience and observation of others but also through information and education. Several countries, including the UK, have introduced national AIDS campaigns which provide public education through the mass media. In TV spots, for example, an outcome expectancy is created that condom use protects from HIV infection. Evaluations of such campaigns have clearly shown that they are highly effective in raising awareness.

According to most theoretical models, however, only those outcome expectancies which are perceived to be of personal importance and relevance are significant for motivating a behavior change. Knowing that AIDS may be a life-threatening condition will not have an impact on someone who is not convinced that this issue may be of importance for them personally. An intervention designer, therefore, faces a dual task. First, one has to ensure that the behavioral consequences of a health-relevant activity are represented cognitively in an accurate way (e.g. 'Condom use gives protection from HIV infection through sexual transmission'). Whether this is achieved depends largely on the credibility of the source of information. Second, the message of the campaign has to be made personal and salient. The recipients of the education campaign should arrive at the conclusion for themselves that a behavior change will lead to better health ('If I use condoms I will be protected from HIV infection through sexual transmission').

However, not all personally relevant outcome expectancies are suitable to develop into salient and, therefore, behaviorally relevant cognitions. For example, Evans (1988), in his school-based smoking prevention campaigns, based his intervention on the assumption that adolescents take more short-term consequences of smoking into consideration (e.g. social acceptance, feeling like a grown-up, coughing, light-headedness, nausea) rather than the long-term effects (lung cancer, cardiovascular disease), which are quite theoretical from a youngster's perspective. In his program, he used monitoring of expiratory carbon monoxide levels to demonstrate, in a drastic way, the difference in concentrations of this toxic gas between smoking students and their non-smoking fellows.

Self-efficacy

Even strong and salient outcome expectancies will not initiate a behavior change, if the person is not convinced of their ability to carry out this behavior. Perceived self-efficacy (derived from Social Learning Theory; Bandura 1997) describes a personal belief that one can successfully perform certain required behaviors, in particular in demanding situations with unfamiliar and difficult characteristics. In relation to obesity, for example, such a cognition could be, 'When I am in good company and someone offers me a sweet I can usually say "No"'. The empirical evidence suggests that self-efficacy is indeed an important determinant of health behaviors. From a health promotion perspective, the issue of how to change such cognitions through educational methods arises.

Bandura (1997) suggests, primarily, three intervention principles:

1 one's own experience
2 behavioral models
3 persuasion.

Mastery experiences, gained through performance accomplishments, are thought to have the greatest impact on establishing and strengthening self-efficacy, because they provide the most information about actual capabilities. Interventions should be designed in a way that enables participants in a program to experience success and to attribute these results to their own effort and competence. Successful interventions use immediate aims and objectives that are challenging yet achievable. Such aims usually take the form of recommendations and, in order to avoid an all-or-nothing thinking pattern, allow for flexibility and even failure. It is important that flexible rather than rigid control governs the design of such a program, as participants have to learn how to cope with a high chance of 'failure' (e.g. giving in to the temptation of having a sweet) by using an appropriate strategy (e.g. compensation for a dietary slip by eating less next time) and not abandoning the whole program in an all-or-nothing fashion.

Quite often, the opportunities to gain experiences oneself are limited. Behavioral role models, whose successful coping behavior can be imitated, can then stand in place of one's own experience. One of the most effective interventions involves the 'self-disclosure' of someone who had to fight with a similar problem. These models then communicate how they coped with the problem and succeeded on the basis of self-regulation capacity. For example, in smoking cessation a motivated smoker might benefit from observing and talking to someone who is a few weeks ahead in the same process. Even when learning by imitation or modeling, it is important to recognize the importance of one's own resources, constructive self-dialogue, positive interpretation of events, and immediate goal setting. In participant modeling, the direct experience and that gained through observing a model are combined to create an intervention strategy which has been found to be particularly effective.

 see D6

In addition to programs which target self-efficacy in relation to specific behaviors and situations, it would appear to make sense from a health promotion and developmental perspective to provide interventions to strengthen young people's self-efficacy on a much more general level and regard self-efficacy as a trait amenable to intervention. Individuals with low self-efficacy are much more likely to imitate undesirable behaviors than those with high self-efficacy. For example, drinking patterns of parents are observed by children who may then imitate them in later life, especially the behavior of the same-sex parent (Heather & Robertson 1997). In adolescence, the drinking behavior of respected older peers may also be imitated and subsequently that of higher status colleagues at work, a phenomenon which might explain the prevalence of heavy drinking in certain professions, such as medicine and journalism. Increasing young people's self-efficacy might help adolescents and, later on in life, adults to be more resilient to the potentially damaging effect of 'bad' models.

Fear appeals

In order to raise awareness and promote healthier living, educational campaigns often use materials designed to induce feelings of threat and anxiety. In the early days of the AIDS epidemic, for example, televised campaigns tended to illustrate in a drastic manner the consequences of unsafe sex and sharing needles in intravenous drug users by showing pictures of patients with full-blown AIDS. Current TV spots in the UK warning of the health risks associated with cigarette smoking use an interview with a smoker stating how much he regretted ever having started. The viewer is informed at the end of the 15-second spot that the person depicted died of lung cancer only 3 weeks after giving the interview.

The record of such fear-arousing messages, however, has not been one of convincing success. Most research today suggests that informational campaigns based on fear can be effective, but only if they do not arouse too much fear. What is required for fear appeals to motivate people to initiate a behavior change is a moderate level of fear induction. Campaigns that arouse either no fear or too much fear are equally ineffective.

But not only the 'dosage' of fear induction is important. Self & Rogers (1990) found that without reassuring people about their ability to cope, attempts to frighten them had negative effects on health behaviors. Job (1988) specifies the circumstances under which fear appeals might be useful in health education campaigns:

- people are fearful before they receive the message
- the fear-arousing event appears imminent
- guidelines are provided on what one should do to reduce the fear (behavior alternatives)
- people begin with a low level of fear that can realistically be reduced by performing a desirable health-related behavior
- the reduction of fear serves as a negative reinforcer.

Well-designed education campaigns can contain such elements of fear appeal, but positive reinforcement is presumably more effective than the use of fear.

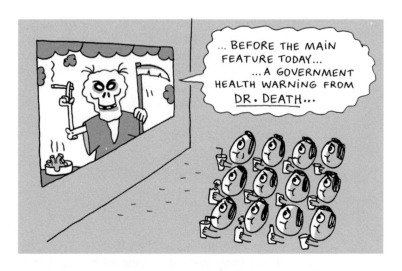

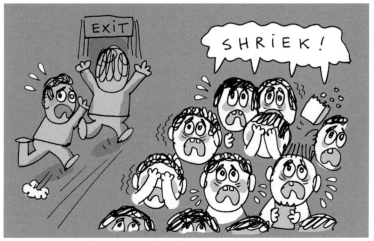

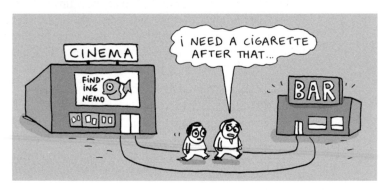

If threat cognitions as a result of fear appeals are effective under these specified circumstances, the question arises as to how they can be changed to create behavior change. In the literature, there are mainly three threat-related aspects that are discussed in the context of intervention programs.

PERCEIVED SEVERITY OF THE PROBLEM

This is determined not only by the available factual knowledge but also by social influence processes (Croyle & Hunt 1991).

PERCEIVED SUSCEPTIBILITY TO THE THREATENING EVENT

Determinants for perceived susceptibility to a specific disorder are current health status, existing early signs and symptoms, family history, and preexisting personal experiences with this disorder. All of these aspects must be targeted in an intervention designed to increase perceived susceptibility.

PERCEIVED TEMPORAL CLOSENESS

As early as 12 years of age, children are aware of the health risks of tobacco smoking. Nevertheless, a substantial proportion of children at that age start smoking. Fear of the long-term consequences (lung cancer, cardiovascular disorders) does not seem to make a lot of difference. Of central importance to the beginning of tobacco smoking are the short-term consequences of smoking, in particular the social consequences. Perceived social pressure to smoke seems the single most important cause for the onset of smoking. Apparently, there is an association between threat cognition and smoking behavior, except that it works in a different direction than most health educators would like. Smoking is not stopped because of adverse long-term health consequences but is initiated because of anticipated social rejection by peers if one fails to do so. This example illustrates how health-related anxieties can compete with fears of social rejection in controlling behavior.

BEHAVIORAL INTERVENTIONS TO CREATE CHANGE IN EATING HABITS, PHYSICAL ACTIVITY, AND WEIGHT CONTROL

Healthy diet

Most health education programs designed to support a healthy diet embark on large-scale information campaigns relying on the assumption that information and knowledge will lead to behavior change. This so-called information appeal is frequently supplemented by vivid descriptions of the health risks associated with an unhealthy diet (fear appeal). As important as information and fear appeals are in appropriate doses, they only constitute the prerequisite to what is supposed to become a long-lasting behavior change.

A popular theme for health education campaigns in the 1980s and 1990s was the diet–heart hypothesis. This is based on evidence that coronary heart disease is associated with raised cholesterol levels, high blood pressure (essential hypertension), and a diet high in salt (sodium). For every 1% change in serum cholesterol levels, there is a 3% change in the likelihood of developing coronary heart disease. A long-term (5-year) change of 5–6 mmHg in diastolic blood pressure (which has been linked to sodium intake) can reduce the chances of stroke by 35–40% and of coronary heart disease by 20–25%. Clearly, the adoption of a prudent diet can reduce the incidence of cardiovascular morbidity.

Foreyt et al (1979) compared four interventions:

1 a leaflet with information on salt and cholesterol
2 instructions on how to eat healthily
3 behavior modification with group discussion
4 a combination of all three.

All four interventions were successful initially in lowering participants' cholesterol levels, but failed to do so on follow-up. In a more recent Australian study (Owen et al 1990), a large group of participants (12 000) were screened for their cholesterol level and then given one of three interventions:

1 brief advice
2 advice plus reminder 4 weeks later
3 in addition to (2), entry into a raffle.

At 4-month follow-up a retest was offered but uptake of this offer did not differ between groups.

There are more examples of studies evidently showing an overall failure of health education campaigns in changing people's eating habits. It is not our view that such campaigns are redundant. Rather, they need to be modified with respect to a number of aspects. The first of the following suggestions seems to be common sense but is apparently difficult to achieve.

HEALTH PROMOTION MESSAGES MUST BE SIMPLE, CLEAR, AND CONSISTENT

Unfortunately, dietary health communications have been the opposite on many occasions, creating much confusion. One example is the controversy over 'the right kind of fat' (butter or margarine). For many years it was believed that butter was the main culprit in raising cholesterol levels and, therefore, was unhealthy. The health-conscious consumer switched to margarine. Then it was claimed that the *trans* fatty acids contained in processed fats, such as margarine, could be equally unhealthy. The consumer switched back to butter. Confusion and mistrust of health messages were the consequence of such conflicting messages.

Another example concerns the recent bovine spongiform encephalopathy (BSE) crisis in the UK and Europe. BSE (also known as 'mad cow disease') is a central nervous system infection affecting cattle. However, at the same time as the BSE crisis, some people developed a new form of Creutzfeldt–Jakob disease ('variant CJD') and exposure to BSE-infected beef was the most likely explanation. Consumers were subsequently confronted with the entire spectrum of recommendations, ranging from warnings against biscuits (because they contained gelatin from processed beef) to 'don't eat beef on the bone', to 'beef is healthy and nutritious', with a British health minister declaring into the camera that he would buy his grandchild a burger any time while biting heartily into one.

We concede that health education campaigns using the mass media share the same problems as any other communication of scientific knowledge to the general public. Results from epidemiological studies and clinical or laboratory trials very often don't convert easily into simple, clear, and consistent recommendations. It is the onerous task of the health education campaign designer to translate scientific probabilities into behavioral instructions that are understood by the target audience. Dietary guidelines are usually formulated in terms of nutrients. Consumers buy and eat food and so they need to be able to translate recommendations about nutrients into how best to purchase foods. Effective nutritional health promotion involves the collaboration of nutritionists, psychologists, epidemiologists, educators, journalists, medical doctors, industrialists, and legislators.

EARLY INTERVENTIONS ARE IMPORTANT

Interventions to change people's eating habits have to take into account that food preferences are acquired in childhood and, once established, are likely to be long lasting and resistant to change. Arguably this would underline the importance of establishing sound nutritional practices in childhood, as a basis for lifelong healthy eating. In this respect, it is interesting to note that the use of schools as sites for the introduction of interventions is being exploited with some success in programs promoting improved cardiovascular health. Programs typically include regular lessons on nutrition and increased numbers of physical education lessons and are introduced early in children's school careers. Measured benefits of such programs include reductions in blood pressure and cholesterol concentrations, as well as increased nutritional and health knowledge (Gore et al 1996). While such programs can be beneficial, their impact is increased when the family is also involved in the intervention. A school and home educational program should involve schoolwork, with associated homework/parental activities. Children with higher family involvement showed the greatest increase in their reported consumption of grain, lower reported intake of cholesterol, and strongest intentions for good nutritional practices in the future (Edmundson et al 1996).

FLEXIBLE CONTROL IS PREFERABLE TO RIGID CONTROL

Nutritional advice provided in health education campaigns should explain the frequent occurrence of dietary 'slips' and offer behavioral alternatives to compensate for them. Rigid rules are difficult to comply with over a long period of time, e.g. 'I must not eat butter'. There is evidence from research on eating disorders that such bans of certain foods tend to focus cognitive activity on these foods and, therefore, to increase the preference for them. The result is often a dietary slip and subsequently the abandonment of the program in an all-or-nothing fashion (known in the clinical literature as counter-regulation; also a part of the self-efficacy concept). Goals in dietary health promotion programs should be realistic so that participants can experience success and learn how to cope appropriately with 'breaking the rules'. Only then will such interventions have a chance to lead to long-term behavior change.

A related concept has been described by Fieldhouse (1996). He proposes five characteristics of successful dietary innovations:

- the perceived advantage of change
- compatibility with existing values and needs
- simple to understand and use
- 'trialability' (experimentation with new behaviors)
- observability (the degree to which the outcomes are visible to others).

Physical activity

There is now an impressive body of literature confirming the benefits of regular physical activity for both physical and mental health (Astrand 1992). The Centers for Disease Control and Prevention (CDC) and the American College of Sports Medicine (ACSM) concluded in a joint report that evidence from cross-sectional epidemiological surveys, as well as controlled experimental studies, suggests that physically active adults tend to develop and maintain better physical health (Pate et al 1995). The report further concludes that prolonged vigorous exercise is not necessary to achieve these benefits and recommends an increase in everyday physical activity, amounting to a total of at least 30 minutes' activity at an intensity corresponding to brisk walking. This activity level should be well within the grasp of most people.

It is puzzling, therefore, that physical activity levels in the general population are well below this recommended intensity and drop-out rates from exercise programs continue to be high, particularly amongst those who would benefit most (i.e. cardiac patients, obese individuals). Data from Europe and the USA suggest that the majority of people start to exercise at one point during their lives, but only a minority succeed in turning this behavior into a lifelong habit. Low levels of physical activity in the general population are, therefore, not so much due to a lack of motivation to start but a result of difficulties in maintaining exercise behavior.

 see B4, B5

The National Institute of Health (NIH) Consensus Development Panel (1996) suggests that a predicament of most exercise programs is the – intentional or unintentional – promotion of the common misperception that vigorous continuous activity is necessary to gain exercise-related health benefits. With the best of intentions, health education programs to promote physical activity have tended in the past to prescribe rigid exercise regimens that may have minimized the chances to develop a sense of self-efficacy and mastery. In addition, most people who start an exercise program have quite unrealistic expectations as to what exercise can accomplish and how long it is going to take to achieve this goal. Frustration and abandonment of such a program are very often the end-result.

Accurate information on the effects of exercise and realistic goal setting may be regarded as the prerequisites of any successful health education program to promote physical activity. A number of other factors, however, may prove to be crucial in maintaining exercise behavior.

VARIETY IS THE SPICE OF LIFE

Exercise can take many forms: resistance training versus aerobic training, alone or in company, outdoors or indoors, with or without music, competitive or non-competitive, to name but a few alternatives. Participants in any program should be encouraged to explore the range of different types of physical activity to find out which suits them best. Guidelines on the suitability of particular forms of exercises for specific target populations should be considered where appropriate, particularly for those with preexisting illnesses (ACSM 1997). Of prime importance, however, for changing a newly acquired skill into a lifelong habit is whether the activity is experienced as enjoyable.

FLEXIBLE CONTROL INSTEAD OF RIGID RULES

Exercise takes time and has to be fitted into everyday activities. As we have discussed in the previous part of this chapter concerning a healthy diet, flexible rules to allow for compensation of missed exercise sessions strengthen one's sense of control over the target behavior, help to avoid all-or-nothing coping strategies, and thus increase adherence to an active lifestyle.

ROLE MODELS

The model character of anyone involved in administering a health education campaign to promote physical activity should not be underestimated. Therapists or health campaigners promoting a behavior that they are evidently not engaged in themselves are not very convincing. On the other hand, this model character provides a powerful intervention tool enabling the program participant to combine the direct experience of exercise and that gained through observing the (therapist) model (i.e. participant modeling).

In their review of randomized controled trials of physical activity promotion programs, Hillsdon et al (1995) summarize five characteristics of effective trials:

1 home-based programs
2 unsupervised, informal exercise
3 frequent professional contact
4 walking as the promoted type of exercise
5 moderate-intensity exercise.

In support of point (3), they also note that the character of the interaction between the professional and the client may be more important than the actual behavioral technique.

Weight control

Health education interventions to promote weight loss have tended in the past to concentrate on changes in dietary regimens based on caloric restrictions. Evaluations of the effectiveness of such programs show, however, that only about 15% of participants succeed in maintaining their reduced weight over a 5-year period (Ayyad & Andersen 2000). The vast majority of overweight or obese participants in these programs regain their original weight not long after the end of the intervention or in some cases even more. This unsatisfactory situation has led to the criticism of 'traditional' weight loss programs and their almost exclusive focus on weight reduction. As supporters of the so-called 'Health at any size paradigm' (H@AS; Miller & Jacob 2001) point out, the sole focus on calorie restriction might in fact contribute to the development of disordered eating behavior (restrained eating, yo-yo dieting, binge eating) and result in an increase in health risk.

More promising are multimodal strategies that combine nutritional education, interventions to increase physical activity, and training in behavioral techniques, such as cognitive restructuring, stimulus control, self-monitoring, and reinforcement of desired behaviors. Some of the health benefits associated with a healthy diet and increased physical activity are in fact independent of weight loss (e.g. improvements in cardiorespiratory fitness and blood lipid profiles, reductions in plasma insulin concentrations, and increased insulin sensitivity). As this approach uses a combination of healthy eating strategies and interventions to promote higher levels of physical activity, all the factors important for health education campaigns discussed in the previous two parts of this chapter apply to health campaigns for the overweight and obese.

Successful as such multimodal strategies may be in promoting better health and reduced weight in obese individuals, effective methods of health promotion and behavior change are needed at a population level. As childhood obesity is one of the strongest predictors of obesity in adulthood, interventions to tackle this problem at an early developmental stage would appear to be particularly promising. An example of such an intervention is a home-based program called 'PowerKids' (www.powerkids.de; Ellrott et al 2000). PowerKids is based on behavioral principles and designed for obese and overweight 8–12 year old children. The 12-week outpatient program is carried out in the children's families. Using a token economy concept, children playfully learn how to decrease dietary fat intake and to reduce physical inactivity. Rather than rapid weight loss, it is the aim of this program to stabilize newly acquired healthy eating habits and increase self-confidence as a basis for long-term success. Results from a first evaluation (Ellrott et al 2000) are promising, in that the completion rate in a sample of 141 overweight children was 70%, despite the fact that no further support was provided. Children's body mass index decreased, on average, by 0.5 standard deviation scores.

CONCLUSION AND FUTURE DEVELOPMENTS

Health education programs are designed to prevent illness by creating the conditions for people to be motivated to adopt certain behaviors and a healthy lifestyle. While health education programs can work at an individual or group level, health education campaigns are directed toward larger communities. Campaigns disseminating information only are generally ineffective, as are programs that use fear appeals, when they do not provide behavior alternatives that allow for fear reduction or support self-efficacy and outcome expectancies.

In recent years, people have increasingly used the Internet to seek health information, to communicate with others who have a similar disease or illness, to receive health promotion advice, and to communicate with health-care advisers. CD-ROM and DVD-ROM technologies also support the delivery of multimedia programs for health promotion that are interactive, entertaining, and graphically rich. An illustration of the use of this approach is provided by Baranowski et al (2003): a multimedia game promoting the consumption of fruit juice and vegetables resulted in a significant increase in the consumption of these foods in a large sample of children from diverse ethnic and socio-economic backgrounds. While the advancement of 'eHealth' (Ahern et al 2003) offers a huge potential for health education and promotion, systematic evaluations of the quality and effectiveness of these technology-based programs are still required. However, the introduction of programs, such as the 'Health e-Technologies Initiative' (Ahern et al 2003), is a significant step towards the scientific evaluation of cost, cost-effectiveness, and overall quality of eHealth applications that are currently in use for health behavior change and chronic disease management.

References

Ahern D K, Phalen J M, Mockenhaupt R E 2003 Science and the advancement of eHealth: a call to action. American Journal of Preventive Medicine 24:108-109

American College of Sports Medicine (ACSM) 1997 Exercise management for persons with chronic diseases and disabilities. Human Kinetics, Champaign

Astrand P O 1992 Why exercise? Medicine and Science in Sports and Exercise 24:153-162

Ayyad C, Andersen T 2000 Long-term efficacy of dietary treatment of obesity: a systematic review of studies published between 1931 and 1999. Obesity Reviews 1:113-119

Bandura A 1997 Self-efficacy: the exercise of control. Freeman, New York

Baranowski T, Baranowski J, Cullen K W et al 2003 Squire's Quest! Dietary outcome evaluation of a multimedia game. American Journal of Preventive Medicine 24:52-61

Croyle R T, Hunt J R 1991 Coping with health threat: social influence processes in reaction to medical test results. Journal of Personality and Social Psychology 60:382-389

Edmundson E, Parcel G S, Perry C L et al 1996 The effects of the child and adolescent trial for cardiovascular health intervention on psychosocial determinants of cardiovascular disease risk behavior among third-grade students. American Journal of Health Promotion 10:217-225

Ellrott T, Lichtenstein S, Pudel V et al 2000 PowerKids: a new cost-effective behavioral approach in the treatment of childhood obesity. Obesity Research 8:46S

Evans R I 1988 Prevention of smoking in adolescents: conceptualization and intervention strategies of a prototypical research program. In Maes S, Spielberger C D, Defares P B et al (eds) Topics in health psychology. Wiley, Chichester, pp 107-125

Fieldhouse P 1996 Food and nutrition: customs and culture. Stanley Thornes, Cheltenham

Foreyt J P, Scott L W, Mitchell R E et al 1979 Plasma lipid changes in the normal population following behavioral treatment. Journal of Consulting and Clinical Psychology 47:440-452

Gore C J, Owen N, Pederson D et al 1996 Educational and environmental interventions for cardiovascular health promotion in socially disadvantaged primary schools. Australian and New Zealand Journal of Public Health 20:188-194

Heather N, Robertson I 1997 Problem drinking. Oxford University Press, Oxford

Hersey J C, Klibanoff L S, Lam D J et al 1984 Promoting social support: the impact of Calofornia's 'Friends Can Be Good Medicine' campaign. Health Education Quarterly 11:293-311

Hillsdon M, Thorogood M, Anstiss T et al 1995 Randomised controlled trials of physical activity promotion in free living populations: a review. Journal of Epidemiology and Community Health 49:448-453

Job R F 1988 Effective and ineffective use of fear in health promotion campaigns. American Journal of Public Health 78:163-167

Miller W C, Jacob A V 2001 The health at any size paradigm for obesity treatment: the scientific evidence. Obesity Reviews 2:37-45

NIH Consensus Development Panel on Physical Activity and Cardiovascular Health 1996 Physical activity and cardiovascular health. Journal of the American Medical Association 276:241-246

Owen N, James R, Henrikson D et al 1990 Community cholesterol screenings: the impact of follow-up letters and incentives on retest rates and biometric changes in follow-up screenings. American Journal of Health Promotion 5:58-61

Pate R R, Pratt M, Blair S N et al 1995 Physical activity and public health: a recommendation from the Centers for Disease Control and the American College of Sports Medicine. Journal of the American Medical Association 273:402-407

Perry C L, Jessor R 1985 The concept of health promotion and the prevention of adolescent drug abuse. Health Education Quarterly 12:169-184

Self C A, Rogers R W 1990 Coping with threats to health: effects of persuasive appeals on depressed, normal, and antisocial personalities. Journal of Behavioral Medicine 13:343-357

World Health Organization (WHO) 1981 Global strategy of health for all by the year 2000. WHO, Geneva

Environmental and social strategies

Brian Oldenburg and Nicola Burton

INTRODUCTION

Given the importance of social and environmental influences as determinants of health behaviors and health across the life course, it is also important to consider the role of social and environmental change methods in the health behavior change process. Such methods involve a complex array of factors and variables that arise from the need to consider the change process at multiple levels, such as individuals, social and family networks, organizations, and society. It is also necessary to consider the health behavior change process across different settings including the home and family, educational and school settings, workplaces, health-care settings, as well as the wider community. Often different change strategies are implemented simultaneously across these different levels and settings.

Social and environmental-level strategies should complement those strategies targeting more individual-level influences and can include introducing particular programs or services, changes in policies or regulations, changes in the roles and functions of particular personnel, environmental modifications, use of the media, governmental policies and legislation, facilitating specific relations among people, and a variety of other initiatives.

This chapter provides an overview and examples of how health behavior change programs can be used to target and influence the physical, information, policy, and social environment in settings such as schools, the workplace, and the broader community. The *physical environment* refers to the presence, characteristics, and location of facilities relevant to those behaviors being targeted for change. The *information environment* includes sources of information and education that are relevant to understanding and influencing the desired behaviors. The *policy environment* includes policies, procedures, rules, and regulations relevant to the behavior and how these can be implemented and enforced. The *social environment* includes

 see C2

 see C5

 see C4

the subjective norms, social connections, and social support provided by family, friends, significant others, community members, and health professionals. This chapter also includes a broader discussion of the challenges involved in using such strategies to change health behaviors.

TARGETING THE SCHOOL AS A SETTING

Schools provide a well-established setting for behavior change programs reaching children, adolescents, and their families, to address age-specific health issues, such as child behavior problems, smoking, teenage pregnancy, and substance use. Schools also have trained staff, policies, and environments that can support such an approach. Social and environmental strategies in this setting may target the physical environment, social reinforcement, peer leaders, social norms, service provision, and local ordinances.

In the South East Asia region, the United Nations Children's Fund (UNICEF) has supported many governments to target the school physical environment to address helminth infection in schools. Through the Water, Environment, and Sanitation (WES) program, strategies aim to improve the number and hygiene status of school toilets and hand-washing facilities, provide safe drinking water, and develop policies relevant to the cleanliness of facilities (Luong 2003). In developed countries, strategies targeting the school physical environment include the provision of kid-safe playgrounds and equipment, sunshade areas, waste receptacles, insect control, and well-lit and ventilated classrooms (St Leger 1999).

Policies can be introduced to promote physical and psychological health within the school setting. Nutrition and food safety policies (integrated with national food and nutrition policies) can support and provide resources to supplement nutrition, rectify micronutrient deficiencies, and ensure appropriate food safety practices (WHO 1997). Governmental policies can prohibit the sale of tobacco and alcohol products to young people and can also prohibit the use of tobacco products by school staff and visitors (WHO 1997). Policies may also relate to the provision of specific services to support the health of students and staff, such as immunization, counseling, medical and nursing care, and psychological and social support services. Other policies to address health issues in the school setting can include sun protection (e.g. 'no hat, no play'), equity issues (e.g. access to subjects irrespective of gender), and classroom behavior management (e.g. use of corporal punishment) (St Leger 1999).

Social and environmental strategies are an integral component of many school-based anti-bullying interventions, with activities implemented at the level of the individual, classroom, and school. Programs aim to restructure the school environment so as to remove the positive and increase the negative consequences of bullying, via clear and firm rules against such behavior and the creation of a warm and positive school environment. The Bergen Anti-bullying Program precipitated many other international programs with strategies such as student assertiveness and conflict mediation skills training, establishing relevant class rules, introducing classroom activities to increase awareness and coping skills, training for playground supervisors and increased supervision in playgrounds, improvements in playground equipment, peer support schemes, and developing school policies addressed specifically at bullies and their targets (Smith & Ananiadou 2003).

The Child and Adolescent Trial for Cardiovascular Health (CATCH) implemented socio-environmental strategies targeting the school-based food service, physical activity opportunities, and tobacco control policies to promote long-term cardiovascular health in young people in America (Perry et al 1992). As part of CATCH, the Eat Smart School Nutrition program aimed to provide tasty, lower fat, and lower sodium meals and addressed menu planning, food purchasing, recipe modification, preparation, production, presentation, and promotion via a manual and training for food service managers at schools. The CATCH Physical Education (PE) program aimed to increase the amount of enjoyable physical activity during PE classes, with specialist training and resources for teachers in methods to maximize the number of students involved in physical activity during classes and to increase the amount of available class time for activity. The CATCH Smart Choices program provided guidelines on how to establish, implement, and evaluate tobacco use prevention policies for students and teachers on school grounds.

Barriers to implementation in the school setting

Typically, schools have a detailed and mandated curriculum and behavior change programs can be seen as competing with educational and administrative activities and disrupting a highly regulated system. Therefore, the degree to which behavior change programs are viewed as consistent with the service role of the school will influence the receptiveness and commitment to the strategies implemented (Linney 1989).

Programs with a social and environmental emphasis require the support of the educational system, school principal, teachers, parents, and sometimes the wider community. While collaboration with the school community is very important, this is often very time consuming and complicated. Furthermore, as teachers have a high level of professional autonomy in their classrooms, they can both support the design and implementation of such strategies or compromise the fidelity of a program (Linney 1989).

TARGETING THE WORKPLACE AND WORK ORGANIZATIONS AS A SETTING

The use of social and environmental strategies in the workplace setting to influence health behaviors aims to improve those aspects of the workplace and workplace culture that support desired behaviors while at the same time reducing workplace barriers to such behaviors. Historically, environmental programs in the workplace tended to focus on safety initiatives, such as reducing injury-related hazards and exposure to harmful substances. More recently, however, programs have focused on the characteristics of the workplace that are relevant for promoting health and preventing chronic disease.

The Australian National Workplace Health Project (NWHP) implemented a variety of socio-environmental strategies to promote health behaviors of physical activity, fruit and vegetable and low fat consumption, appropriate alcohol consumption, and smoking cessation (Simpson et al 2000). Box D8.1 provides a summary of some of the specific intervention components. Strategies for the physical environment included modifying the amount, availability, and appeal of health-enhancing facilities and options, such as adding low-fat, high-fiber food choices to vending machines and removing cigarette vending machines. Strategies for the information environment included posters, point-of-purchase messages, and take-home messages in employees' pay slips about healthy behavior choices. Strategies for the policy environment involved consideration of existing policies relating to employee health and the inclusion and implementation of specific statements about organizational support for healthy behaviors, such as restricting smoking and alcohol consumption.

The Brabantia project included screening of each employee for work-related wellness risks (Maes et al 1998). The screening information was used to create socio-environmental profiles for worksite production units and provided a basis for a 'wellness committee' to propose modifications to the work organization and environment that were implemented and evaluated in consultation with employees (Maes et al 1998). In one area, these modifications included increased worker authority over the rate and sequence of the production process, task rotation, improved ergonomic conditions, increased opportunities for social contacts among workers, and training staff to be multiskilled, thereby changing the organizational structure from a product to a functional orientation (Maes et al 1998).

The Working Well Trial included strategies targeting the social environment to change worksite norms relating to nutrition and smoking (Biener et al 1999). In addition to education programs, printed information, and smoking control activities, contests were held to encourage employees to learn about the dangers of tobacco smoke, support a smoker trying to quit, and understand the benefits of smoking cessation. To complement individual-level nutrition interventions, employees

Box D8.1   Core components of the Australian National Workplace Health Project (NWHP) Socio-Environmental Strategies to Promote Health-Enhancing Behaviors within the Workplace

Physical

Put up display racks and bulletin boards promoting healthy behaviors.

Addition of low-fat, high-fiber food items in vending machines and canteens.

Improve display of healthy food choices in canteens.

Increase amount, availability, and appeal of on-site exercise equipment.

Identify and promote local facilities, e.g. gyms, playing fields.

Increase non-smoking areas.

Remove cigarette vending machines.

Restrict access to alcohol at work.

Information

Induction package for all new employees.

Rotating poster series in key locations.

Newsletter and pay slip promotion of healthy behaviors, e.g. quick-and-easy 'bring-your-own lunches', on-site and local physical activity facilities, local quit smoking services, employee assistance programs.

Point-of-purchase information in canteens and on vending machines.

Magazines on healthy living purchased and placed in lunch areas.

Policy

Review existing policies for relevant statements related to healthy behaviors.

Encourage diet-specific statements, e.g. 'canteen staff will be trained/encouraged to follow health promotion guidelines'.

Encourage exercise-specific statements, e.g. 'the workplace promotes regular physical activity through the provision of, or arrangements with, on-site or local facilities'.

Encourage more restrictive smoking policies.

Encourage stricter enforcement of no-smoking policies.

Relaunch smoking policies, emphasizing the health-promoting benefits.

Encourage stricter enforcement of alcohol policies.

Relaunch alcohol policies, emphasizing health-promoting benefits.

used traditional family recipes, modified them to meet nutritional guidelines, prepared the foods, and then shared them at worksite taste tests and recipe contests.

Barriers to implementation in the workplace setting

The challenge for worksite-based programs is to implement socio-environmental behavior change strategies without adversely affecting productivity or profits (Oldenburg & Harris 1996). Most employers can only afford to devote organizational resources to socio-environmental behavior change programs when this provides some benefit to the organization, such as reduced medical costs, enhanced productivity, and/or enhanced company image (O'Donnell & Harris 1994). However, research evidence on the effectiveness of environmental and structural changes in the workplace to promote behavior change is still only emerging.

Few worksite studies have provided definitive evidence that health behavior change programs are a cost-effective means of decreasing health-care costs. The imprecision in estimating the economic and productivity costs of ill health often leads to an overstating of likely benefits and the dollar value of many indirect benefits of socio-environmental initiatives, such as improved social and emotional functioning of employees, is difficult to cost (Shephard 2002). Participation of employees, employers, and relevant stakeholders, such as union representatives, during the planning, implementation, and evaluation process is essential to gain support and commitment for socio-environmental strategies. However, the participation by senior and union personnel can also be interpreted as coercive and compromising individuals' rights (Shephard 2002). An integral part of program planning therefore is to identify strategies to gain and maintain access to the worksite, build support within the workplace, and develop and win the commitment of employees (e.g. Harris et al 1999).

TARGETING THE COMMUNITY AS A SETTING

Implementation of social and environmental strategies in the broader community aims to target those social settings and physical environments where behaviors occur, so that the norms in relation to particular behaviors and the environmental conditions supporting those behaviors are improved. Community-wide programs target entire populations or population subgroups using media, policy, or legislative action, at a regional or national level, and often in conjunction with many of those other methods already discussed in relation to other settings, such as the school and workplace.

The North Karelia Project (Puska et al 1995) was implemented in Finland in response to concern about Finland, and the North Karelia region in particular, having one of the highest international rates of cardiovascular disease at that time. The basic goals of the project were to:

- distribute information to make the community aware of the relationships between health behaviors and health outcomes
- provide persuasive messages to motivate people to make lifestyle and other changes to improve health
- provide training and support for individuals to make lifestyle changes
- give social support to help maintain lifestyle changes
- make changes in the environment to stimulate, facilitate, and maintain lifestyle change
- utilize existing community organizations to promote and support lifestyle change in the community
- provide improved preventive services to identify risk factors and appropriate interventions and treatment.

Information-based strategies included the distribution of bulletins, leaflets, posters, signs, and stickers in the community, as well as newspaper and radio articles (McAlister et al 1991). Public meetings about cardiovascular risk factors and their management were coordinated by local community-based organizations. Endorsements for health messages were obtained from prestigious organizations, such as the WHO, and opinion leaders, such as respected medical and other experts (Neittaanmaki et al 1980).

One major environmental goal was to increase the availability of low-fat foods. Local manufacturers were involved, with the main county dairy promoting low-fat dairy products and a local sausage factory developing a new product that replaced meat and fat content with mushrooms. Increased local production of berries and vegetables was encouraged, with education and training provided to farmers, as well as changes to institutional policies, to create markets for local products (e.g. purchase of orange juice by schools and hospitals) (Kuusipalo et al 1986). An informational and persuasive campaign was conducted to promote nutritional and economic incentives for consuming locally grown vegetables and berry products.

To facilitate healthy nutritional practices, the North Karelia Project collaborated with leaders of a local housewives' association to run community classes to teach women how to prepare healthy meals that were economical, enjoyable, and socially acceptable. These meals were promoted as increasing work capacity, conserving family and community resources, and consistent with a more traditional diet. Families were also invited to attend these sessions, so as to create social reinforcement.

Social modeling was further provided by a national television program showing people receiving behavioral counseling and skills training for healthy behaviors (Puska et al 1987). This campaign was complemented by trained volunteers providing explicit social reinforcement in their social networks for attention to and imitation of the television models. Additional social reinforcement was provided with a lottery offered to smokers to win a trip to Hawaii, with the reward provided if they became a non-smoker.

The provision of preventive services in North Karelia was reorganized to increase the responsibility assigned to local public health nurses and establish new offices at community health centers. Other environmental modifications included the promotion of smoke-free environments, which led to national tax legislation – there were increases in tobacco taxes that included a specific allocation to support health promotion campaigns on a national scale.

Examples of socio-environmental strategies implemented in other community-based health behavior change programs have included targeting policies and ordinances, merchant policies and practices, and enforcement practices; these form the basis of many tobacco control programs. The Tobacco Policy Options for Prevention (TPOP) program aimed to reduce youth access to tobacco and utilized a community activation approach to establish ordinances, such as bans on tobacco vending machines and self-service merchandising, a licensing fee to cover compliance checks, unannounced compliance checks at all retail outlets by a designated enforcement agency, and a graduate civil penalty scheme against license holders who violated age-sale laws (Blaine et al 1997).

Barriers to implementation in the community setting

Often the results of implementing community-based socio-environmental strategies are disappointingly small in comparison to the efforts required to implement such strategies. One reason for this is the unrealistic expectations created by individual-level approaches to behavior change that can yield greater magnitude of change, although in fewer individuals (Sorenson et al 1998). However, the magnitude of the results of community-based strategies must be judged according to population-level effects; therefore, using clinical significance alone as the standard for interpretation of results is inappropriate (Sorenson et al 1998).

Desired and sustained behavior change outcomes in the broader community can often take several years to achieve, with the precise causal pathways being difficult to disentangle from many other programs and activities addressing the same or related behaviors. Therefore, successful changes in socio-environmental exposures are difficult to evaluate in terms of their impact on incidence at a population level. Moreover, the majority of community-based behavior change programs do not have the resources to conduct long-term follow-up and last for less than 1 year (Freudenberg et al 2000).

MEASUREMENT OF THE CHANGE PROCESS

Measurement of the impact and outcomes following the implementation of social and environmental strategies can be objective, where there is direct observation of any change, or subjective, which relies on participant perceptions of change. Methods of data collection can include environmental audits, participant surveys, and key informant interviews.

Environmental audits involve direct observation of the relevant features of the environment and are typically conducted before and after the intervention to assess potential change. The Checklist for Health promoting Environments at Work (CHEW), for example, can be used to assess the observable characteristics of worksite buildings and properties, and features of the observable information environment and immediate neighborhood that could potentially influence health behaviors (Oldenburg et al 2002).

Community-level indicators (CLIs) are based on observations of aspects of the community and may evaluate socio-environmental change (Cheadle et al 2000). CLIs for promotion of physical activity, for example, include policies which address physical education in school curricula, the proportion of local budget per capita devoted to physical activity resources, the proportion of health-care providers routinely advising patients to be physically active, the miles of walking and cycle trails per capita, observations of usage of community-based activity facilities, availability of worksite facilities to support physical activity, such as bike racks and showers, and membership in physical activity organizations (Cheadle et al 2000).

Self-administered participant surveys are a common means of assessing participant perceptions of socio-environmental change. Worksite programs may include employee survey questions about perceptions of organizational, supervisor, and co-worker support for the targeted behaviors. Community-based surveys can be used to assess perceptions of the availability and accessibility of products or facilities. School-based surveys can be used to assess teachers' knowledge and implementation of policies and procedures. Surveys may be administered by telephone, mail, or using other strategies, such as dissemination via key individuals or organizations.

The use of interviews with key informants involves face-to-face interviews with key stakeholders associated with the socio-environmental change. In the workplace, this may include senior managers to assess relevant worksite policies and their implementation and use. School-based programs may access teachers, parent and citizen committees, or senior education-based personnel to assess their perceptions of the social environment within the school.

STRENGTHS AND CHALLENGES OF IMPLEMENTING SOCIAL AND ENVIRONMENTAL STRATEGIES TO PROMOTE BEHAVIOR CHANGE

Targeting social and environmental influences of behavior in defined settings, such as work organizations, schools, and the broader community, is consistent with a *population-based* approach to behavior change. With this approach, social and environmental strategies aim to reduce the average levels of risk in large numbers of individuals by targeting the conditions that contribute to problems at the individual level. As discussed by Rose (1994), population-based approaches have the potential to be radical and powerful. Such strategies also move beyond 'blaming' individuals for their behavior and acknowledge the salience of social, environmental, and cultural influences on behavior.

Social and environmental approaches to behavior change, however, can be limited by their acceptability, feasibility, and costs. For example, a strategy such as introducing legislation to limit behavior may compromise individual choice. Individuals passively exposed to such strategies in the broader community or within a particular setting may not perceive the intervention components as relevant to them nor perceive themselves as active program participants working towards a specific behavior change outcome.

 see A3

Where specific actions are required by the individual to initiate and maintain behavior change, such changes are more likely to be adopted if they are not complex, have minimal impact on social relations, are easily reversible, require only modest time and resource commitment, and involve minimal risk and uncertainty (Rogers 1995). Accordingly, social and environmental strategies often have very limited adoption because of their complexity, irreversibility, need for extensive resources and commitment, and degree of uncertainty. Changes in social relations and environments are often complex, requiring the introduction of new programs or services, changes in policies or regulations, changes in the roles and functions of particular personnel, use of the media, governmental policies and legislation, as well as coordination of a variety of other individual-level initiatives. Programs incorporating these various elements require considerable resources, large budgets, and an extended period of time for implementation and evaluation, and may therefore not be easily reversible if the desired outcomes are not achieved. The evidence base supporting various program components is also often far from compelling.

Typically, social and environmental strategies are implemented in 'real-world' communities and other settings and are therefore subject to 'real-world' issues and limitations. Compared to individual-level behavior change programs, there is generally less control over activities, there are a large number of potential participants, and numerous limitations and restrictions to deal with. Widespread programs are costly and require extensive planning, coordination, liaison, and monitoring. The challenge, therefore, is to provide sufficient reach and program exposure to a population or target group that is physically, geographically, and socially diverse. There is also the challenge to coordinate activities to avoid unnecessary duplication and 'participant overload'. Consequently, consultation and collaboration are required with many stakeholders, which is time consuming. Collaboration with stakeholders not directly involved in the behavior change program as part of their core business can be particularly challenging.

CONCLUSION AND FUTURE DIRECTIONS

Behavior change researchers and practitioners have increasingly come to recognize the strong links between behavior and aspects of individuals' social and physical environment. Ecological models of behavior change focus on the interrelationships among the intrapersonal, social, cultural, and environmental influences of behavior (Sallis & Owen 2002), and provide a useful framework for facilitating the design, implementation, and evaluation of socio-environmental change strategies to promote health (Stokols 1992, 1996).

Social and environmental influences are ubiquitous and more work is needed to identify relevant salient variables and ways to assess and influence them (Sallis & Owen 2002). Research is needed to demonstrate that socio-environmental variables add to our explanation of variance in behavior beyond that of individual-level variables. We need a better understanding of the relevant social and environmental barriers and facilitators of behavior change across a range of behaviors, population subgroups, and settings. More research is needed to demonstrate that strategies targeting socio-environmental factors are effective in changing behavior and maintaining change.

As research and practice evidence regarding the interconnectedness between individual behavior and social and physical environments continue to accumulate, so the traditional lines of delineation between different professional and other roles will also need to change. It is becoming more important to work across disciplines and sectors in order to develop, implement, and evaluate more innovative and effective approaches to behavior change that address satisfactorily the multiple social, environmental, and other influences on health and health behaviors. Behavior change researchers and practitioners need to work together more cooperatively and collaboratively on this endeavor to achieve social and environmental change.

References

Biener L, Glanz K, McLeraan D et al 1999 Impact of the Working Well Trial on the worksite smoking and nutrition environment. Health Education and Behavior 26:478-494

Blaine T M, Forster J L, Hennrikus D et al 1997 Creating tobacco control policy at the local level: implementation of a direct action organizing approach. Health Education and Behavior 24:640-651

Cheadle A, Sterling T D, Schmid T L et al 2000 Promising community-level indicators for evaluating cardiovascular health-promotion programs. Health Education Research 15:109-116

Freudenberg N, Silver D, Carmona J M et al 2000 Health promotion in the city: a structured review of the literature on interventions to prevent heart disease, substance abuse, violence, and HIV infection in US metropolitan areas 1980-1995. Journal of Urban Health – Bulletin of the New York Academy of Medicine 77:443-457

Harris D, Oldenburg B, Owen N 1999 Australian National Workplace Health Project: strategies for gaining access, support, commitment. Health Promotion Journal of Australia 9:49-54

Kuusipalo J, Mikkola M, Moisio S et al 1986 The East Finland berry and vegetable project: a health related structural intervention programme. Health Promotion 1:385

Linney J A 1989 Optimizing research strategies in the schools. In: Bond L A, Compas B E (eds) Primary prevention and promotion in schools. Sage, Newbury Park, pp 50-76

Luong T V 2003 Deworming school children and hygiene intervention. International Journal of Environmental Health Research 13(suppl):S153

Maes S, Verhoeven C, Kittel F et al 1998 Effects of a Dutch worksite health program: the Brabantia Project. American Journal of Public Health 88:1037-1041

McAlister A, Orlandi M, Puska P et al 1991 Behavior modification in public health: principles and illustrations. In: Holland W W, Detels R, Knox E G (eds) Oxford textbook of public health. Oxford Medical Publications, London

Neittaanmaki L, Koskela K, Puska P et al 1980 The role of lay workers in community health education in the North Karelia Project. Scandinavian Journal of Social Medicine 8:1

O'Donnell M P, Harris J S 1994 Health promotion in the workplace. Delmar Publishers, New York

Oldenburg B, Harris D 1996 The workplace as a setting for promoting health and preventing diseases. Homeostasis 5:226-232

Oldenburg B, Sallis J, Harris D et al 2002 Checklist of health promotion environments at worksites: development and measurement characteristics. American Journal of Health Promotion 16:288-295

Perry C L, Parcel G S, Stone E et al 1992 The Child and Adolescent Trial for Cardiovascular Health (CATCH): overview of the intervention program and evaluation methods. Cardiovascular Risk Factors 2:36-44

Puska P, McAlister A, Niemensivu H et al 1987 A television format for national health promotion: Finland's 'Keys to Health'. US Public Health Reports 102:263

Puska P, Tuomilehto J, Nissinen A et al 1995 The North Karelia Project. Twenty year results and experiences. Helsinki University Printing House, Helsinki

Rogers E M 1995 Diffusion of innovations, 4th edn. Free Press, New York

Rose G 1994 The strategy of preventive medicine. Oxford University Press, Oxford

Sallis J, Owen N 2002 Ecological models. In: Glanz K, Lewis F M, Rimer B K (eds) Health behavior and health education: theory, research and practice, 3rd edn. Jossey-Bass, San Francisco, pp 462-484

Shephard R J 2002 Issues in worksite health promotion: a personal viewpoint. Quest 54:67-82

Simpson J, Oldenburg B, Owen N et al 2000 The Australian National Workplace Health Project: design and baseline findings. Preventive Medicine 31:249-260

Smith P K, Ananiadou K 2003 The nature of school bullying and the effectiveness of school-based interventions. Journal of Applied Psychoanalytic Studies 5:189-209

Sorensen G, Emmons K, Hunt M K et al 1998 Implications of the results of community intervention trials. Annual Review of Public Health 19:379-416

St Leger L H 1999 The opportunities and effectiveness of the health promoting primary school in improving child health – a review of the claims and evidence. Health Education Research 14:51-69

Stokols D 1992 Establishing and maintaining healthy environments: toward a social ecology of health promotion. American Psychologist 47:6-22

Stokols D 1996 Translating social ecological theory into guidelines for community health promotion. American Journal of Health Promotion 10:282-298

World Health Organization (WHO) 1997 Promoting health through schools. World Health Organization, Geneva

Mediated communication

Michael Slater

INTRODUCTION

Few tasks are more challenging than trying to influence human behavior via mass media. We are all familiar with the difficulty of influencing behavior of the people who are closest to us, who have the greatest reason to listen to what we have to say, and to whom we have nearly unlimited access. It is clearly not an easy thing to influence behavior at second hand, via media messages that have been generated to appeal to masses of people as against a single, idiosyncratic human being, without the ability to directly and individually respond to reservations and doubts. Nonetheless, such influence clearly is possible, for better (as in public health campaigns) and for worse (as in the case of tobacco marketing).

Use of mediated communication (television, radio, the Internet, posters, newspapers, etc.) to change health behaviors is widespread in both industrialized and less developed nations (Hornik 2002a). Recent metaanalyses of such campaigns in the USA suggest that they do often succeed in influencing health-related attitudes and behavior, though effect sizes, especially for resistant behaviors, such as smoking, are typically quite small (Snyder & Hamilton 2002). Even assuming small effect sizes, the relative efficiency of reaching millions of people via mass media can render them a potentially highly cost-effective means of influencing health behaviors (Hornik 1989).

INDIVIDUAL-LEVEL BEHAVIOR CHANGE AND MEDIATED COMMUNICATION

The strategic, theory-based use of mass media

Too often, naïve health practitioners or public health officials will respond to public needs for health information or behavior change by asking for a brochure or poster. What rational person, after all, would fail to change their behavior once the risks involved are pointed out?

Professional communicators sometimes refer to this as the 'octopus' strategy – the reflex of squirting ink blindly at a problem. The reality, of course, is that many people are unlikely to even attend to the poster or pick up the brochure, dismissing them as irrelevant or believing that the behaviors recommended are ineffective or too difficult to carry out (McGuire 2001).

i see B5

The Stages of Change or Transtheoretical Model (Prochaska et al 1992) is widely used as a basis for understanding individual behavior change. Figure D9.1 illustrates how major theories of behavior change relevant to mediated communication, such as the Theory of Reasoned Action (Ajzen & Fishbein 1980), Social Cognitive Theory (Bandura 1997), and attitude accessibility (Fazio et al 1989), can be conceptually integrated using a transtheoretical framework.

These relationships and their implications for media-based health behavior change have been discussed in detail elsewhere (Slater 1999). To briefly summarize: mass media have obvious utility for persons who are uninformed or are in denial regarding a health risk (or in precontemplation); media campaigns can be very efficient at increasing the salience of health issues through increased exposure (Fan 2002) and at

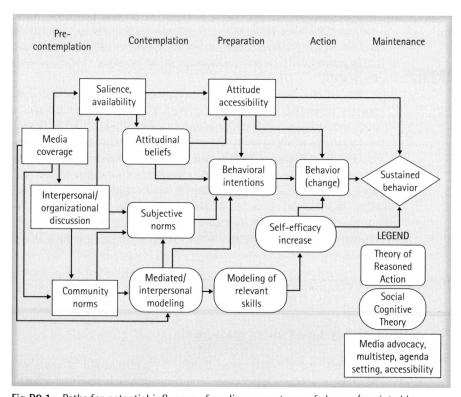

Fig D9.1   Paths for potential influence of media across stages of change (reprinted by permission from Slater 1999)

influencing people by providing new information (Snyder & Hamilton 2002). Such increased salience, particularly if reinforced through continued media exposure and including appropriate situational cues (e.g. AIDS messages regarding condom use that portray intimate situations and discussions), is likely to increase the accessibility of relevant attitudes at the time of behavioral decision (Fazio et al 1989).

In addition, new information conveyed via mass media can be targeted to people who are in the 'contemplation' stage, i.e. aware of the health risk and weighing the costs and benefits of behavior change. This new information, consistent with the Theory of Reasoned Action (Ajzen & Fishbein 1980) and Theory of Planned Behavior (Ajzen 1991), can focus on those attitudinal beliefs most closely linked to relevant behavioral intentions. For example, beliefs that condoms are ineffective in preventing AIDS or that they interfere with sexual performance can be directly addressed in the message content.

Social Cognitive Theory (Bandura 1997) and the Theory of Planned Behavior (Ajzen 1991) emphasize the importance of self-efficacy or the belief that one can successfully carry out a given behavior in bridging the gap between attitudes and actual behavior change. Media, especially audiovisual media, such as television or the Internet, lend themselves to showing models similar to target audience members successfully enacting the skills needed to carry out the new behavior. For example, AIDS messages that show women successfully negotiating use of condoms with a prospective sexual partner are likely to increase women viewers' self-efficacy and likelihood of enacting the behavior (Maibach & Cotton 1995).

The most difficult determinants of behavior to address via the media are perceived social norms and actual social pressures, or subjective norms in the Theory of Reasoned Action terminology (Ajzen & Fishbein 1980). To some extent it may be possible to influence perceptions regarding such norms by modeling desirable norms in narrative media messages (Singhal & Rogers 1999). A more direct approach of reporting actual behavioral norms that contradict widely held misperceptions has been used with some apparent success to reduce 'binge' drinking on American college campuses (Perkins 2003). Media can also convey support of national leaders and other influential people for new health behavioral norms that can impact both policy and individual behavior, as has taken place in Thailand, one of the few AIDS control success stories (Rogers & Singhal 2003).

Segmenting the audience for health information and the role of formative research

Audience segmentation, or identifying and prioritizing relatively homogeneous audience subgroups, is fundamental to behavior change communication (Slater 1995). There are a variety of research tools with which to conduct audience segmentation, ranging from extensive survey research to create composite psychobehavioral profiles (Maibach et al 1996) to literature searches and key informant interviews; the appropriate level of research is a function both of how well known audiences are with respect to a given behavior and the time, expertise, and money available to the campaign planner (Slater 1995). The Stages of Change Model is itself a kind of segmentation strategy, focusing attention on systematic differences between readiness to engage in behavior change and associated barriers to change. However, it should be noted that there are likely to be distinctive subaudiences within any given stage, with distinctive barriers to behavior change and different media use preferences that should result in distinctive media intervention strategies (Slater 1999).

Formative research – research intended to identify audience segments, profile their knowledge, beliefs, and barriers to behavior change, and to pretest messages tailored to such segments – is an essential element of any communication-based behavior change effort (Atkin & Freimuth 2001). Surveys can be used to help develop segmentation schemes, to describe patterns of beliefs and attitudes, and to provide a baseline for evaluation research. Focus groups are widely used to explore the beliefs and perceptions of audience segments (though limits on generalizability should be kept in mind) and to iteratively test messages designed to address the beliefs and perceived barriers of that segment. Few investments in a media behavior change effort are more rewarding (or more sobering) than showing proposed messages to members of the intended audience in a focus group and getting their candid, in-depth reactions.

Tailoring messages for audience segments

There are a variety of strong theory-based models for developing messages for various audience segments (Maibach & Parrot 1995). For example, research in the elaboration-likelihood model of persuasion suggests that for persons in the precontemplation stage, messages must be simple, short, and cognitively undemanding and may depend heavily on credible or attractive sources (Petty & Cacioppo 1986). Messages consistent with the Theory of Reasoned Action and Planned Behavior may be carefully calibrated to influence key attitudinal beliefs for people weighing the costs and benefits of behavior change (Capella et al 2001). Messages seeking to influence behavior change to reduce exposure to risk can be developed utilizing research into effective versus ineffective messages concerning health risks (Witte et al 2001). Other authorities point out that some audiences (such as many adolescents) are not very risk averse and that message design must take into account tendencies such as arousal and novelty seeking (Palmgreen et al 2001).

As noted above, modeling can be used in media messages to teach skills needed to enact behavior change and to increase self-efficacy (Bandura 1997, Maibach & Cotton 1995). Use of narrative messages may be especially effective in encouraging behavior change with resistant audiences (Singhal & Rogers 1999). In tailored messaging, an audience segmentation algorithm is developed that permits segmenting audience members based on several segmentation variables. Highly targeted messages are then created through computer programs that can typically generate over 100 possible combinations of distinctive messages into a single customized newsletter. Such customized newsletters have been found to be more successful than traditional print media in influencing health behavior change (Kreuter et al 2000).

The reader charged with responsibility for using mediated communication in health interventions is urged to review sources cited here and available communication planning resources (CDC 2001, US DHHS 2002) for guidance in developing segmentation schemes and appropriately tailored messages. These resources also provide step-by-step guides for channel selection and evaluation efforts.

Channel selection

Selection of appropriate media channels – flyers, posters, television ads, radio, newsletters, newspaper coverage of special events, etc. – is another critical communication planning decision. Three factors usually shape this decision.

The first factor is the stage of change or level of involvement of members of an audience segment. Detailed, technical information typical of many print channels is likely to be ignored by persons who do not consider the information personally relevant or a high priority (Johnson 1997). Use of television and radio ads, news coverage, and highly visible posters make more sense. Conversely, if important audience segments are known to be actively seeking information regarding a topic (e.g. cancer prevention and treatment), access to hotlines and websites that can provide authoritative and detailed information becomes a high priority (Rice & Katz 2001), and other mass media may serve largely as a means to publicize the availability of the information research to those interested audiences. Interactive media can be designed to maximize the likelihood of behavior change for audiences who are motivated, or obliged, to make use of them (Buller et al 2001).

The second factor is audience preference. Use of television ads with an audience that has little access to television or watches programs other than the ones on which the ads are placed represents a waste of time and money. An important task in formative research (usually best achieved through surveys) is to identify the media channels preferred by each audience segment of interest.

The third factor, of course, is resource limitations: money, time, and expertise. Paid television ads are available only for the best-funded efforts. On the other hand, visually and dramatically engaging special events, skillfully staged and promoted to the media, may inexpensively result in the kind of extensive media exposure that would be impossible to buy at any cost. Flyers and posters, with intelligently designed and pretested content, distributed widely to locations frequented by one's intended audience, can be quite effective. And, of course, where money is limited, there is a natural tendency to focus on media that existing staff members are already experienced in developing. Care should be taken, of course, that audience member needs and not prior experience drive channel selection (i.e. don't do a brochure or newsletter just because someone on staff knows how to produce them).

Exposure

It is not enough to do an effective job of characterizing one's audiences and developing appropriate messages responsive to audience members' concerns and barriers. If people do not receive an adequate level of exposure to the messages, they are unlikely to have an impact. Many otherwise well-conceived media campaign efforts may have failed for just this reason (Hornik 2002b, Snyder & Hamilton 2002). Complicating this problem is the difficulty of ascertaining in advance what a required level of exposure might be. Advertisers are able, by tracking audience responses as a function of advertising expenditure, to compute the level of expenditure required to maintain a given level of audience awareness. Most health campaigns do not pay for advertising space and have no ability to track exposure in such a way.

Therefore, it is incumbent on the health communication practitioner to try to maximize exposure, usually through use of multiple and reinforcing communication strategies. Posters might be seen in a health clinic or at schools, public service announcements (PSAs) heard on the radio, messages stamped on grocery bags at a local market, brochures handed out by a doctor or nurse, even stamped on rulers or key chains given away as promotions. Ingenuity in maximizing exposure among intended audiences on a limited budget is as important as thoughtful research and creativity in message development.

Evaluation

Evaluation is a fundamental element of behavior change campaigns employing mediated communication. Formative research, used for planning interventions and developing messages, has been briefly discussed already. Process evaluation is normally employed as a management

Table D9.1 Attitude–behavior segmentation matrix

Audience segment	Relevant objective	Concerns/ obstacles	Message to address such concerns	Channels appropriate to audience and message	Evaluation
Segment 1					
Segment 2					
Segment 3					
Segment 4					

tool to ensure plans are being carried out and, if the process evaluation resources permit, to assess preliminary data regarding impact on objectives and to shift resources from unsuccessful initiatives to those that appear to have more impact (Rice & Foote 2001).

Summative or outcome evaluation is used to assess the extent to which a communication intervention achieved desired objectives. Evaluation of mediated interventions can pose exceptional methodological challenges, given the wide and often hard-to-control reach of mass media and possibly varying criteria for effectiveness (Hornik 2002c, Salmon & Murray-Johnson 2001). A planning matrix may be used to facilitate the integration of these elements into a comprehensive plan (see Table D9.1); a checklist is also provided in Box D9.1.

COMMUNITY-LEVEL INTERVENTION EFFORTS AND MASS MEDIA

Critics sometimes point out that intervention campaigns typically involve a government agency or non-governmental organization (NGO) pursuing its vision of health objectives without explicit policy input from the people whom the campaign hopes to influence (Salmon 1989). Community-based interventions, in contrast, involve representatives of communities in communication, identifying objectives and strategies before the intervention plan is finalized and implemented (Bracht 1999).

There is some evidence that such community-based efforts can successfully shift health behaviors throughout a community or region. One

---

Box D9.1   Checklist for mediated communication interventions

- Define health problem.
- Determine resources/obstacles/opportunities.
- Obtain community/stakeholder inputs.
- Define measurable objectives.
- Identify distinctive audience segments to be addressed (using stages of change and other theoretical frameworks as needed).
- Conduct formative research (surveys, focus groups, literature search, and/or key informant interviews) with each priority segment to determine relevant concerns, obstacles, benefits desired, media channels, and sources preferred.
- Build planning matrix to guide message development, channel strategy, and evaluation.
- Develop channel strategy appropriate to audiences and to content, given available financial and message development resources, as well as plan for rollout of communication effort.
- Work with creative team to develop message concepts and storyboards.
- Test messages with appropriate market segments using focus groups or theater testing; obtain feedback from key community and other stakeholders.
- Revise, retest if needed, produce and distribute messages.
- Monitor exposure to campaign messages and effects of messages if possible; adjust strategies as needed.
- Summative evaluation: assess what worked and what didn't, take lessons into next effort.

---

of the most successful examples of such efforts has taken place in North Karelia, Finland, in which very high cardiovascular risks have been reduced largely through changes in diet (Vartiainen et al 2000).

However, it is important to temper enthusiasm for the potential of community-based approaches with a realistic appraisal of associated obstacles and challenges. Often, communities suffer from significant social conflicts, based on economic class, caste, religion, and ethnicity. Building consensus and support for a behavior change norm can be difficult and interventionists may confront difficult political and ethical issues in such a community environment. For example, health behavior change that empowers women may be highly controversial among community leadership in a traditionalist culture, making consensus building a problematic exercise, and may even place community members cooperating with an intervention effort at risk.

Even without substantial dissension within a community, communities vary considerably in their ability and willingness to engage in a behavior change effort. Some researchers argue that communities move through a stages of change process, as do individuals. Community readiness to engage with a problem behavior, from this perspective, must not only be assessed, but the nature of coalition building efforts and communication approaches should vary depending on where communities fall on the readiness continuum (Slater et al 2000). For the community as for the individual, one size does not fit all.

MASS MEDIA AND SOCIAL POLICY CHANGE

Some critics (Wallack et al 1993) criticize communication and social marketing efforts intended to change individual behaviors, rather than social and economic policies that may help create the public health problems. Alternatively, one may view the relationship between individual behavior and social policy as a continuum rather than as an opposition. As noted earlier, communication to encourage individual behavior change, to a considerable extent, impacts relevant opinions and concerns in a national population (Fan 2002). Mass communication research suggests that such salience, by influencing perceptions of public opinion, can also impact policy makers and other influential people (Price & Roberts 1987). Other recent research also suggests that news coverage of substance use risks impacts individual behavior not directly but via the impact of news coverage on public policy (Yanovitzky & Bennett 1999).

Public health advocates, then, can use the mass media to influence public opinion and public policy. This approach has been referred to in public health circles as 'media advocacy' (Wallack et al 1993) or 'behavioral journalism' (McAlister & Fernandez 2002). One of the most attractive elements of such media advocacy approaches, as noted earlier, is that ingenious use of events, visuals, and arresting individual experiences or research-based facts can result, at very little cost, in widespread media coverage with an impact that would be impossible to achieve by directly spending any amount of cash (Wallack et al 1999).

CONCLUSION

The public health practitioner would be wise to approach use of mass media and other mediated communication with a sober optimism. Successful use of mediated communication takes a considerable investment in thought, planning, and in formative research to understand one's audiences. Success is unlikely without understanding how to segment audiences into more meaningful and reasonably homogeneous subgroups, identifying the issues and barriers to behavior change, characterizing people in those segments, and assessing their level of attention and the type of media they are likely to use. Even if these are adequately characterized and theoretically appropriate message strategies are developed, success is still uncertain. There is still the creative challenge of designing messages consistent with these theoretical models to which people will respond as intended. One has to be very lucky to get that right on the first try; that is why message pretesting is so crucial to a successful communication effort. Even with good formative research, good planning, good messages, and good pretesting, attitude or behavior change is unlikely if one is unable to generate enough exposure to these messages among a target audience.

These are cautions to encourage careful implementation and are not intended to discourage such initiatives. The benefits of well-conducted media-based campaigns are considerable. They have tremendous reach and typically have low costs relative to such reach. They can create a climate of concern and attention that facilitates efforts of health providers when they give direct advice to patients. They can raise public and policy maker concern and impact policies relevant to public health. And, with good research, good planning, good execution, and sometimes a touch of good luck, they can help change health-related behavior for the better.

References

Ajzen I 1991 The theory of planned behavior. Organizational Behavior and Human Decision Processes 50(2):179-211

Ajzen I, Fishbein M 1980 Understanding attitudes and predicting social behavior. Prentice-Hall, Englewood Cliffs

Atkin C K, Freimuth V S 2001 Formative evaluation research in campaign design. In: Rice R E, Atkin C K (eds) Public communication campaigns. Sage, Thousand Oaks, pp 125-145

Bandura A 1997 Self efficacy: the exercise of control. Freeman, New York

Bracht N (ed) 1999 Health promotion at the community level, 2nd edn. Sage, Newbury Park

Buller D B, Woodall W G, Hall J R et al 2001 A web-based smoking cessation and prevention program for children aged 12 to 15. In: Rice R E, Atkin C K (eds) Public communication campaigns. Sage, Thousand Oaks, pp 357-372

Capella J N, Fishbein M, Hornik R C et al 2001 Using theory to select messages in anti-drug campaigns: reasoned action and media priming. In: Rice R E, Atkin C K (eds) Public communication campaigns. Sage, Thousand Oaks, pp 214-230

Centers for Disease Control (CDC) 2001 Communication at CDC, in CDCynergy, Interactive Health Communication Program Planning CD-ROM. Available online at: www.cdc.gov/cdcynergy/

Fan D P 2002 Impact of persuasive information on secular trends in health-related behaviors. In: Hornik R C (ed) Public health communication: evidence for behavior change. Lawrence Erlbaum Associates, Mahwah, pp 251-264

Fazio R H, Powell M C, Williams C J 1989 The role of attitude accessibility in the attitude-to-behavior process. Journal of Consumer Research 16:280-288

Hornik R C 1989 Channel effectiveness in development communication programs. In: Rice R E, Atkin C K (eds) Public communication campaigns. Sage, Newbury Park, pp 309-330

Hornik R C (ed) 2002a Public health communication: evidence for behavior change. Lawrence Erlbaum Associates, Mahwah

Hornik R C 2002b Evaluation design for public health communication programs. In: Hornik R C (ed) Public health communication: evidence for behavior change. Lawrence Erlbaum Associates, Mahwah, pp 385-405

Hornik R C 2002c Public health communication: making sense of contradictory evidence. In: Hornik R C (ed) Public health communication: evidence for behavior change. Lawrence Erlbaum Associates, Mahwah, pp 1-22

Johnson J D 1997 Cancer-related information seeking. Hampton Press, Cresskill

Kreuter M, Farrell D, Olevitch L et al 2000 Tailoring health messages: customizing communication with computer technology. Lawrence Erlbaum Associates, Mahwah

Maibach E W, Cotton D 1995 Moving people to behavior change: a staged social cognitive approach to message design. In: Maibach E W, Parrott R L (eds) Designing health messages: approaches from communication theory and public health practice. Sage, Newbury Park, pp 41-64

Maibach E W, Parrott R L (eds) 1995 Designing health messages: approaches from communication theory and public health practice. Sage, Thousand Oaks

Maibach E W, Maxfield A, Ladin K et al 1996 Translating health psychology into effective health communication: the American healthstyles audience segmentation project. Journal of Health Psychology 1:261-277

McAlister A L, Fernandez M 2002 'Behaviorial journalism' accelerates diffusion of healthy innovations. In: Hornik R C (ed) Public health communication: evidence for behavior change. Lawrence Erlbaum Associates, Mahwah, pp 315-326

McGuire W J 2001 Input and output variables currently promising for constructing persuasive communications. In: Rice R E, Atkin C K (eds) Public communication campaigns. Sage, Thousand Oaks, pp 22-48

Palmgreen P, Donohew L, Lorch E et al 2001 Television campaigns and adolescent marijuana use: tests of sensation seeking targeting. American Journal of Public Health 91:292-295

Perkins W H 2003 The social norms approach to preventing school and college age substance abuse. Jossey-Bass, San Francisco

Petty R E, Cacioppo J T 1986 Communication and persuasion: central and peripheral routes to attitude change. Springer Verlag, New York

Price V, Roberts D F 1987 Public opinion processes. In: Berger C R, Chaffee S H (eds) Handbook of communication science. Sage, Newbury Park, pp 781-816

Prochaska J O, DiClemente C C, Norcross J C 1992 In search of how people change: applications to addictive behaviors. American Psychologist 47:1102-1114

Rice R E, Foote D R 2001 A systems-based evaluation planning model for health communication campaigns in developing countries. In: Rice R E, Atkin C K (eds) Public communication campaigns. Sage, Thousand Oaks, pp 146-167

Rice R E, Katz J E 2001 The Internet and health communication: experiences and expectations. Sage, Thousand Oaks

Rogers E M, Singhal A 2003 Combating AIDS: communication strategies in action. Sage, Thousand Oaks

Salmon C T 1989 Campaigns for social improvement: an overview of values, rationales, and impacts. In: Salmon C T (ed) Information campaigns: balancing social values and social change. Sage, Thousand Oaks, pp 19-53

Salmon C T, Murray-Johnson L 2001 Communication campaign effectiveness: critical distinctions. In: Rice R E, Atkin C K (eds) Public communication campaigns. Sage, Thousand Oaks, pp 168-180

Singhal A, Rogers E M 1999 Entertainment-education: a communication strategy for social change. Lawrence Erlbaum Associates, Mahwah

Slater M D 1995 Choosing audience segmentation strategies and methods for health communication. In: Maibach E W, Parrott R L (ed) Designing health messages: approaches from communication theory and public health practice. Sage, Newbury Park, pp 186-198

Slater M D 1999 Integrating application of media effects, persuasion and behavior change theories to communication campaigns: a stages of change framework. Health Communication 11:335-354

Slater M D, Kelly K, Edwards R 2000 Integrating social marketing, community readiness, and media advocacy in community-based prevention efforts. Social Marketing Quarterly 6:125-137

Snyder L, Hamilton M 2002 Meta-analysis of U.S. health campaign effects on behavior: emphasize enforcement, exposure, and new information, and beware the secular trend. In: Hornik R C (ed) Public health communication: evidence for behavior change. Lawrence Erlbaum Associates, Mahwah, pp 357-383

US Department of Health and Human Services (DHHS), National Cancer Institute 2002 Making health communication programs work. Available online at: cancer.gov/pinkbook

Vartiainen E, Jousilahti P, Alfthan G et al 2000 Cardiovascular risk factor changes in Finland, 1972-1997. International Journal of Epidemiology 29(1):49-56

Wallack L, Dorfman L, Jernigan D 1993 Media advocacy and public health. Sage, Newbury Park

Wallack L, Woodruff K, Dorfman L et al 1999 News for a change: an advocate's guide to working with the media. Sage, Thousand Oaks

Witte K, Meyer G, Martell D P 2001 Effective health risk messages. Sage, Thousand Oaks

Yanovitzky I, Bennett C 1999 Media attention, institutional response, and health behavior change: the case of drunk driving, 1978-1996. Communication Research 26:429-453

Social marketing

Gerard Hastings, Elinor Devlin,
and Lynn MacFadyen

INTRODUCTION

i see C5

The Framework Convention on Tobacco Control is testament to the power of marketing. It is the first international treaty specifically designed to constrain the marketing of a product because it is known to have such an important impact on health behavior. Similarly, the World Health Organization (WHO) recognizes the power that marketing has to influence health behavior in its well-publicized critiques of alcohol, tobacco, and food marketing.

But this coin has another side. If marketing can be used by commerce to influence health-damaging consumer behavior, it can also be used in the non-profit sector to encourage health-improving behavior. In this chapter we will explore the potential for marketing to work in this beneficial way. The chapter begins by considering the ideas and theories underpinning the discipline. Social marketing planning is then examined step by step. The principle of exerting influence further 'upstream' by targeting stakeholders is then discussed, as are the benefits of relational thinking and ethical issues.

IS IT POSSIBLE TO SELL BROTHERHOOD LIKE SOAP?

The unique feature of social marketing is that it takes learning from the commercial sector and applies it to the resolution of social and health problems. The logic is that the Nikes and Coca Colas of this world are ultimately concerned with influencing behavior. They want people to start buying their products, buy more of them, stop buying someone else's, and so on. Social marketers argue that we should both criticize this activity when it does harm, for example in the hands of the tobacco industry, but also learn from it when the opportunity exists to do good.

Social marketing is concerned with the application of marketing knowledge, concepts, and techniques to enhance social as well as economic ends. It is also concerned with the analysis of the social consequences of marketing policies, decisions, and activities. (Lazer & Kelley 1973)

This thinking dates back to 1951, when Wiebe suggested that we could consider selling brotherhood like soap. For the first time, people began to think seriously that methods used very successfully to influence behavior in the commercial sector might transfer to a non-profit arena. Wiebe evaluated four different social change campaigns and concluded that the more similarities they had to commercial marketing, the more successful they were.

In 1971, Kotler & Zaltman developed this thinking into a recognizable discipline, coining the term 'social marketing' and defining it as:

... the design, implementation, and control of programs calculated to influence the acceptability of social ideas and involving considerations of product planning, pricing, communication, distribution, and marketing research.

Social marketing did not go unchallenged. Arnold & Fisher (1996) describe how the emerging discipline was flanked on the one hand by marketing 'apologists' who wanted to keep marketing clearly defined within the firm and on the other by 'reconstructionists' who were pushing for an even broader, macro marketing perspective.

Social marketing ideas were innovative and made distinct changes to the practice of what was then almost exclusively called health education. In the early 1980s, for example, the idea of pretesting communication materials with the target audience prior to use was new to health professionals (Leathar & Hastings 1987, US DHHS 1980) and the suggestion that this research should be cyclical, action oriented, and substantially ethnographic was quite revolutionary (Leathar & Hastings 1987). Similarly, the idea that social advertising alone could not do the job, that it had to be embedded in the broader approach of social marketing, came as a revelation (Hastings & Haywood 1991). Branding and imagery even began to impinge on the world of public health (Leathar & Hastings 1987).

Underpinning this was the idea that not just the target but the health promoter might – and should – be getting something out of their interventions (Hastings & Haywood 1991), which was so new to the health sector that even in the mid 1990s it was still being seen by some as heresy (Buchanan et al 1994).

Social marketing thought has continued to develop, as discussed later in this chapter, extending both laterally to address social change and temporally to consider relational as well as transactional approaches.

THEORY IN SOCIAL MARKETING

Social marketing is a way of thinking about and managing social change. It is not a theory in itself, but it does make use of theory. In essence, a focus on behavior change poses three questions for social marketers.

1 Where are people in relation to a particular behavior?
2 What factors cause this positioning?
3 How can they be moved in the desired direction?

Theory helps answer these questions by building on previous understanding and research. Specifically, Stages of Change or the Transtheoretical Model can help answer the first question, Social Cognitive Theory the second, and Exchange Theory the third. The first two theories are discussed elsewhere in this book so we will focus on Exchange Theory here.

 see B5, B2

Exchange Theory has its foundations in psychology and economics (Housten & Gassenheimer 1987) and assumes that we are need-directed beings with a built-in inclination to try and improve our lot. In order to increase consumers' readiness to change, therefore, social marketers must provide them with something beneficial in exchange. In this sense, exchange involves the transfer of tangible or intangible items between two or more social actors (Bagozzi 1979). Kotler (2000) suggests five prerequisites are required for exchange to take place.

1 There are at least two parties.
2 Each party has something that might be of value to the other party.
3 Each party is capable of communication and delivery.
4 Each party is free to accept or reject the offer.
5 Each party believes it is appropriate or desirable to deal with the other party.

Central to these assumptions is the notion that the exchange must be mutually beneficial.

However, within the social marketing domain, the benefits customers can derive are often more ambiguous than in commercial marketing. In commercial marketing, goods are often exchanged for money – utilitarian exchange – whereas social marketing usually involves the mutual transfer of psychological, social, or other intangible entities – symbolic exchange. This type of exchange can make the job of the social marketer more problematic. For instance, it is more difficult to 'sell' benefits that the consumer may never see, e.g. not getting cancer or not contracting sexually transmitted diseases.

Nonetheless, the notion of exchange provides an invaluable discipline: if we want to change someone's behavior we have to see things from their point of view, understand why they do what they currently do, and determine what would motivate them to change. Or as social marketers express it, we need to be 'consumer oriented'.

SOCIAL MARKETING PLANNING

Social marketing offers a powerful method of facilitating voluntary behavior change. It has been used successfully to encourage people to eat more healthily (Lefebvre et al 1995), recycle (Thøgersen 1997), avoid and treat leprosy (Williams et al 1998), avoid psychoactive substances or use them more sensibly (Lavack 1999, Murray & Douglas 1988), and practice safer sex (Fishbein et al 1997).

Every marketing enterprise worthy of the name begins with a marketing plan (Kotler et al 1999). This addresses four questions (Wilson & Gilligan 1997).

- Where are we now? (strategic analysis)
- Where do we want to be? (strategic direction and strategy formulation)
- How might we get there? (strategic choice)
- How can we ensure arrival? (strategic implementation and control)

This planning process can also be applied in social marketing (Andreasen 1995, Kotler & Andreasen 1996).

As can be seen in Figure D10.1, a marketing plan comprises standard steps that guide the marketer through accepted best practice and so maximizes the chance of success in a particular intervention. More fundamentally, the plan also provides a progressive process of learning about the market and its particular exchanges; it drives our consumer orientation.

This learning takes place within particular initiatives. For example, a systematically produced and carefully researched anti-smoking intervention for school children will enable social marketers to improve their understanding of school children and their desires and thereby to enhance the intervention.

The learning process also takes place between interventions. The social marketer will be able to use the lessons learned from one initiative as a basis for future projects. Thus the process is not just progressive but cyclical. Hence the 'return arrow' in Figure D10.1. Furthermore, the development of understanding is not restricted to repeated anti-smoking interventions. For example, social marketing efforts in quite different areas, such as recycling or road safety, may well provide useful insights.

The next part of this chapter will examine the social marketing plan step by step.

Strategic analysis

Social marketing does not take place in a vacuum; a mix of macro and micro environmental factors has to be considered. This is illustrated in Figure D10.2. The former comprise political, economic, social, and technological forces (Andreasen 1995), which can present both opportunities (e.g. technical advances in nicotine replacement therapy) and

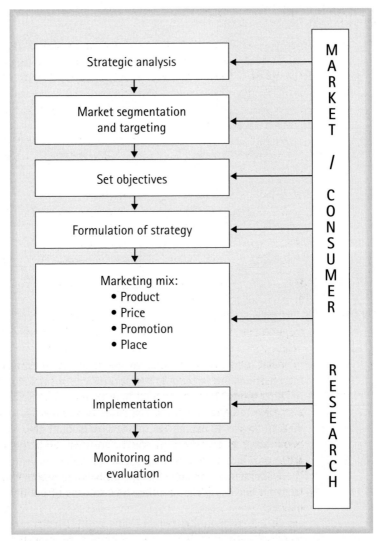

Fig D10.1 A social marketing plan (reprinted with permission from Hastings & Elliott 1993)

threats (e.g. a government which refuses to accept any link between poverty and ill health). They are generally very difficult to change. The micro environment, comprising customers, suppliers (e.g. research agencies), competitors (e.g. the tobacco industry), distributors, and funders, is slightly more controllable and again presents both opportunities and threats. These external forces have to be plotted against the social marketing organization's internal strengths and weaknesses.

The basic purpose of strategic analysis is then to ensure that opportunities are exploited and threats avoided by harnessing the organization's strengths and minimizing its weaknesses.

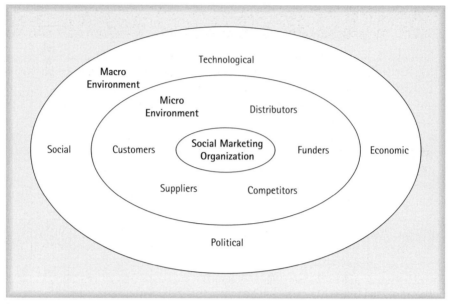

Fig D10.2   The marketing environment

Social marketers also have to ask strategic questions about what interventions are needed. Is the priority youth smoking, drink driving, or spina bifida? Decisions about how these problems are to be tackled also have to be made; in the last case, for example, is there a need for dietary advice to would-be mothers or should the target be bread manufacturers and the behavior the fortification of flour? Case Study D10.1 outlines this dilemma. Social marketers have to engage with these agenda-setting and strategic problem definition issues if they are to avoid becoming the mindless foot soldiers of politicians and policy makers.

Market segmentation and targeting

Successful marketing operates by offering optimum satisfaction of consumer needs (Kotler et al 1999). In theory, to do this properly, every individual needs to be treated differently and make a unique offering. Clearly this would be impractical. Instead, there is a compromise and people are grouped according to the similarity of their needs (Brassington & Pettitt 1997). A decision is then made as to which is (are) the most appropriate group(s) of consumers around whom to organize the marketing effort. In short, the population is 'segmented' into 'target markets' (Brassington & Pettitt 1997, Evans 2001, Frain 1986, Wilson & Gilligan 1997).

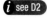

Case Study D10.1   The case of spina bifida

Spina bifida – a potentially fatal birth defect – can be prevented if women consume adequate quantities of vitamin B folate before conception and during the early stages of pregnancy. Social marketers may decide to target on an individualistic level, informing women of the risks and advising them to eat foods, such as broccoli and Brussels sprouts, that are rich in folates or alternatively market folic acid supplements. However, given that many pregnancies are unplanned, this approach will be ineffective among a significant proportion of the target audience (for example, in 2001 50% of pregnancies in Britain were unplanned). In the USA, the problem has been tackled by adopting a more upstream approach. Since 1998 all US wheat, rice, and corn have been fortified with folic acid. The Food and Drug Administration (FDA) ordered the measures after research showed that only about 25% of women of child-bearing age regularly consume enough folic acid in the form of a vitamin supplement.

The measure worked. By 1999 the Centers for Disease Control and Prevention (CDC) found that the average red blood cell folate concentration had increased by over 50% (BMJ 1999). And by 2001, CDC were able to show a decline in spina bifida and anencephaly rates (Spina Bifida Association of America). In this case, therefore, a strategic social marketing analysis suggests that the best approach is to target policy influencers and makers like CDC and the FDA, rather than individual consumers, and encourage them to change their behavior in favor of fortification.

Having chosen the segmentation variables and divided the population into groups, the next task is to decide which segments will become targets (Patron 1998). Three principles guide this decision. First, the target should be *substantial*, i.e. big enough to warrant attention (Dibb et al 1994, Kotler et al 1999). In commercial terms, it must be capable of generating sufficient profit; in behavior change terms, it must be capable of having a significant impact on the problem being tackled. Second, it must be *accessible* (Dibb et al 1994, Kotler et al 1999) – viable channels of communication and service delivery must exist. In drugs prevention, school children are, for example, likely to be much more accessible than young adults. Third, the target should be *actionable* – one that the marketer is capable of serving (Dibb et al 1994, Kotler et al 1999). There is no point in having a big and accessible target if there is nothing to offer them or they are likely to be impervious to any initiatives.

Setting objectives

Once the problem and target(s) have been determined, the next step is to set objectives (Kotler & Andreasen 1996). 'Good' objectives are valuable for two reasons. First, they ensure that a clear understanding and consensus about the intent of the intervention are developed by all those involved. This includes people both within the organization and outside it. For example, if an advertising agency is being used, well-defined and agreed objectives can ensure that they are absolutely clear about what their advertising has to achieve from the outset. Similarly, good objectives facilitate communication with superiors and controlling bodies. This can be particularly important in social marketing where funding agencies or politicians may have to be convinced of the value of an intervention. Second, objectives provide an excellent management tool. They provide a clear focus for intervention design and make it possible to monitor progress and ultimately to measure success.

i see A4

Good objectives are *measurable* (i.e. able to be readily evaluated) and *realistic* (i.e. within the capability of the organization). They are also based firmly on consumer perceptions because they are the only ones who understand the exact nature of a particular behavior and therefore what offerings are most likely to change it. However, it should be noted that whilst consumers are very capable of communicating about their life situations and expressing their needs, they are not experts on marketing or health promotion. It makes sense to ask them how they feel when confronted by a particular message, but not to judge its effectiveness. They are consumers, not consultants. They can provide vital information that will guide professional decision making, but the decisions still have to be made.

Formulating a strategy

Marketing is essentially about getting the right product, at the right price, in the right place, at the right time, presented in such a way as to successfully satisfy the needs of the consumer. (Cannon 1986)

Table D10.1 shows how the commercial marketing mix of product, price, promotion, and place can be adapted for use in social marketing (Andreasen 1995, Kotler & Roberto 1989, MacFadyen et al 2002).

Strategy formulation involves using all the intelligence gained in the first three steps of the planning process – what is known of the market, the target group, and the proposed objectives – to guide the deployment of the mix (Kotler & Andreasen 1996, Kotler et al 1999). Three general points should be noted about the marketing mix.

First, as the name suggests, the four elements (or the four Ps) are often (though not always) used in conjunction with each other.

Second, in operating the mix, the marketer is seeking the best combination of variables to offer their consumers (Kotler et al 1999). This best combination is the one which comes closest to satisfying their needs. This is what Cannon means by the term 'right' in the quote above. Hence, it is essential to monitor the marketing mix continually so it can be designed and developed to meet these needs. For example,

Table D10.1	The social marketing mix (MacFadyen et al 2002)	
Tool	**Definition**	**Types**
Product	The offer made to target adopters	Adoption of idea (belief, attitude, value) Adoption of behavior (one-off, sustained) Distance from current behavior Non-adoption of future behavior
Price	The costs that target adopters have to bear	Psychological, emotional, cultural, social, behavioral, temporal, practical, physical, financial
Place	The channels by which the change is promoted and places in which the change is supported and encouraged	Media channels Distribution channels Interpersonal channels Physical places Non-physical places (e.g. social and cultural climate)
Promotion	The means by which the change is promoted to the target	Advertising, public relations, media advocacy, direct mail, interpersonal

consumer research may show that a particular population is unaware of the benefits of safer sex and so the promotional element of the mix may be given greatest emphasis. However, as the campaign proceeds, awareness may become widespread and the main problem changes to one of condom availability. This is likely to increase the importance of the product element of the mix. In essence, the marketing mix is a multifaceted and flexible means of responding to consumer needs.

Third, as this last example shows, the importance of the different Ps is likely to vary and in some instances individual tools may be of little importance. Social marketers do not use the whole mix on every occasion. It should be seen as a rubric for thinking about your intervention, not a straitjacket to determine it. This thinking also applies to the promotional P. Social marketing is sometimes erroneously equated with social advertising; in fact, this is just one tool which may be important in a particular situation, but equally may not (Stead & Hastings 1996).

Implementation

When it comes to implementation, social marketing has two main ideas to offer: *pragmatism* and *flexibility*. *Pragmatism* means keeping objectives clearly in mind and sticking to them throughout an initiative, even when worthy but unrelated consumer needs emerge. For example, during pretesting of advertising intended to discourage drink driving it may become apparent that the target group does not understand the concept of units of alcohol and how these can be used to monitor intake. The temptation is to divert the initiative to provide what is felt to be much-needed education about units. However, the pragmatism of social marketing suggests that a better approach is to leave this task alone and find a way of communicating about quantities of alcohol – such as pints of beer – that the target does understand. The general desirability of informing the public about units should not be allowed to divert attention from the need to meet specific campaign objectives. Somerset Maugham's comment about the art of writing could equally apply to marketing: 'When you are hunting a fox you have no business to course a hare'.

Flexibility, on the other hand, means using any and every available means (within ethical constraints) to achieve objectives. This may involve altering an initiative in midstream if it is not working or circumstances change. The improved chance of success should, for example, override considerations of project neatness or purity of research design.

Monitoring and evaluation

As Figure D10.1 shows, research is crucial to every step of the marketing plan; it keeps us constantly in touch not just with the progress of our interventions, but also with our target markets and stakeholders. The former provides the conventional benefits of producing relevant, appropriate, and accurately targeted interventions. The latter encourages innovation and originality.

To do this, social marketing research must develop beyond an ad hoc collection of evaluative measures and become a continuous and cyclical *process*. Figure D10.3 illustrates this process. It must also combine qualitative with quantitative methods, recognizing that social science research can never produce certainty, only reduce the uncertainty of our attempts to understand a very complex and ever-changing reality.

Qualitative research can provide an understanding of what is and is not possible and why, as well as giving essential clues to behavior change. It involves informal interviewing with restricted samples. Interviewing may be conducted individually or with small groups of respondents (sometimes called 'focus groups' or 'group discussions'). It will not provide the statistics or accuracy of a quantitative survey. However, it enables the researcher to investigate issues in depth following the priorities and using the language of the target. Motivations, rationalizations, emotions, and associations can all be explored. Complex questioning methods are possible and during an interview the same issue can be approached from several different angles to check consistency of response. Reliability can be enhanced by checking

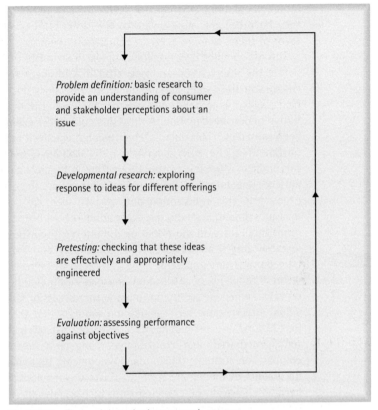

Problem definition: basic research to provide an understanding of consumer and stakeholder perceptions about an issue

Developmental research: exploring response to ideas for different offerings

Pretesting: checking that these ideas are effectively and appropriately engineered

Evaluation: assessing performance against objectives

Fig D10.3   The social marketing research process

responses between interviews and continuing fieldwork until no new data emerge. Extensive probing and exploration are feasible. In essence, qualitative methods add the question 'why' to the 'how many' asked by quantitative procedures.

Quantitative methods, which collect standardized information from large representative samples, providing statistical measures to a calculable degree of accuracy, can also contribute to this depth of understanding. In addition, they play a vital role in evaluating effectiveness. As noted already, the starting point for any evaluation of effectiveness – or outcome evaluation – must be the intervention's objectives. It is not possible to measure achievements without clear original intentions.

At the simplest level, these objectives may be concerned with the targets' reactions to an initiative – whether they are aware of it, have participated in it, understood it, etc. Measuring this is fairly straightforward. Once it is complete, the target audience simply has to be asked the relevant questions (e.g. have they seen the relevant advertising or used a particular service?). Provided the research methodology is sound, reliable data will result. However, given that social marketing is all about behavior change, you may want to measure actual change in the target population; whether, for example, as a result of an initiative, they have become more aware of the benefits of condoms, more in favor of them, or more likely to actually use them.

This is a complex task. It involves at least two stages of research – one before the intervention and one after it – to check for any relevant changes in the target population. If such changes do take place, the next problem is to determine whether they are attributable to the initiative under investigation. A drop in smoking, for example, may have been caused by a particular intervention but equally it may be the result of something else, such as an increase in taxation. The only way round this problem is to use a control group. That is, to select a population that matches the target in every respect except that they have not been exposed to the intervention and to take identical before-and-after measures among both groups. Comparing one set of measures with the other should isolate the effect of the intervention. Thus four separate research stages are required. The complexity and expense of these procedures is very apparent.

i see A4

These problems of attribution and measuring change become most prevalent when we are trying to judge the success or failure of an individual intervention. Social marketing suggests that there is a need to look beyond one-off judgments in research. Instead, it should be long-term, integrated, and constructive. *Long-term* means putting the emphasis on strategic thinking and recognizing that change is likely to be gradual. A metaanalysis of road safety campaigns found that the average change to be expected from such campaigns is less than 10% improvement in the measure, whether it is knowledge, attitude, or behavior (Elliott 1992). *Integrated* means that the evaluation of effectiveness should be seen as only one part of a research function that takes place throughout the development and implementation of initiatives – that evaluation is just one stage in a research process. *Constructive* means that the ultimate purpose of this research process is not just to test interventions but to provide a better understanding of the consumer.

This shifts the research emphasis from elaborate one-off research designs that are costly and time consuming – and often only produce findings long after an intervention is complete – to continuous research or 'tracking studies' that provide regular updates on what is happening in the market place.

Before leaving research and evaluation, it is perhaps worth addressing the issue of cost. The expense involved can be daunting. Three points should guide thinking here. First, research expenditure should be calculated as a percentage of the overall cost of an initiative (including staff costs). Figures of between 10% and 25% are typically applied by commerce. The principle is that, for example, 90% of a budget with research will be spent more effectively than 100% without. Second, research costs can be greatly reduced by doing it 'in house'. Third, if funds are really limited, then qualitative problem definition and developmental research are likely to be more productive than a quantitative outcome evaluation (Elliott 1992).

MOVING UPSTREAM

So far, we have focused on social marketing's ability to influence the voluntary behavior of individuals – to get them to drink sensibly or practice safer sex. However, we know that many behaviors are not completely in the control of the individual – tobacco is addictive, poverty limits our ability to make healthy choices, and the ubiquity of McDonald's can tempt a saint away from dietary guidelines. Furthermore, our discussions of theory and strategic analysis, in this chapter, showed that behavior is strongly influenced by our environment.

 see C, D8

Social marketers recognize this reality and therefore that their efforts may in some instances be best targeted 'upstream' from the final customer, at those who are in a position to change these environmental influences (Hastings et al 2000). Social marketing is ideally suited to bringing about this change, using the standard principles of strategic analysis, consumer orientation, and mutually beneficial exchange. The first determines whose behavior has to change, the second how they feel about the issue, and the third how the behavior change can be turned to their advantage.

RELATIONSHIPS NOT TRANSACTIONS

In the last 10 years, there has been a development in commercial marketing that brings an important new dimension to social marketing. Starting in the business-to-business and service sectors but moving more widely across commerce, the focus has shifted from isolated transactions to a longer term perspective that emphasizes the importance of building mutually beneficial relationships with customers and other stakeholders. Customer satisfaction, trust, and commitment are all crucial considerations here. This thinking has great resonance for social marketers, typically targeting behaviors which are often high involvement (e.g. quitting smoking) and multifaceted (e.g. teen smokers are more likely than their non-smoking peers to misuse drugs and alcohol), and where trust is particularly important (witness the current difficulties in the UK over childhood immunizations where government protestations about the safety of particular vaccines are just not believed (Evans et al 2001)).

'NE Choices', a major 3-year schools-based drugs prevention initiative recently delivered in the north east of England, is a case in point (Case Study D10.2). It adopted a social marketing perspective, focusing on behavior change and using a multifaceted action research design to ensure that the program was quintessentially consumer

Case Study D10.2   NE Choices – a behavior change failure or an incomplete exercise in relationship marketing? (Hastings et al 2002, Stead et al 2000, 2001)

NE Choices was a 3-year drugs prevention intervention built around a high school drama initiative, with additional community, school governor, and parent components. It had four behavioral objectives:

- to reduce prevalence of drug use
- to delay the age of onset of drug use
- to reduce the frequency of drug use among those who use drugs
- to reduce mixing of drugs (including with alcohol) by those who use drugs.

The program adopted a social influences approach, backed by social marketing, and was thoroughly researched with all the stakeholder groups using a design that incorporated a 2-year pilot, along with formative, process, impact, and outcome evaluations. The last comprised a rigorous experimental design.

An action research model meant that the pilot and formative research informed the initial program design and ongoing process, and impact findings guided its development. The result was, therefore, extremely consumer oriented and the young people – as well as other stakeholders – strongly endorsed it. The impact evaluation showed, for example, that the vast majority of children felt the program was enjoyable (89%), thought-provoking (88%), and credible (84%), and that the drama was realistic (79%), and non-didactic (e.g. 88% agreed that 'it encouraged us to speak our own minds'). However, despite three annual follow-ups, the outcome research showed no changes on any of the four behavioral objectives. According to social marketing lore, and the program's own objectives, NE Choices had failed.

A number of explanations could be offered for this: the research may have been insensitive to actual change; the intervention too small to make significant difference to behavior; intermediate measures (which were not taken because of the deliberate emphasis on behavior) may have given more promising results.

Alternatively, it can be argued that from a relational perspective NE Choices had considerable potential.

- There was much evidence of customer satisfaction in the impact evaluation.
- The young people trusted the program and its brand. For example, the last stage of research had to be conducted by mail, as a proportion of the young people had by then left school. The vast majority were prepared to provide contact details and 70% completed the sensitive and complex (40-minute) questionnaire.
- This resulted in the production of a key relationship marketing tool: a comprehensive database for what is an elusive and vulnerable group.

Case Study D10.2   NE Choices – a behavior change failure or an incomplete exercise in relationship marketing? (Hastings et al 2002, Stead et al 2000, 2001)–(continued)

Furthermore, three of the strengths which emerged from the impact evaluation are known to be markers for successful knowledge, attitudes, and behavior change: reaching a range of stakeholders and settings as well as the core customers (Fortmann et al 1995, King 1998, Pentz et al 1997); the successful use of drama in education to engage the audience (Blakey & Pullen 1991, Bouman et al 1998, Denman et al 1995, Orme & Starkey 1998); and being non-didactic (ACMD 1993, Allott et al 1999, Blakey & Pullen 1991, Joseph Rowntree Foundation 1997, Orme & Starkey 1999).

driven. Key stakeholders were also involved to tackle social, as well as individual, determinants of drug use. All the intermediate research findings – formative, process, and impact – were consistently and markedly positive, but the outcome evaluation (even after three annual follow-ups) showed no behavior change. According to both the social marketing canon and the program's own objectives, NE Choices had failed.

However, the program did deliver excellent customer service and built up a marked degree of trust with the young people, as well as other stakeholders. A valuable database of a vulnerable and normally elusive group was also constructed, providing a unique opportunity to develop these putative relationships further. Furthermore, as Case Study D10.2 demonstrates, three of NE Choices' impact evaluation successes are known to be linked to effective knowledge, attitude, and behavior change. This does suggest that, as well as good relationships being established, the first signs of behavior change were also emerging. Arguably, therefore, from a relationship marketing perspective, NE Choices offered a great deal of promise, but transactional thinking cut it off in its prime. As Morgan & Hunt (1994) express it:

Understanding relationship marketing requires distinguishing between the discrete transaction, which has a 'distinct beginning, short duration, and sharp ending by performance,' and relational exchange, which 'traces to previous agreements [and] ... is longer in duration, reflecting an ongoing process.'

NE Choices was judged by the former school of thought, but had the potential to deliver the latter.

ETHICAL ISSUES

Ethical concerns have been raised since Kotler & Zaltman first introduced the concept of social marketing in 1971. This is perhaps not surprising given that social marketers typically deal with entrenched taboo or illegal behaviors and their resolution may involve conflicting views of the interests of the social marketer, the consumer, and wider society (Hastings & MacFadyen 2002).

These ethical considerations arise at every stage of the marketing planning process. Figure D10.4 outlines the ethical dilemmas at each stage.

Social marketers need to decide which behaviors warrant attention and this involves prioritizing certain issues over others. Furthermore, they need to decide which behaviors should be discouraged or endorsed. For instance, there may be moral implications in deciding between teen

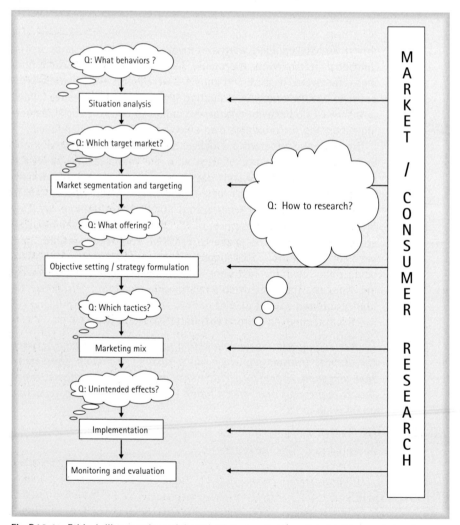

Fig D10.4 Ethical dilemmas in social marketing planning (reprinted with permission from MacFadyen & Hastings 2001)

pregnancy and alcohol abuse and, having chosen the former, about providing safer sex guidelines to those below the age of legal consent.

The decision on which groups to target also raises questions, as it ultimately leads to certain segments being ignored. On the other hand, targeting certain populations may lead to consumers becoming stigmatized, particularly if they are segmented according to such criteria as poverty, disability, or inclination to engage in proscribed behaviors. However, as discussed earlier, all consumers are different and will respond more or less enthusiastically to a particular intervention, so arguably targeting will happen anyway – the question is whether we plan for it or leave it to chance.

Setting objectives and formulating the strategy is also a controversial area. The notion of exchange which is central within social marketing can lead to compromises by setting modest objectives and employing harm reduction strategies which may be viewed as defeatist and unethical.

The design of the social marketing mix can also pose problems. The use of fear-based appeals, for example, can be at best ineffective, at worse disempowering, distressing, and damaging (MacFadyen et al 2002) and social marketing products, like condoms or methadone, create clear ethical dilemmas for some.

 see D7

The Hippocratic injunction to 'first do no harm' raises another potential dilemma. Does sex education encourage promiscuity or hamfisted tobacco youth prevention actually encourage smoking? For example, tobacco industry-run anti-smoking advertising campaigns have been shown to be at best ineffective and perhaps counterproductive (Devlin et al 2002).

Research can minimize such 'collateral' but this brings its own ethical problems, not least because it requires often vulnerable groups to engage with and talk about often difficult and threatening behaviors and issues. Social marketers have two important but often conflicting obligations: to ensure that the research does no harm and, second, that the data obtained are reliable.

Ethical theory can help resolve these problems. Deontological theory, for example, helps us think about the morality of our actions and teleological theory focuses on their consequences. Similarly, codes of conduct can also be helpful, especially when combined with management systems that acknowledge the existence and legitimacy of these dilemmas.

CONCLUSION

Commercial marketing influences us all on a daily basis; social marketing harnesses this power to bring about beneficial behavior change. It recognizes that strategic analysis, a consumer and stakeholder orientation, and systematic planning, all driven by constructive and timely research, can work as well for the WHO as for Nike. Increasingly it also recognizes that this is more complex than stimulating one-off actions,

often requiring the development of long-term mutually beneficial
relationships between social marketer and stakeholder.

References

Advisory Council on the Misuse of Drugs (ACMD) 1993 Drug education in
schools: the need for a new impetus. HMSO, London

Allott R, Paxton R, Leonard R 1999 Drug education: a review of British
government policy and evidence on effectiveness. Health Education
Research Theory and Practice 14(4):491-505

Andreasen A 1995 Marketing social change. Jossey-Bass, San Francisco

Arnold M, Fisher J 1996 Counterculture, criticisms and crisis: assessing the
effect of the sixties on marketing thought. Journal of Macromarketing
16:118-133

Bagozzi R P 1979 Toward a formal theory of marketing exchange. In: Ferrell O C,
Brown S W, Lamb C W (eds) Conceptual and theoretical developments in
marketing. American Marketing Association, Chicago

Blakey V, Pullen E 1991 You don't have to say you love me: an evaluation of a
drama-based sex education project for schools. Health Education Journal
50(4):161-165

BMJ 1999 Fortification of flour raises folate levels in US women, says CDC.
British Medical Journal 318:1506

Bouman M, Maas L, Kok G 1998 Health education in television entertainment
– 'Medisch Centrum West': a Dutch drama serial. Health Education
Research Theory and Practice 13(4):503-518

Brassington F, Pettitt S (eds) 1997 Segmenting markets. In: Principles of
marketing. Pitman Publishing, London, ch 5

Buchanan D R, Reddy S, Hossain Z 1994 Social marketing: a critical appraisal.
Health Promotion International 9(1):49-57

Cannon T 1986 Basic marketing. Principles and practice. Holt, Rinehart and
Winston, London, p 37

Denman S, Pearson J, Moody D et al 1995 Theatre in education on HIV and
AIDS: a controlled study of schoolchildren's knowledge and attitudes.
Health Education Journal 54(1):3-17

Devlin E, MacFadyen L, Hastings G et al 2002 evaluation of the industry
funded 'Youth Smoking Prevention' (YSP) campaign. Proceedings of the 3rd
European Conference on Tobacco or Health, Warsaw, June

Dibb S, Simkin L, Pride W M 1994 Marketing concepts and strategies, 2nd edn.
Houghton Mifflin, Boston

Elliott B 1992 Road safety mass media campaigns: a meta analysis. Federal
Office of Road Safety, Department of Transport and Communications, ACT,
Canberra

Evans M 2001 Market segmentation. In: Baker M J (ed) The marketing book,
4th edn. Butterworth-Heinemann, Oxford

Evans M, Stoddart H, Condon L et al 2001 Parents' perspectives on the MMR
immunization: a focus group study. British Journal of General Practice
51:904-910

Fishbein M, Guenther-Grey C, Johnson W et al 1997 The Aids Community Demonstration Projects. Using a theory-based community intervention to reduce AIDS risk behaviours: the CDC's AIDS Community Demonstration Projects. In: Goldberg M E, Fishbein M, Middlestadt S E (eds) Social marketing. Lawrence Erlbaum Associates, New Jersey

Fortmann S P, Flora J A, Winkleby M A et al 1995 Community intervention trials: reflections on the Stanford Five-City Project experience. American Journal of Epidemiology 142(6):576-586

Frain J 1986 The principles and practice of marketing. Pitman, London

Hastings G B, Elliot B 1993 Social marketing in practice in traffic safety. In: Marketing of traffic safety. OECD, Paris, pp 35-53

Hastings G B, Haywood A 1991 Social marketing and communication in health promotion. Health Promotion International 6(2):135-145

Hastings G B, MacFadyen L 2002 The limitations of fear messages. Tobacco Control 11:73-75

Hastings G B, MacFadyen L, Anderson S 2000 Whose behavior is it anyway? The broader potential of social marketing. Social Marketing Quarterly VI(2):46-58

Hastings G B, Stead M, MacKintosh A M 2002 Rethinking drugs prevention: radical thoughts from social marketing. Health Education Journal 61(4):347-364

Housten F S, Gassenheimer J B 1987 Marketing and exchange. Journal of Marketing 51:3-18

Joseph Rowntree Foundation 1997 Young people and drugs. Available online at: www.jrf.org.uk/knowledge/findings/socialpolicy/sp133.asp

King A C 1998 How to promote physical activity in a community: research experiences from the US highlighting different community approaches. Patient Education and Counselling 33(1suppl):S3-S12

Kotler P 2000 Marketing management. Prentice-Hall, Upper Saddle River

Kotler P, Andreasen A R 1996 Strategic marketing for non profit organizations, 5th edn. Prentice-Hall, Upper Saddle River

Kotler P, Roberto E L 1989 Social marketing: strategies for changing public behavior. Free Press, New York

Kotler P, Zaltman G 1971 Social marketing: an approach to planned social change. Journal of Marketing 35(July):3-12

Kotler P, Armstrong G, Saunders J et al 1999 Principles of marketing, 2nd edn. Prentice-Hall, Upper Saddle River

Lavack A M 1999 De-normalisation of tobacco in Canada. Social Marketing Quarterly. Special Issue: Innovations in Social Marketing Conference Proceedings V(3):82-85

Lazer W, Kelley E 1973 Social marketing: perspectives and viewpoints. Irwin, Homewood

Leathar D S, Hastings G B 1987 Social marketing and health education. Journal of Services Marketing 1(2):49-52

Lefebvre R C, Doner L, Johnston C et al 1995 Use of database marketing and consumer-based health communication in message design. In: Maibach E, Parrott R (eds) Designing health messages. Sage, Newbury Park

MacFadyen L, Hastings G B 2001 First do no harm: the case for ethical considerations in social marketing. Presentation at Academy of Marketing

Science 10th Biennial World Marketing Congress – Global Marketing Issues at the Turn of the Millennium. Cardiff University, Cardiff, 28 June–1 July

MacFadyen L, Stead M, Hastings G B 2002 Social marketing. In: Baker M J (ed) The marketing book, 5th edn. Butterworth-Heinemann, Oxford

Morgan R M, Hunt S D 1994 The commitment-trust theory of relationship marketing. Journal of Marketing 58(July):20-38

Murray G G, Douglas R R 1988 Social marketing in the alcohol policy arena. British Journal of Addiction 83:505-511

Orme J, Starkey F 1998 Evaluation of HPS/Bristol Old Vic Primary Drug Drama Project 1997/98. Full report. Faculty of Health and Social Care, UWE, Bristol

Orme J, Starkey F 1999 Young people's views on drug education in schools: implications for health promotion and health education. Health Education 4(July):142-152

Patron M 1998 Advances in segmentation. Admap, July

Pentz M A, Mihalic S F, Grotpeter J K 1997 Blueprints for violence prevention. Book One – The Midwestern Prevention Project. University of Colorado, Boulder, Colorado

Spina Bifida Association of America. Available online at: www.sbaa.org/html/sbaa_folic.html

Stead M, Hastings G B 1996 Advertising in the social marketing mix: getting the balance right. In: Goldberg M, Fishbein M, Middelstadt S (eds) Social marketing: theoretical and practical perspectives. Lawrence Erlbaum Associates, New Jersey

Stead M, MacKintosh A M, Eadie D R et al 2000 NE Choices: the development of a multi-component drug prevention programme for adolescents. Home Office Drugs Prevention Advisory Service (DPAS) Paper 4. Home Office, London

Stead M, MacKintosh A M, Eadie D R et al 2001 NE Choices: the results of a multi-component drug prevention programme for adolescents. Home Office Drugs Prevention Advisory Service (DPAS) Paper 14. Home Office, London

Thøgersen J 1997 Facilitating recycling: reverse-distribution channel design for participation and support. Social Marketing Quarterly IV(1):42-55

US Department of Health and Human Services (DHHS) 1980 Pretesting in health communication. US Department of Health and Human Services, Maryland

Wiebe G D 1951 Merchandising commodities and citizenship in television. Public Opinion Quarterly 15(Winter):679-691

Williams P G, Dewapura D, Gunawardene P et al 1998 Social marketing to eliminate leprosy in Sri Lanka. Presented at Innovations in Social Marketing Conference, Washington, June

Wilson R M S, Gilligan C 1997 Strategic marketing management: planning, implementation and control. Butterworth-Heinemann, Oxford

Index

Page numbers in bold indicate the main treatment of a subject

value systems, influence of, 33

walking, facilitation in cities, 144, 147
weight control, education programs, **284–5**
weight reduction, individual differences and, 66
work
    active, 160
    passive, 160

Working Well Trial, 292, 294
workplace
    effort–reward imbalance, 158–9, 163
    health promotion measures, 164
    physical risk factors, 143, 145
    social and environmental strategies, 292–4
    stress in, 155
    stress-control balance, 159–60, 163

Journals of related interest

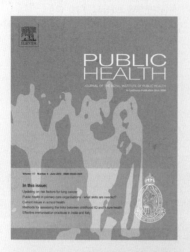

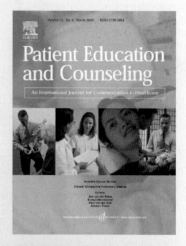

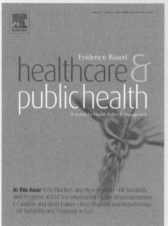

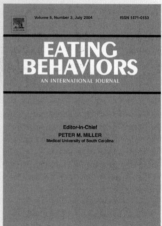